Learning Disabilities

For Churchill Livingstone:

Commissioning editor: Ellen Green
Project manager: Valerie Burgess
Project development editor: Valerie Bain
Design direction: Judith Wright
Project controller: Pat Miller
Illustrator: Lee Smith
Copy editor: Jennifer Bew
Indexer: Janine Fearon
Sales promotion executive: Hilary Brown

Learning Disabilities

Edited by

Bob Gates BEd MSc CertEd DipN RMN RNMH RNT
Sub-Dean and Lecturer in Nursing, School of Health, The University of Hull, Hull, UK

THIRD EDITION

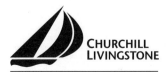
CHURCHILL
LIVINGSTONE

NEW YORK EDINBURGH LONDON MADRID MELBOURNE SAN FRANCISCO TOKYO 1997

CHURCHILL LIVINGSTONE
Medical Division of Pearson Professional Limited

Distributed in the United States of America by Churchill
Livingstone, 650 Avenue of the Americas, New York,
N.Y. 10011, and by associated companies, branches and
representatives throughout the world.

First edition 1986
        Reprinted 1989 (twice), 1990, 1991
Second edition 1993
        Reprinted 1994
        Reprinted 1995
Third edition 1997

ISBN 0 443 05539 4

British Library Cataloguing in Publication Data
A catalogue record for this book is available from the British
Library.

Library of Congress Cataloging in Publication Data
A catalogue record for this book is available from the Library
of Congress.

Note
Medical knowledge is constantly changing. As new
information becomes available, changes in treatment,
procedures, equipment and the use of drugs become
necessary. The editor, contributors and the publishers have,
as far as it is possible, taken care to ensure that the
information given in this text is accurate and up-to-date.
However, readers are strongly advised to confirm that the
information, especially with regard to drug usage, complies
with latest legislation and standards of practice.

The
publisher's
policy is to use
**paper manufactured
from sustainable forests**

Printed by Bell and Bain Ltd., Glasgow

Contents

Contributors

Kathryn Baillie RNMH
Community Nurse, Community Team Learning
Disabilities, Hull and Holderness Community
Health NHS Trust, Hull, UK
17. Helping agencies for the family

Owen Barr BSc RGN RNMH CNMH ADDipED
PGCertCoun
Lecturer in Nursing, Learning Disabilities
Option Leader, Community Learning
Disabilities Nursing, School of Health Sciences,
University of Ulster, Coleraine, Northern Ireland
16. Interventions in a family context

Rhona Billington MSc RNMH RMN DipN CertEd RNT
Lecturer/Practitioner, School of Health, The
University of Hull, Hull, UK
5. Ethics

Jim Clutterbrook RNMH
Community Nurse, Community Team Learning
Disabilities, Hull and Holderness Community
Health NHS Trust, Hull, UK
17. Helping agencies for the family

Glynn Connolly RNMH MHSM CertHMS
Manager, Strut House, Lincoln, UK
8. Accessing services

Mary Dearing RNMH
Community Nurse, Community Team for
Children and Adolescents with Learning
Disabilities, The Children's Centre, Hull, UK
17. Helping agencies for the family

David Dickinson BA MSc(EdPsych) PGCE AFBP
CPsychol
Principal Educational Psychologist, County
Offices, Newland, Lincoln, UK
7. Education

Linda Dickinson BEd(Hons)
Learning Support Teacher, County Offices,
Newland, Lincoln, UK
7. Education

Rita Ferris-Taylor MSc DipCSLT CertEd
CertTrainingDevelopment
Lecturer, Kensington and Chelsea Further
Education College; National
Tutor, Makaton Vocabulary Development
Project; Freelance Training Consultant, UK
12. Communication

Bob Gates BEd MSc CertEd DipN RMN RNMH RNT
Sub-Dean and Lecturer in Nursing, School of
Health, The University of Hull, Hull, UK
1. Understanding learning disability
9. Behavioural difficulties

Rachel Gladden
Student Nurse on BSc Nursing Sciences
(Learning Disabilities) course, The School of
Health, The University of Hull, UK
Appendix

Allyson Kent RNMH CNLDCert
Community Nurse, Community Team Learning
Disabilities, Hull and Holderness Community
Health NHS Trust, Hull UK
17. Helping agencies for the family

David Lewis RNMH RNT CertEd CertCouns
CSLAFoundCert
Senior Lecturer, Division of Social Work,
Learning Disability and Mental Health,
University of Hertfordshire, UK
13. Leisure

Steven McNally RMN RNMH MSc CertEd
Lecturer Practitioner, School of Health Care
Studies, Oxford Brookes University, Oxfordshire
Learning Disability NHS Trust, UK
14. Representation

Peter Oakes BA DipPsych CPsychol
Consultant Clinical Psychologist, The University
of Hull, Hull and Holderness Community
Health NHS Trust, UK
15. Sexual and personal relationships

Janice Phillips *DipLearning Disabilities*
Care Manager, Horizon Trust, Hertfordshire, UK
13. Leisure

John D. Pougher MA BA RNMH RGN FBIS
Quality Development Co-ordinator, Hull and
Holderness Community Health NHS Trust,
Hull, UK
4. Providing quality care

Caron Swann MEd CertEd RNMH
Tutor, School of Health, The University of Hull,
Hull, UK
3. Development of services

Ian M. Tweddell RNMH
Clinical Team Manager, Community Team
Learning Disabilities, Hull and Holderness
Community Health NHS Trust, UK
17. Helping agencies for the family

Debbie Vernon BSc RNMH RGN
Graduate Teaching Assistant, School of Health,
The University of Hull, Kingston-upon-Hull, UK
6. Health

Eileen Wake BA RNMH RGN RSCN
Tutor, Professional Studies Division, School of
Health, The University of Hull, Hull, UK
11. Profound and multiple disability

Debbie Watson RNMH PGDipHealthEd CertEd
Tutor, School of Health, The University of Hull,
Hull, UK
2. Causes and manifestations

Jane Wray BA HETC RGN
Research Assistant, School of Health, The
University of Hull, Hull, UK
10. Complementary therapies

Preface

It is with considerable pride that I write the preface for the third edition of *Learning Disabilities*, although it would be thoughtless of me to begin writing it without first thanking Eamon Shanley and Thomas Starrs for the second edition of the book, which served as a model of excellence for the third edition.

This edition has been divided into three sections: 'Understanding Learning Disability and Service Provision', 'Helping People Towards Independence' and 'Supporting the Family in Learning Disabilities', providing three crucial focal points for the text. The text has been expanded to include new chapters on complementary therapies, health, education, leisure and representation. Also, there is now a substantial appendix covering the social policy and mental health legislation which have affected the lives of people with learning disabilities.

The contributors to the third edition represent people from practice and academic backgrounds who, while belonging to different professions and agencies of care, all share a common commitment and vision: to advance understanding and knowledge of learning disabled people and their families.

Each chapter contains a number of reader activities. The character and purpose of the activities vary: some are intended to encourage the reader to reflect on an issue in greater depth than the text permits, while others are designed to act as a prompt to undertake an associated activity, or to encourage discussion between readers and their peers. Overall, the activities are designed to give the text an interactive feel.

This book arrives at a tremendously important time for learning disability nurses. The assumption that the NHS and Community Care Act (DoH 1990) would make the contribution of the learning disability nurse redundant has been proved erroneous. Nurses in this specialism have regrouped and can now be found using their knowledge base and practising their skills in a variety of different care settings, including the National Health Service, social services, and the independent and voluntary sectors. Learning disability nurses can also be found occupying specialist practitioner clinical nurse roles, as well as working as community care managers and assessment officers. They have had to be adaptable. The Cullen Report's (DoH 1991) conclusion that learning disability nurses were 'facility independent' has proved to be prophetic. The NHS and Community Care Act (DoH 1990) has forced learning disability nursing to face some harsh truths about its direction and its level of competence to deliver health and social care to people with learning disabilities in a variety of different contexts.

Learning disability nursing is now responding to this challenge with confidence and the contribution of this book to the debate is to articulate the role of the learning disabilities nurse. However, its primary aim is to provide a useful standard text on a range of issues in learning disabilities for diploma and degree courses, and to present the information in a way that readers find informative and accessible in directing their study and professional development.

Lincoln 1996   B.G.

REFERENCES

DoH 1990 NHS and Community Care Act. HMSO, London
DoH 1991 Caring for people: the implications for mental handicap nursing (Cullen Report). HMSO, London

1

Understanding learning disability and service provision

1

Understanding learning disability

B. Gates

INTRODUCTION

This chapter serves as an overall introduction, both to help the reader understand what learning disability means, and to make sense of subsequent chapters. It is assumed that the primary intended audience – diploma students in learning disabilities branch programmes of Project 2000 courses – will already have encountered the term learning disabilities, and will also have had some practical experience of working with such people.

Before exploring in any depth what learning disabilities might mean, it is worth noting that the Department of Health (1995) has recently estimated that mild learning disability may affect as many as 20 people in every 1000 of the population, and that a further three to four in every 1000 will have a severe learning disability; the latter group of people, they suggest, will need frequent support with some aspect of daily living. Given that these numbers have been estimated, it might be argued that there already exists clear criteria to identify the presence of learning disability. Such an assumption is simplistic, and may account for the fact that statutory providers of services for such people frequently underestimate the size and resource requirements of this group of people (Turner et al 1995).

UNDERSTANDING LEARNING DISABILITIES

How we understand learning disabilities is a

most interesting and perplexing question for people engaged in the care of people with learning disabilities. This section attempts to illustrate that, although many health and social care professionals speak with some confidence about what constitutes learning disability, from a theoretical perspective and at an operational level it is not at all clear whether this is what they are in fact referring to. This point should not be confused with the continuing debate about how people with learning disabilities are referred to, but is rather a more sophisticated definitional issue that is of the utmost importance in calculating the size of the relevant population and any subsequent analysis of their needs, along with any attendant social and/or health resource requirement predictions. Learning disability has been identified using a number of different classifications, and these have included legislative definitions, intellectual ability and social ability. Professionals also attempt to categorize learning disability by causation. This approach is not discussed here; for further information see Chapter 2.

Classifying learning-disabled people using legislative definitions

Throughout history many societies have attempted to describe learning disabilities through the use of legislative definitions. This section only deals with such attempts as have been used in the United Kingdom, and in particular in England during this century.

The Mental Deficiency Act (1913) defined four categories (Malin et al 1980):

- Idiots – so deeply defective in mind from birth or from an early age as to be unable to guard themselves against common physical dangers.
- Imbeciles – persons who, although not as defective as idiots, are still incapable of managing their own affairs.
- Feeble-minded – not as defective as imbeciles, but requiring care, supervision and control for their own protection or for the protection of others.

- Moral defectives – people who from an early age display some permanent mental defect coupled with strong vicious or criminal propensities, on whom punishment has little or no effect.

In 1927 the Mental Deficiency Act defined mental defectiveness (people with learning disabilities) as 'a state of arrested or incomplete development of mind existing before the age of eighteen years, whether arising from inherent causes or induced by disease or injury'.

In 1959 a new Mental Health Act was passed that defined new terms: subnormality and severe subnormality:

- Severe subnormality – a state of arrested or incomplete development of the mind which includes subnormality of intelligence and is of such a nature or degree that the patient is incapable of living an independent life or of guarding himself against serious exploitation, or will be so incapable when of an age to do so.
- Subnormality – a state of arrested or incomplete development of mind, not amounting to severe subnormality, which includes subnormality of intelligence, and is of such a nature or degree which requires, or is susceptible to, medical treatment or other special care or training of the patient.

By 1983 yet another Mental Health Act introduced two more new terms:

- Mental impairment – a state of arrested or incomplete development of the mind (not amounting to severe mental impairment) which includes significant impairment of intelligence and social functioning and is associated with abnormally aggressive or seriously irresponsible conduct on the part of the person concerned.
- Severe mental impairment – a state of arrested or incomplete development of mind which includes severe impairment of intelligence and social functioning and is associated with abnormally aggressive or seriously irresponsible conduct on the part of the person concerned.

It can be seen from the nature of these definitions that this legislation was intended to apply to those people with learning disabilities who demonstrated 'aggressive' behaviour, and further that such behaviour might warrant admission to an appropriate setting for compulsory treatment and/or assessment. This piece of legislation effectively prevented most people with learning disabilities from being categorized under mental health legislation. It is interesting to note that although such legislative definitions were developed in order to categorize people with learning disabilities, they themselves were dependent upon other criteria to establish its presence. It would appear that throughout this century the following factors have at one time or another been present in legislative definitions of learning disabilities:

- Low intelligence
- Social incompetence
- Needing treatment
- Affected from an early age (usually before 18)
- Unable to guard themselves against danger
- Criminal tendencies and/or aggressive behaviour
- Incomplete or arrested development of the mind.

These factors may be important in helping us understand the nature of learning disabilities, although as will be shown in later chapters, the value base of at least some of them reflects contemporary attitudes towards people with learning disabilities at various stages of our history.

Classifying learning-disabled people using intellectual ability

Apart from legislation, since the beginning of this century measured intelligence has been used as

Activity 1.1

To what extent do you think that the definitions identified above have helped to shape negative societal attitudes, if they exist, toward people with learning disabilities?

another criterion upon which to judge whether someone has a learning disability. However, there is a considerable diversity of opinion as to just what intelligence is. This chapter will not explore this issue in any depth, but an assumption is made that intelligence is something to do with the ability to solve problems, and that this ability, or the lack of it, can be measured; one way of doing this is by intelligence tests. Intelligence tests enable a comparison to be made of the ability of an individual to complete a range of standardized tests, against a large and representative sample from the general population. The origin of such tests can be traced to the turn of this century, when Alfred Binet, in France, was asked to produce a method of identifying and separating children who were congenitally mentally retarded from those who were environmentally disadvantaged; the former were to be viewed and treated as ineducable. Clearly, it is important that the sample used for comparison will be of a similar chronological age to the individual being tested. The score an individual attains can be converted into a percentile, so that it can be seen how that individual compares with others in the general population. Normally this figure is converted to an intelligence quotient (IQ), which is still used as means of identifying learning disabilities. Intelligence tests seek to compare the mental age of an individual against their chronological age, and this is achieved by using the following formula:

$$\frac{\text{Mental age}}{\text{Chronological age}} \times 100 = \text{IQ}$$

Chronological age is the actual age of an individual, and mental age refers to the developmental stage that the individual has reached, compared to others of a similar age. If the number reached by dividing mental age by chronological age is multiplied by 100, then one arrives at the IQ. Not surprisingly, given the nature of this formula, if one was to continue to use it throughout an individual's life then their IQ would progressively diminish; therefore, the formula is probably only of use until the chronological age of about 18. If the reader wishes to study both the concept of intelligence and the history associated with IQ, they should consult Gross (1991).

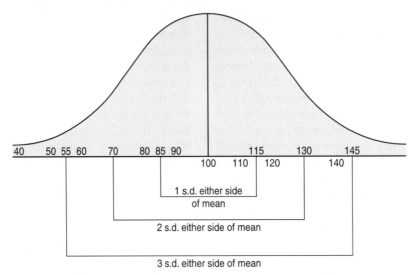

Figure 1.1 The normal distribution curve of intelligence.

If an assumption is made that intelligence is present in the population, and further that it is evenly distributed, then it should be possible to measure how far an individual moves away from what constitutes 'normal'. This so-called normal distribution of intelligence can be demonstrated diagrammatically (Figure 1.1). It can be seen from this that some people will have an IQ above normal, and some below.

Intelligence tests have been widely used by psychologists since their inception, but were especially popular in the 1950s, 1960s and 1970s. However, there is now a widespread view that there are many limitations in their use, including their validity in measuring intellectual ability, along with an uncomprehensive reliability for the identification of learning disabilities. However, despite the criticisms, if intelligence tests are used appropriately and by properly trained technicians, they can provide a relatively objective measure of intellectual ability which, if used in conjunction with other criteria, can be extremely useful in identifying learning disabilities.

Classifying learning-disabled people using social ability

Another universally used criterion for the identification of learning disabilities is that of social competence. This refers to the ability of an individual to adapt to the changing demands made by society (Mittler 1979). At a superficial level the identification of adaptive, and therefore maladaptive, behaviour sounds relatively straightforward and unproblematic, because if people are socially incompetent and do not respond well to changing societal demands, one could simply label them as having learning disabilities. Further, this would be relatively easy to establish on the basis of the individual performing significantly below what might be considered normal. However, there are a number of problematic issues in relation to using social competence to identify learning disabilities. First, social incompetence is to be found in a wide cross-section of people, not just those with learning disabilities: consider, for example, people with chronic mental health problems or those from ethnic minority groups. Secondly, there is the issue of expectation and the attendant concept of the self-fulfilling prophecy: assume that an individual has been identified as having learning disabilities on the basis of measured social incompetence; do you think this individual genuinely has learning disabilities, or is the social incompetence merely an artefact of a hospital setting in which they spent their formative years? Such a finding is not beyond the realms of credibility. It is only relatively recently that the large learning disability hospitals have been closing, and over the years thousands of people with learning disabilities were segregated from society in institutions, where they led very devalued lifestyles. Opportunities for the development of social competence were few and far between; even when opportunities arose, they were often perverted attempts to create some kind of social reality in the institutional setting. In short, the expectations of people in these environments were low, and therefore it is not unreasonable to assume that their development of social competence was reduced. A further problem in using the criterion of social competence is being able to separate out causes other than learning disability, for example communication, hearing and vision problems. However, despite these criticisms, social competence remains a globally used criterion for the identification of learning disabilities.

What is learning disability?

It should be remembered that the term learning disability is relatively new in the United Kingdom. It is used to describe a group of people with significant developmental delay that results in arrested or incomplete achievement of the 'normal' milestones of human development. These relate to intellectual, emotional, spiritual and social aspects of development. Significant delays in the achievement of one or more of these

milestones may lead to a person being described, defined or categorized as having learning disabilities. It is worth bearing in mind that the term is not one that is used internationally. Until recently the term 'mental handicap' was much more frequently used, but it was felt that it purveyed a negative image of this group of people. In a relatively recent study by Nursey, Rhode and Farmer (1990) it was shown that parents and doctors had preferences in the words that they chose to use when referring to people with learning disabilities. This study, using a questionnaire, established that both parents and doctors preferred the term mental handicap or learning difficulties. However, it is interesting that doctors were more inclined to accept the words dull, backward and developmentally delayed.

In the USA the term mental retardation is widely used for the classification of learning disability, based on the World Health Organization Classification of Mental and Behavioural Disorders (WHO 1993). This uses the term mental retardation to refer to 'a condition of arrested or incomplete development of the mind, which is especially characterised by impairment of skills manifested during the developmental period which contributes to the overall level of intelligence, i.e. cognitive, language, motor and social abilities'.

The World Health Organization has organized the degree of disability (retardation) according to how far an individual moves away from the normal distribution of IQ for the general population,

Activity 1.2

Consider the following list of terms which are commonly associated with people with learning disabilities.

Intellectual disability
Learning disability
Learning difficulty
Mentally subnormal
Severely mentally subnormal
Mentally retarded
Mentally impaired
Mentally defective
Spastic

Idiot
Imbecile
Moron
Cretin
Benny

Are you aware of other terms that are in general use?

Which of these terms do you think is the most acceptable to people in general?

Do you think that any of them is capable of creating a negative image concerning this group of people?

as discussed earlier. Using this system, an individual who consistently scores less than two standard deviations of an IQ test, i.e. a measured IQ of less than 70, would be said to be mentally retarded (see Figure 1.1). It is generally accepted that if an individual's IQ is consistently below 50, then the term 'severe mental retardation' is used. Those whose IQ is in the range 50–70 are generally identified as having a 'mild mental retardation', and those with an IQ of between 71 and 84 are said to be on the borderline of intellectual functioning. It might be argued with some justification that the above is not actually very helpful. Luckasson et al (1992) have provided a much more useful framework for operationalizing and understanding the nature of learning disability. They have identified the different levels of support that a person may require, based on need rather than forcing someone into a predetermined category of administration.

TERMS AS LABELS

One of the problems in deciding which term to use is the possibility that it may become a label, conjuring up a negative image. The use of labels for people with learning disabilities has in the past served as a way of segregating this group from society. Clearly, the sustained use of a label, coupled with any consequent negative imagery, can result in people being perceived as deviant and therefore devalued citizens. Wolfensberger (1972) has demonstrated the particular negative effects that may occur when people become marginalized as deviants, and has identified eight social role perceptions of people with learning disabilities (Figure 1.2). Such perceptions may be understood as follows:

• **Subhuman.** Throughout history, and in many different cultures, people with learning disabilities have often been viewed as subhuman. Evidence of such a belief can be found in relatively contemporary literature: for example, in relation to absolute, complete or profound idiocy, Tredgold and Soddy (1956) have said:

In this condition we see humanity reduced to its lowest possible expression. Although these unfortunate creatures are, indeed, the veritable

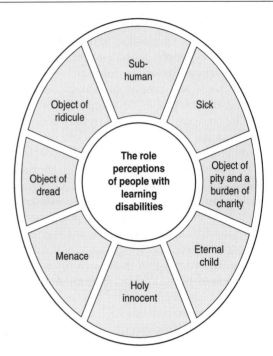

Figure 1.2   Role perceptions of people with learning disabilities (after Wolfensberger 1972).

offspring of *Homo Sapiens*, the depth of their degeneration is such that existence – for it can hardly be called life – is on a lower plane than that of even the beasts of the field, and in most respects may be described as vegetative (Tredgold & Soddy 1956).

In the last century and at the beginning of this one there was a strong eugenics movement, where segregation and the search to prevent deterioration of the human race were seen as very important. Mittler (1979) has commented:

The late Victorians were so haunted by the spectre of a declining national intelligence that they pursued a ruthless segregationist policy which led to many thousands of people being identified as mentally handicapped and incarcerated in asylums and colonies. The fact that their names were later changed to hospitals does not alter the fact that they were sited and designed to meet the needs of the time to segregate the handicapped from the rest of society and to do everything possible to prevent them from multiplying (Mittler 1979).

Such a perception of learning disabilities is further evidenced in this century, and has included attempts to rid society of people with learning disabilities. For example, as early as 1924 in Nazi Germany, Adolf Hitler, in *Mein Kampf*, had commented:

Defective people must be prevented from propagating equally defective offspring . . . For, if necessary, the incurably sick will be pitilessly segregated – a barbaric measure for the unfortunate who is struck by it, but a blessing for his fellow men and posterity.

This attitude was even reinforced in material for schoolchildren. Reflect on the following mental arithmetic problem that was set for German children in 1936:

A mentally defective person costs the republic 4 Reichmarks per day, a cripple 5.50 Reichmarks . . . 300 000 persons are being cared for in public mental institutions. How many marriage loans at 1000 Reichmarks per couple could be annually financed from the funds allocated to these institutions? (Independent Television Corporation 1993).

The reader may think that the examples given are only of historical interest, and that we now live in a society that values people with learning disabilities as equal citizens; however, consider the following example from recent media coverage. In a recent *Guardian* newspaper article (Toolis 1996) the plight of a young woman with Down syndrome was discussed at length. The young woman, Jo, was reported to have a 'hole in the heart' and therefore required a heart and lung transplant. However, the article reported that no centre will accept anyone with Down syndrome as a patient. Indeed, the medical director of one such transplant centre is recorded as saying:

As a doctor I see that my main aim is to make people live, and to become independent human beings that will live a fulfilled life . . . I have grave doubts as to whether, however good a Downs sufferer is, they will ever be able to lead a totally independent life. And in view of the shortage of organs, I feel that my priority, if asked to make a decision between a normal person and a Downs patient, is to go for the one who can become that independent person (Toolis 1996).

For further information concerning the influence of the eugenics movement on people with learning disabilities see Köbsell (1993).

- **Sick.** Following the establishment of the National Health Service came the medicalization of some services offered to people with learning disabilities, resulting in hospital provision being seen as the most appropriate way to care for such people. A natural consequence was the development of a whole 'adult' nursing-oriented approach to caring for people based upon the medical model of care. Although it is clear that people with learning disabilities do face particular challenges to their health that are not always met very well by generic services, this does not mean that they are sick, and services should not be constructed for them to meet this distorted role perception.

- **Holy innocent.** A consistent perception of people with learning disabilities, throughout history, is that they are in some way innocent of original sin, and because of this enjoy some form of special relationship with the deity, perhaps as recompense for their disability.

- **Eternal child.** This is probably the most commonly encountered perception of people with a learning disability, and can prevent such people being allowed to 'grow up'. This often manifests itself in carers not allowing adults with a learning disability to take risks, and make their own choices, or even giving them childlike clothes or toys that are not appropriate to their age.

- **Object of pity and burden of charity.** Because the person with a learning disability is perceived as not enjoying the 'normality' of being human, it is common to find people who feel pity for them, with such intensity that they are ascribed the need for charity – to be looked after. In some countries the church has had a historical involvement in the care of people with a learning disability, and this is evidenced by charitable homes to care for them. Such a perception may assume that the needs of people with learning disabilities are met in return for submission and gratitude.

- **Object of ridicule.** There is some historical evidence that people with a learning disability were used as 'fools' and jesters in court entertainment (Williams 1985). The perception that such people with learning disabilities are in some way 'stupid', 'thick' or 'incompetent' is still prevalent in our own society, and it is often thought not inappropriate to ridicule them. In this context the

THE FEEBLE-MINDED

OR THE

HUB TO OUR WHEEL OF VICE, CRIME AND PAUPERISM

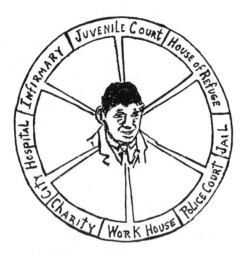

Cincinnati's Problem

Figure 1.3   'Cincinnati's Problem': cover of a pamphlet distributed to show the views held on people with learning disabilities *circa* 1915. Reproduced with permission from the University of California Press, © 1994 The Regents of the University of California (Trent 1994).

reader might find it worthwhile to read John Steinbeck's (1937) classic book entitled *Of Mice and Men*.

• **Menace.** Even today people with learning disabilities are perceived as a menace. It is common to find initiatives for the relocation of such people from hospital to community settings beset with problems of neighbour complaints. These complaints typically concern a drop in the value of their own property, or people 'wandering around' who may get into trouble with the police. Interestingly, but not surprisingly, this notion of people with learning disabilities as being menacing in some way has developed over a long period of time. For example, Trent (1994), on tracing the history of learning disability in America, reproduced some written comments made by the Cincinnati

Juvenile Protective Association in 1915, to the effect that:

The moron group is the most serious menace to society. The idiot and the imbecile, because of their low degree of intelligence, are easily recognised. They usually do not look normal and often are physically repellent. The moron, however, can pass as normal among lay-men (Trent 1994).

The perception of menace presented to society by people with learning disabilities is well illustrated by Figure 1.3, which featured on a pamphlet entitled *The Feeble-Minded* that was distributed in Cincinnati in 1915. This demonstrates the universality of such a perception early in this century. The notion of someone passing as normal, even though they were not, in a society and time when segregation and eugenics were high on the agenda, merely fuelled the notion of learning-disabled people as a menace.

• **Object of dread.** Because of this perception of learning disability, when a child is either born or diagnosed as having a learning disability it is often regarded as a punishment. Prospective parents view the possibility of having such a child with dread. As Bannerman and Lindsay (1994) have argued, 'A family's investment in and expectation of their children is often very high and the arrival of a child with a disability may be the end of dearly held dreams about what that child would achieve in life.'

It is apparent that people with a learning disability are not perceived in the same way as other people in society, and this may be accounted for partly by the images and attitudes that society holds toward this group of people; this in part is brought about by the effects of labelling and the creation of a deviant group. The next section briefly explores some historical information about learning disabilities: it is interesting to note how the imagery has changed very little over the centuries. Subsequent chapters, where appropriate, provide relevant historical information; for example, Chapters 3, 7 and 8 and Appendix 1 provide a highly relevant and useful summary of legislation and social policy that has affected people with learning disabilities during this century. For further information concerning the history of labelling in learning disability the reader should refer to Williams 1978, Ryan & Thomas 1987, and Hastings & Remington (1993).

HISTORICAL INFORMATION

It must be remembered that whenever historical aspects of learning disabilities are written about, the issue is often confused with the broader history of mental health. Also it is not unusual to find conflicting opinions as to how one should interpret the data. For example, Gilbert (1985) found that in the Judaeo-Hellenistic world people with learning disabilities were often perceived as gifts from the Gods, and were therefore treated with kindness. Later, mediaeval periods abounded with folklore explanations for learning-disabled children. For example, in much of Europe the idea of 'changelings' was common. Here it was believed that a child would be stolen by fairies and replaced with a changeling (said to be a fairy child), and therefore it was important for parents to be kind to the changeling because the fairies still had their own child. By 1325 there was an Act that sought to make a clear distinction between people with mental health problems and those with learning disabilities (*De Praerogativa Regis 1325*). This Act made provision for the ways in which their properties should be dealt with: fools were to have them protected, whereas lunatics were to have them protected until they recovered. By 1689 Locke had attempted to make a qualitative distinction in the ways in which these two distinct groups of people thought. He said:

In short herein seems to be the difference between idiots and madmen, that madmen put wrong ideas together, and so make wrong propositions, but argue and reason from them; but idiots make very few or no propositions and reason scarce at all (Locke 1689).

Following the agricultural and industrial revolutions came the introduction of a variety of institutions to rid the streets of our new and industrial cities of the rogues, madmen, cripples and outcasts. Such groups were treated with compassion despite the desire to see them moved on. This was a period of philanthropy, where asylums, colonies and retreats were built for practically any subgroup of humanity that did not quite belong to society. Unfortunately, this phil-

anthropic attitude turned harsh, towards an all-pervasive attitude of segregation to purify humankind, especially of the defective. In 1869 Galton wrote his first important piece of work on eugenics. He had studied the families of eminent people and had concluded that it would be possible to produce a gifted race of men, by manipulating marriages through several consecutive generations. All that was required was the removal and total segregation of people with learning disabilities from society. In 1904 a Royal Commission was set up to advise on the needs of the 'mentally defective' population. Bannerman and Lindsay (1994) have distilled the four major recommendations from this Commission:

- People who were mentally defective needed protection from society, and indeed from themselves.
- All mentally defective people should be identified and brought into contact with caring agencies.
- Mentally defective people should not be condemned because of their condition.
- A central organizing body should be established to work with the local caring agencies who would be responsible for the care of individual people.

The commission led to the enactment of the 1913 Mental Deficiency Act. This was a most interesting piece of legislation, which introduced compulsory certification of 'defectives' admitted to institutions; clearly, it served to segregate people with a learning disability from society at large. However, it must be acknowledged that at this time there was still a eugenics movement, originating from the mid-19th century.

The desire to segregate people with a learning disability from the rest of society resulted in large numbers of institutions being built. The idea of segregation appeared to have been universally prosecuted during this period. It is, however, possible to find something positive in the 1913 Act, and this was the separation of learning disability from mental illness. Until this time people with mental health problems and those with learning disabilities were often cared for in the same institution. It is interesting to note that the Act placed the management and responsibility for the care of people with a learning disability with local authorities. It is also interesting that the asylums which developed during the end of the last and the beginning of this century, did not become hospitals as we know them until the emergence of the National Health Service in 1946. In a sense, the health service as a major provider of care for people with a learning disability occurred almost by chance. This shift in responsibility and the subsequent model of care have led to a continuing and unhelpful argument as to the most appropriate agency and / or model for care provision, i.e. a social or a health model of care. The next major piece of mental health legislation to affect people with a learning disability was the 1959 Mental Health Act, which replaced previously used terminology with the terms mental subnormality, severe mental subnormality, mental disorder and psychopathic disorder. This Act required local authorities to provide both day and residential care for people with a learning disability. It also made provision for voluntary attendance at a hospital, rather than compulsory certification. The importance of this should not be underestimated, as it reflected a fundamental shift in the attitudes of legislators, if not society as well. This Act provided new definitions (see earlier in the chapter) for what we now refer to as learning disabilities; however, it perpetuated the apparent need for mental health legislation for people with learning disabilities. During the 1960s a series of scandals was reported concerning the care of such people in the large hospitals. In 1971 the then Labour Government published an extremely significant document in the history of learning disability; known as *Better Services for the Mentally Handicapped* (DHSS 1971), this promoted a model of community care, with a significant reduction in the number of hospital beds and a corresponding increase in local authority provision. This shift in responsibility resulted in the Griffiths Report (1988), the Government's White Papers *Caring for People* (1989a) and *Working for Patients* (1989b) and the 1990 National Health Service and Community Care Act. This series of reports, White Papers and subsequent legislation was evidence of the final move from hospital to community care for peo-

ple with learning disabilities. It is important to note that the National Health Service and Community Care Act (1990) also made local authorities responsible for acting as lead agents in the provision of care packages for people with learning disabilities. For a comprehensive analysis of current legislation and its impact on the ways in which care is provided, the reader is advised to consult Malin (1994). Readers with a special interest in the historical study of learning disability should refer to Lazerson (1975) and Trent (1994).

The case histories presented in Case studies 1.1, 1.2, 1.3 and 1.4 are authentic. They represent a number of people who may be described by some professionals as having learning disabilities.

MODELS TO EXPLAIN LEARNING DISABILITY

Clarke (1986) has commented that 'Learning dis-

 Case study 1.1

A small child

Ayesha is 8 years of age and is said to have profound learning disabilities with associated physical disabilities. She is the youngest member of a large Indian immigrant family who settled in this country some 7 years ago. Her birth followed a normal and uneventful pregnancy and there were no difficulties associated with her delivery. By the age of 6 months, however, there were noticeable abnormalities in her psychomotor development. Both the arm and the leg on one side of her body failed to develop properly, and her parents noticed a progressive stiffness and rigidity to her muscles. Following an outpatient visit to the local paediatrician, cerebral palsy was diagnosed and the parents were told that other aspects of her development might be affected. This prediction was indeed correct: Ayesha failed to develop any self-help skills or communication skills, and showed no sign of developing any motor coordination or the ability to walk. She remained incontinent of urine and faeces and required to be changed on a regular basis. At the age of 3 she was assessed by an educational psychologist, who thought that she had profound learning disabilities with complex needs, and would require special schooling to meet those needs. She has attended the same school since she was 5 but appears to have made little or no progress. Her teachers and parents report her as a happy and contented child who needs total care.

Case study 1.2

A young man

David is 19 years old and lives with foster parents, having been removed from his natural family because of an incestuous relationship with his younger sister. Little is known of his early childhood because of conflicting reports from his natural family and his foster parents. It is known that he was slow, and this resulted in his attending a school for children with special needs. He left school at 17 and attended a course on basic numeracy and literacy at a local further education (FE) college for people with special needs. During his two terms at college he was desperately unhappy, seldom spoke to his peers, and failed to settle in. His foster parents, through his general practitioner, referred him to a local community learning disabilities team as they thought this might help David enjoy a better quality of life. A community learning disability nurse, along with an occupational therapist, visited the foster parents at home to assess David's level of disability and then establish how the team could assist the family, if at all. Following the initial meeting and assessment it soon transpired that David and his foster parents were encountering a number of problems. For example, David would return from college and run straight to his bedroom, where he would masturbate for hours on end. This had resulted in considerable soreness and bleeding to his penis, and a subsequent visit to his GP. At home David refuses to wash either himself or his clothes, or take part in any domestic duties. David complains that he hates college and that he feels frustrated that he can't get a girlfriend or manage his private affairs. At the same time he hates being with his foster parents and wants to leave home and set up his own flat.

 Case study 1.3

A woman

Jill is 38 years of age; she is an obese woman described as having severe learning disabilities associated with extremely complex behavioural difficulties. She attends a resource centre run by the local authority and receives respite care from an independent provider of services for people with learning disabilities. Jill has little verbal communication, although many of the people who know her feel she understands 'a good deal more than she lets on'. For most of the time Jill is well behaved, she smiles, laughs and is good company for those around her. For some, so far unexplained, reason she sporadically demonstrates very difficult behaviour, including screaming, stripping herself of clothes, soiling herself, and attacking any of her carers, including her parents if she is at home. She has a history of epilepsy that appears to be well controlled by drugs. She is able to walk, dress and toilet herself. However, her self-help skills are quite limited and she does not enjoy learning new ones, this sometimes being a reason for her difficult behaviour.

A sociological perspective

Kurtz (1981) has provided a theoretical insight on learning disability using a sociological approach to explain its nature. He has suggested that individuals in any society are occupants of a status attached to their role in that society. He has promoted the work of Guskin (1963), who noted that people with learning disabilities tend to play very generalized roles in society. Such roles, he suggested, emphasized the inability of such people to undertake functional activities adequately. The functional activities referred to were everyday experiences; for most people these include going to work, taking care of oneself, behaving in an acceptable way, and managing one's own finances. The issue here is that it was suggested that people with learning disabilities could not perform these activities adequately. Of particular interest was the question whether the cause of such inability could be identified. Was the inability caused by the learning disability, or was it a consequence of behaving in the ways that people expected them to? Guskin (1963) suggested that:

. . . one could hypothesise non achievement orientation, dependency behaviour, and

ability has been a source of speculation, fear, scientific enquiry for hundreds of years. It has been regarded in turn as an administrative, medical, eugenic, educational and social problem'.

As briefly outlined earlier in the chapter, quite how we understand learning disabilities is a perplexing question. Possibly because of this, it is not surprising that the way in which learning disability has been catered for throughout history has to some extent reflected the theoretical perspectives in vogue at the time. This next section will provide a very brief overview of two different theoretical perspectives that are commonly associated with learning disability. For a fuller account of other perspectives the reader is advised to refer to Gates and Beacock (1996).

Case study 1.4

Two older people
Henry (68) and Martha (71) share a community home for people with learning disabilities. They were both admitted to a large (now closed) learning disability hospital on the edge of a large city. They were both discharged from the hospital some 5 years ago, after being resident there for over 35 years. Both have a full range of communication skills and both can read and write, albeit not very well. They are able to wash and dress themselves, and pretty much care for all other aspects of independent living, with the exception of cooking and household chores. The home where they live is run by the local authority, who provide day care staff to assist the couple in this respect. They both enjoy a full social life and relish their bingo nights. Henry likes to go the pub by himself two nights a week, and enjoys putting some money on the horses. Martha has close connections with a local church group and attends a weekly open evening for senior citizens. The only problem that they have encountered is local children, who frequently hang around the area and taunt Henry and Martha when they see them. Martha attempts to ignore them, but Henry loses his temper and shouts and screams, and then cries; this always makes the children laugh, and they then run off before they get into trouble. Unfortunately, it takes Henry some time to calm down, and some time after such events he can be found wandering around the housing estate, shouting at any children he meets. On at least two occasions the police have been called; they have informed the local community learning disabilities nurse, who has managed to defuse the situation.

Activity 1.3

Spend some time reading case histories 1.1–1.4. Who do you think has learning disabilities, if anyone. In determining this, identify what criteria you are using to make your decision.

rebelliousness as patterns of behaviour determined by previous and present interactions with people who have role concepts of the defective emphasising inability, helplessness, and lack of control, respectively.

Kurtz (1981) further argued that, because of the ways in which learning disability had been perceived, two important images of such individuals emerged in the United States. These were:

- the person with a learning disability as a sick person
- the person with a learning disability as a developing person.

He suggested that the first of these images was chiefly held by medicine, whereas the second was held by educators, psychologists and possibly parents. In conclusion, sociological approaches to learning disabilities have focused on the role of this group of people within society. It is suggested that because of the images that society holds, expectations of their role are limited; in this sense, Dexter (1958) has argued that learning disability is a creation of society.

A psychological perspective

Psychology is concerned with the study of human behaviour and, as some human behaviour is deemed abnormal, a branch of study concerned specifically with the study of abnormal behaviour has developed, known as abnormal psychology. Like learning disabilities, abnormal behaviour is difficult to define, so there is a need to identify criteria in order to distinguish abnormal from normal behaviour (Atkinson et al 1990). Generally speaking, abnormal behaviour is identified by the following:

- Deviation from statistical norms
- Deviation from social norms
- Maladaptive behaviour
- Personal distress.

This chapter has already described how intelligence tests are used to establish whether people deviate from statistical norms in relation to their measured intelligence. In the United States a category system has been used for the identification of abnormality; this is known as the *Diagnostic and Statistical Manual of Mental Disorders*, and approximates to the International System of the World Health Organization (identified earlier in this chapter). The system comprises a number of diagnostic categories that are themselves comprised of subclassifications. Using this system an individual is evaluated against a number of dimensions, from which developmental disorders, such as learning disability, can be identified. In the pursuit of identifying deviation from social norms, extensive use has been and is made of a large number of maladaptive behaviour assessment formats; for further information see Chapter 9 or Sparrow et al (1984).

ROLE OF THE LEARNING DISABILITIES NURSE

Within the specialty of learning disabilities nursing the promotion of health and social wellbeing is seen as the ultimate goal of nursing intervention. Health, as a concept, is viewed holistically to include all the dimensions of being fully human. Health has been defined by Beck et al (1988) as including dimensions of being such as biological, educational, spiritual, cultural and social. They have stated that:

Holistic health philosophy includes a primary focus on health promotion, or health as a positive process, rather than the absence of disease, it is a dynamic active process of continual striving to reach one's own balance and highest potential. Health involves working towards optimal functioning in all areas. The process varies among people and even within individuals as they move from one situation and life stage to another, and is contingent on personal needs, imbalances and individual perceptions of reality. (Beck et al 1988).

This definition is useful because of its inclusiveness, in that it incorporates the notion of health and social wellbeing. In this final section the nurse's role in achieving health and social wellbeing will be explored.

Baldwin and Birchenall (1993) have suggested that the role of the learning disabilities nurse is multidimensional in nature and comprises six key role areas:

- Clinician
- Helper/counsellor
- Advocate/adviser
- Manager/leader
- Teacher/educator
- Therapist.

They have further suggested that the nurse is in an ideal position to practise nursing at different levels of role:

- **Primary role** At this level it was suggested that the nurse would provide 'hands-on' care.
- **Secondary role** At this level the nurse would coordinate care at a very practical level, using other members of the multidisciplinary team and/or lay carers.
- **Tertiary role** At this level nurses would plan services at the 'macro' level, which might possibly equate to the role of care manager.

More recently, Rose and Kay (1995), reporting on the outcome of a recent report into learning disabilities nursing (DOH 1995), identified eight key roles for the learning disabilities nurse:

- **Assessment of need** This is seen as a crucial first step in identifying the needs of an individual. Nurses have a legitimate involvement in helping identify people's lifestyles in order to predict their health needs. Nurses will be aware of the need to use assessment tools and methods that have high reliability and validity.
- **Health surveillance** Learning disability nurses will work with a range of healthcare professionals, either directly or indirectly, to monitor and promote health and thereby contribute to the wellbeing of individuals. This involvement is particularly important in the areas of nutrition, sleep, posture, psychological wellbeing, accident prevention, health, lifestyle, medication for epilepsy or mental health problems.
- **Enhanced therapeutic skills** Some people with learning disabilities have very complex needs and/or display behaviours that make them vulnerable to abuse from others. Such people will require access to and support from nurses who are able to implement a range of psychotherapeutic approaches to enhance their wellbeing.
- **Developing personal competence** Using her knowledge of human development and the processes involved in learning, the nurse can facilitate the growth of personal competence in people with learning disabilities. Helping

people to learn through skilful teaching is a legitimate role of the nurse, and contributes to a sense of self-control and empowerment.

- **Management and leadership** Nursing often provides a focus for the delivery of care to people with learning disabilities. Therefore, it is not unusual to find nurses leading teams of professionals from a range of backgrounds. There is clearly a need for team managers to have advanced people management skills; these are now an integral component of pre- and post-registration nursing courses.
- **Enhancement of quality service** There is evidence (DOH 1993) that nurses contribute to improving clinical standards and service audit, because of their specialist knowledge and skills in this area. It is also acknowledged (National Health Service Executive 1994) that nurses can make an important contribution to the setting of standards and advising on issues of importance in the contracting process.
- **Enablement and empowerment** People with learning disabilities are at great risk of becoming devalued and disadvantaged. Nurses can assist people in accessing services or by advocating for them (see Chapter 14; also Gates 1994).
- **Coordination of services** It must be acknowledged that no single discipline can meet all the needs of learning-disabled people. Often there is a need for someone to coordinate the input of the various disciplines and adopt the role of key worker. Although not exclusively a feature of nursing, this role is often adopted in practice, especially in community and residential patterns of care.

These eight key roles can be shown diagrammatically (Figure 1.4).

Rose and Kay (1995) also identified five areas of service provision upon which nurses may have a significant impact. These include:

- Child health
- Adult health
- Independent sector provision
- Local authority services
- Services for people who challenge services.

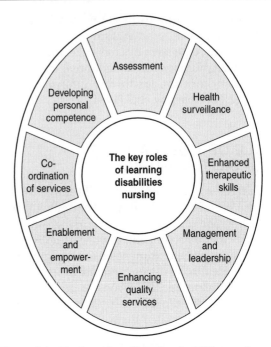

Figure 1.4   The key roles of learning disabilities nursing.

Learning disability nurses may be found in all of the above settings; they may also be regarded as 'facility independent' (DOH 1991), that is, learning disability nurses care for, work with and support people with learning disabilities where they are, and therefore their role is not dependent upon the agency of care. Despite minor differences in the articulation of the role of the learning disabilities nurse, from the sources identified above it is clear that there is a degree of consensus that enables this role to be defined as follows:

To skilfully assess the social and health care needs of people with learning disabilities, and/or their families, in order to assist them to live as independently as possible. The nurse will achieve this by marshalling her skills as manager, enabler and coordinator of services, and will demonstrate that her evidence based interventions lead to health maintenance and/or gain. The nurse will practise her craft work autonomously yet interdependently with other colleagues from a variety of other academic disciplines and service agencies in a variety of settings, in partnership with people with learning disabilities to assist them to lead valued life styles. This role will require her to develop and refine her knowledge and competence in a range of skills in order to meet the changing needs of people with learning disabilities.

It is suggested that this definition is grounded in the learning disability nursing literature, along with the professional and theoretical frameworks identified within the wider literature of nursing. Having defined their role, it should be noted that learning disabilities nurses do not own the sole franchise on caring for this group of people: it is necessary to use the knowledge and skills of a number of different academic and professional disciplines. However, what is unique about learning disabilities nursing is that it combines practice-oriented courses along with a vocational element located in higher education. This combination enables students to develop into practitioners who can provide care at a very practical level, as well as at more sophisticated levels of care management.

Nurses from this specialty will encounter learning-disabled people with particular challenges to their health (DOH 1995), which include:

- Communication problems
- Hearing problems
- Eyesight problems
- Obesity and poor cardiovascular fitness
- Behaviour problems
- Epilepsy
- Psychiatric illness
- Respiratory problems
- Orthopaedic and other problems of mobility.

These health problems are explored in more detail later in the book, providing direction for nurses to help ameliorate these aspects of health and/or identify how they may be improved.

CONCLUSION

This chapter sets out to provide an introduction to the book along with an exploration as to what learning disability means, and it is hoped that the reader now appreciates the complexity of deciding just what learning disability is, without making arbitrary decisions, especially for those who are often described as having a mild learning disability. It has also been demonstrated that people with learning disabilities have been viewed both positively and negatively throughout history, and such perceptions have affected their lifestyles and opportunities. The contribution that nursing may make to the lives of people with learning disabilities has also been outlined, but it must be remembered that in this branch of nursing the specialist input of other disciplines is often essential. People with learning disabilities are among the most vulnerable in society, and because of this they are often exploited. If all those involved in the care of people with learning disabilities could convince others of the potentially important contributions such people could make, then perhaps society would be more tolerant and caring. If nursing has any impact upon changing perceptions, this will be a significant and important contribution to the acceptance of people with learning disabilities as equal and valued members of society.

REFERENCES

Atkinson R L, Atkinson R C, Smith E E, Bem D J, Hilgard E R 1990 Introduction to psychology, 10th edn. Harcourt Brace Jovanovich London
Baldwin S, Birchenall M 1993 The nurse's role in caring for people with learning disabilities. British Journal of Nursing 2(17): 850–855
Bannerman M, Lindsay M 1994 Evolution of services. In: Shanley E, Starrs T (eds) Learning disabilities. A handbook of care. Churchill Livingstone, Edinburgh
Beck C M, Rawlins R D, Williams S R 1988 Mental health psychiatric nursing – a holistic life cycle approach. C V Mosby, London
Clarke D 1986 Mentally handicapped people living and learning. Baillière Tindall, London

Department of Health and Social Security 1971 Better services for the mentally handicapped. HMSO, London
Dexter L 1958 A social theory of mental deficiency. American Journal of Mental Deficiency 62: 920–928
DOH 1989a Caring for people: community care in the next decade and beyond. Cm. 849. HMSO, London
DOH 1989b Working for patients. Cm. 555. HMSO, London
DOH 1991 Caring for people: The implications for mental handicap nursing. (Cullen Report.) HMSO, London
DOH 1993 Targeting practice: the contribution of nurses, midwives and health visiting. HMSO, London
DOH 1995 Continuing the commitment: the report of the learning disability nursing project. HMSO, London

DOH 1995 The health of the nation: a strategy for people with learning disabilities. HMSO, London

Galton F 1869 Hereditary genius. MacMillan, London

Gates B 1994 Advocacy: a nurse's guide. Scutari Press, Middlesex

Gates B, Beacock C 1996 Dimensions of learning disability. Baillière Tindall, London

Gilbert P 1985 Mental handicap: a practical guide for social workers. Business Press International, Surrey

Griffiths R 1988 Community care: agenda for action. HMSO, London

Gross R D 1991 Psychology: the science of mind and behaviour. Hodder and Stoughton, London

Guskin S 1963 Social psychologies of mental deficiency. In: Ellis N (ed) Handbook of mental deficiency. McGraw-Hill, New York

Hastings R P, Remington S 1993 Connotations of label for mental handicap and challenging behaviour: a review and research evaluation. Mental Handicap Research 6(3): 237–249

Independent Television Corporation 1993 Führer: seduction of a nation. Independent Television Corporation, London

Köbsell S 1993 Testing, testing: the new eugenics. Disability, Pregnancy and Parenthood International 4: 11–13

Kurtz R 1981 The sociological approach to mental retardation. In: Brechin A, Liddiard P, Swain J (eds) Handicap in a social world. Hodder and Stoughton, Suffolk

Lazerson M 1975 Educational institutions and mental subnormality: notes on writing a history. In: Begab M Richardson SA (eds) The mentally retarded and society: a social science perspective. University Park Press, Baltimore

Locke J 1689 An essay concerning human understanding. Basset, London

Luckasson R, Coulter D, Polloway E et al 1992 Mental retardation. Definition, classification and systems of support. AAMR, Washington DC

Malin N, Race D, Jones G 1980 Services for the mentally handicapped in Britain. Croom Helm, London

Malin N 1994 Development of community care. In: Malin N (ed) Implementing community care. Open University Press, Buckingham

Mittler P 1979 People not patients: problems and policies in mental handicap. Methuen, London

National Health Service Executive 1994 Building a stronger team – the nursing contribution to purchasing. NHSE, Leeds

Nursey N, Rhode J, Farmer R 1990 Words used to refer to people with mental handicaps. Mental Handicap 18(1): 30–32

Rose S, Kay B 1995 Significant skills. Nursing Times 6(91): 63–64

Ryan J, Thomas F 1987 The politics of mental handicap. Free Association Books, London

Sparrow S, Balla D, Cicchetti V 1984 Vineland Adaptive Behaviour Scores. Interview edn. Survey Form Manual. American Guidance Service, Minnesota

Steinbeck J 1937 Of mice and men. Heinemann, London

Toolis K 1996 A Heart for Jo. Weekend Guardian 10 August 1966 18–23

Tredgold R F, Soddy K 1956 A textbook of mental deficiency, 9th edn. Baillière Tindall, London

Trent J 1994 Inventing the feeble mind: a history of mental retardation in the United States. University of California Press, Berkeley

Turner S, Sweeney D, Hayes L 1995 Developments in community care for adults with learning disabilities: a review of 1993/94 community care plans. HMSO, London

WHO 1993 Describing developmental disability. Guidelines for a multiaxial scheme for mental retardation (learning disability), 10th revision. World Health Organization, Geneva

Williams P 1978 Our mutual handicap: attitudes and perceptions of others by mentally handicapped people. Campaign for Mentally Handicapped People, New York

Williams P 1985 The nature and foundations of the concept of normalisation. In: Kracos E (ed) Current issues in clinical psychology. Clinical psychology 2. Plenum, New York

Wolfensberger W 1972 The principle of normalisation in human management services. National Institute of Mental Retardation, Toronto

FURTHER READING

Alaszewski A 1986 Institutional care and the mentally handicapped: the mental handicap hospital. Croom Helm, London

Audit Commission for Local Authorities England and Wales 1986 Making a reality of community care: a report by the audit commission. HMSO, London

Ayer A, Alaszewski A 1984 Community care and the mentally handicapped: services for mothers and their mentally handicapped children. Croom Helm, London

Barber P 1987 (ed) Using nursing models series: mental handicap: facilitating holistic care. Hodder and Stoughton, London

Beardshaw V 1981 Conscientious objectors at work: mental hospital nurses – a case study. Social Audit, London

Blunden R, Allen D (eds) 1987 Facing the challenge: an ordinary life for people with learning difficulties and challenging behaviour. Kings Fund Centre, London

Booth T, Booth W 1994 Parenting under pressure: mothers and fathers with learning difficulties. Open University Press, Buckingham

Craft M 1985 Classification, criteria, epidemiology and causation. In: Craft M, Bicknell J, Hollins S (eds) Mental handicap: a multidisciplinary approach. Baillière Tindall, London

Deacon J J 1974 Tongue tied: fifty years of friendship in a subnormality hospital. MENCAP, London

Department of Health 1992 Social care for adults with learning disabilities (Mental Handicap LAC (92)(15). HMSO, London

Department of Health and Social Security 1984a Helping mentally handicapped people with special problems. HMSO, London

Department of Health and Social Security 1984b Mental handicap: progress, problems and priorities. Cmnd 4663 HMSO, London

Department of Health and Social Security 1985 The role of

the nurse for people with a mental handicap. CNO 855. HMSO, London

English National Board for Nursing Midwifery and Health Visiting 1985 Caring for people with a mental handicap: a learning package for nurses. ENB, London

Gostin L 1985 The law relating to mental handicap in England and Wales. In: Craft M, Bicknell J, Hollins S (eds) Mental handicap: a multidisciplinary approach. Baillière Tindall, London

Henderson V 1966 The nature of nursing. Macmillan, London

Malin N 1990 Services for people with learning disabilities. Routledge, London

Malin N (ed) 1994 Implementing community care. Open University Press, Buckingham

Open University 1987 Mental handicap: patterns for living. Open University Press, Milton Keynes

Owens G, Birchenall P 1979 Mental handicap – the social dimensions. Pitman, London

Reid A 1982 The psychiatry of mental handicap. Blackwell Scientific, Oxford

Rutter M 1995 The roots of mental handicap. Medical Research Council News 20–23

Segal S 1984 Society and mental handicap: are we ineducable? Costello, Guildford

Sines D 1988 Towards integration: residential care for people with a mental handicap in the community. Harper and Row, London

Todd M, Gilbert T 1995 Learning disabilities: practice issues in health settings. Routledge, London

Wright K, Haycox A, Leedham I 1994 Evaluating community care: services for people with learning difficulty. Open University Press, Buckingham

2

Causes and manifestations

D. Watson

INTRODUCTION

The reasons for learning disability are frequently sought and yet only partial answers have been found since the first attempts to define the condition were made. Since the beginning of history, in even the simplest of societies, assumptions have been made about the causes of learning disabilities, and in England, statutory mention of people with such disabilities dates back to the reign of Edward 1 (1272–1307), when the first attempts to distinguish between people who had learning disabilities and people who had mental health problems were made (Clarke & Clarke 1974).

Learning disabilities can be described as an umbrella term under which all affected individuals are described as having varying degrees of impairment of intellectual and social function-

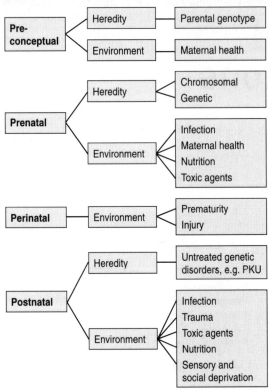

Figure 2.1   Causative factors of learning disabilities by time.

ing. Learning disabilities are diverse and may be the result of a range of causative factors. Such conditions are manifested during the different stages of the developmental process — preconceptual, prenatal, perinatal and postnatal – and can be described as being genetic or environmental in nature (Fig. 2.1).

It is difficult to state the precise number of people who have a learning disability, but it is estimated that approximately 20 in every 1000 of the population will have a mild learning disability and that three or four per 1000 will be diagnosed as having a severe learning disability (Health of the Nation 1995). Even if there were a more precise method of establishing these numbers, the actual number of known causes would still remain small because of the diverse and complex aetiologies of the various conditions.

An understanding of the potential causes and manifestations of learning disabilities is essential for professionals working with such individuals,

allowing them to assess and plan, in partnership with the individuals concerned, appropriate health and social care programmes that may ameliorate some of the adverse aspects of their condition. However, it must be emphasized that labelling an individual with a particular condition can have a negative effect, and carers should avoid this as the individual may not possess or display all of the known characteristics and traits associated with the condition: they should therefore be thought of as unique and assessed as such. An understanding of the causes and manifestations of learning disabilities will also assist the professional conducting research into the prevention of the primary and secondary causes of such disabilities, and be of benefit when offering counselling and support to parents or potential parents.

The birth of an individual with learning disabilities may be the result of genetic action, environmental influences or a mixture of the two. Figure 2.1 illustrates the causative factors implicated in learning disabilities and locates them in the developmental process.

INHERITANCE

Variation between individuals is a biological rule, resulting in the variety of the human species. Genetics could be described as the branch of science that is concerned with the study of heredity, i.e. the passing on of characteristics from parents to offspring.

Every human being originates as the result of the union of two gametes, the ovum and the sperm. The resultant individual is one of a kind, with a unique genotype. The individual's genetic makeup, or genome, represents the two sets of genetic instructions received, one from each parent.

Chromosomes

Each human cell contains 23 pairs of chromosomes, each pair consisting of one chromosome from each parent. During mitosis the cell replicates, ensuring that the same chromosomal pattern is achieved in each new daughter cell. The exception to this is in the gametes, where only one set of 23 chromosomes, one from each original pair, is represented. These will join to make up 23 pairs of chromosomes in the newly formed embryo.

Every chromosome is divided into loci, which contain the particular gene substance that determines the individual's inherited characteristics. Dutton (1975) likened the relationship between chromosomes and genes to that of a string of beads, with the string being the chromosome and the individual beads representing genes.

Of the 23 pairs of chromosomes, pairs 1–22 can be matched and are described as autosomes. Pair 23 is known as the sex chromosomes. In the female these are matched and referred to as XX. In the male they are not matched and are referred to as XY. The chromosomes are numbered from 1 to 23 according to the Denver System, with the largest pair being number 1 and the smallest being number 22; pair 23 are the sex chromosomes (Fig. 2.2). Another method of organizing chromosomes is to place them in one of seven groups labelled A – G according to size and shape. This enables the description of normal and abnormal karyotypes.

Genes

Genes are the units of heredity: they reside upon the chromosome and are responsible for many different traits, such as hair and eye colour. Like chromosomes they are matched (for the most part), and matched genes that are on the same locus of a homologous chromosome are called alleles. Therefore, when an individual inherits from each parent the same allelic form of a particular gene they are described as homozygous for that gene locus. However, if different alleles are present they are described as heterozygous. When a particular allele, when present in the heterozygote, gives rise to an obvious physical characteristic it is described as dominant. However, if the particular characteristic only appears in the individual when they are homozygous for the gene, it is described as recessive.

The individual's hereditary characteristics may then be described as chromosomal if they can be linked to one or more of the 23 pairs of identified chromosomes, and genetic if they are determined by one or more of the genes that reside upon those chromosomes. For example, an individual's sex is determined by a chromosomal hereditary characteristic (chromosome 23), whereas eye colour is identified as being caused by one or more genes and is referred to as genetic.

CHROMOSOME ABNORMALITIES

Chromosomal abnormalities are estimated to be the cause of approximately one-third of the 50% of learning disabilities which are attributable to genetic factors (Mueller & Young 1995).

Autosomal

The incidence of autosomal abnormalities has been calculated and is reproduced in Table 2.1 (Mueller & Young 1995).

Autosomal abnormalities may be subdivided into three main categories:

1. Abnormality of number. Here there may be a loss (or more commonly a gain) of one or more chromosomes, for example Down syndrome, or trisomy 21, where there is an extra chromosome in pair 21, or Edwards

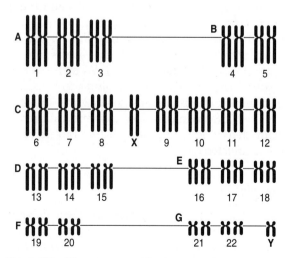

Figure 2.2 Chromosomes of the human male.

Table 2.1 Incidence of autosomal abnormalities in the newborn

Abnormality		Incidence per 10000 births
Trisomy	13	2
	18	3
	21	15

Table 2.2 Incidence of sex chromosome abnormalities in the newborn

Abnormality		Incidence per 10000 births
Female births	45,XO (Turner syndrome)	1
	47,XXX (Triple X syndrome)	10
Male births	47,XXY (Klinefelter syndrome)	10
	47,XYY (XYY syndrome)	10

syndrome, which has an extra chromosome present in pair 16, 17 or 18.

2. Abnormality of structure. Here there may be a loss of part of a chromosome (deletion) or a rearrangement (translocation) of the chromosomal material. For example, *Cri-du-chat* syndrome has a deletion of the short arm of chromosome 5. In Down syndrome an extra segment of chromosome may have been rearranged and attached to one of the following pairs: 13, 15, 21 or 22.

3. Mosaicism. Here individuals have cells with different numbers of chromosomes. This may occur as non-disjunction, or the accidental loss of a particular chromosome, usually during the first few cell divisions following fertilization. Mosaicisms for autosomes do occur, but are encountered more frequently on sex chromosomes. Examples of mosaicism are Down syndrome and Klinefelter syndrome.

Sex chromosome abnormalities

As with autosomes, additions and deletions to the sex chromosomes may occur. Primary non-disjunction, if it occurs during the formation of the ova or the spermatozoa, gives rise to a gamete with an extra X or Y chromosome. Sex chromosome abnormalities can be divided into four main subgroups:

XO Turner syndrome
XXX Triple X syndrome
XXY Klinefelter syndrome
XYY syndrome.

The incidence of sex chromosome abnormalities in the newborn has been calculated and is reproduced in Table 2.2 (Mueller and Young 1995).

MANIFESTATIONS OF AUTOSOMAL DISORDERS

Down syndrome

Down syndrome was first described in 1866 by Dr Langdon Down, from whom it derives its name. However, the chromosomal basis of Down syndrome was not established until 1959, when Lejeune and his colleagues discovered that people who had Down syndrome had 47 chromosomes, the extra chromosome residing with autosome 21 (trisomy 21).

The overall incidence of Down syndrome is approximately 1 in 650 to 1 in 700 (Mueller & Young 1995). The relationship between maternal age and the incidence of Down syndrome is well documented: in women aged 25 years and younger the incidence is under 1 in 1000, and the risk does not rise above that of the normal population until around 30 years. At the maternal age of about 40 the risk rises to 1 in 100, and thereafter continues to rise steeply. Paternal age would seem to be of little significance, as studies have shown that over 90% of cases are of maternal origin (Harper 1993). Women over 35 years of age should be offered amniocentesis, and informed of the risk of Down syndrome (Box 2.1). The risk of having further trisomic children is estimated as low, with only a few rare families being affected.

Translocation Down syndrome

This group make up only 5% of all cases of Down syndrome (Harper 1993). Where parents who are chromosomally normal have a child with translocation Down syndrome, the risk of having

Box 2.1   Amniocentesis

Amniocentesis is a prenatal procedure by which the diagnosis of a number of congenital abnormalities, such as chromosomal disorders and open neural tube defects, can be detected. The procedure is usually carried out by a skilled practitioner at an outpatients clinic, at around 15–16 weeks' gestation. The procedure commences with an ultrasound scan to locate the placenta and confirm the gestation (15–16 weeks is the earliest time that a satisfactory sample can be obtained). Then, under a local anaesthetic, a long thin needle is inserted into the amnion (the fluid-filled sac surrounding the fetus) via the mother's abdomen and a sample of the amniotic fluid withdrawn. The sample is then cultured, to provide enough cells for analysis. This process takes about 3–4 weeks, which means that the results are not available until 17–20 weeks' gestation.

Box 2.2   Chorion biopsy

Chorion biopsy is a prenatal diagnosis that is carried out in the first trimester (10–11 weeks' gestation) to detect chromosomal defects and inborn errors of metabolism. Fetal tissue is obtained from the chorionic villi (fingerlike projections of the outermost membrane surrounding the fetus). With the aid of ultrasound, a small tube is inserted through the vagina and cervical canal and guided towards the placenta, where a sample of tissue can be removed. The sample contains large numbers of rapidly dividing cells that allow studies to be carried out within a few hours of sample collection.

another affected child is low. However, chorion biopsy may be offered to diagnose translocation in high-risk cases (Box 2.2).

Characteristics

There are a large number of characteristics associated with Down syndrome and it should be remembered that not all people with this condition exhibit them all. However, the commonly known features usually allow identification of the condition in the neonatal period, with obvious floppiness (hypotonia) being a striking feature. In some cases chromosomal analysis may be the only method of confirming or excluding the condition.

The head is usually brachycephalic (small) and round, with a reduced cranial capacity. The brain appears 'simple' in structure and underweight. The higher brain functions are affected by the structural variations and accompanying malfunctions. However, the level of intellectual impairment varies between individuals. The achievement of developmental milestones may be slower and the child may appear to lag behind its peers, but with early intervention and support the individual may be allowed to work towards the achievement of their maximum potential.

Hair has a tendency to be dry, sparse and fine, with a possibility of recurrent focal alopecia in adulthood.

The face is flat (as is the occiput), and the ears are small with underdeveloped lobes. The eyes are usually upward- and outward-slanting, often with an epicanthic fold on the inner aspect of the upper eyelid. Strabismus, nystagmus and cataracts are common. Brushfield spots can be found flecked throughout the iris, which is often poorly developed. Owing to the lack of the enzyme lysozyme in tears, which acts as an antiseptic, conjunctivitis and blepharitis are common. The bridge of the nose is often poorly developed, and mouth breathing is common. The mouth is often small with a high narrow palate, whereas the tongue has a tendency to be large with horizontal fissures. As a result of this particular anatomy the mouth tends to be held open, with the tongue protruding. There is delayed development of the teeth, with an abnormality in their size, shape and alignment. Mouth breathing increases the risk of respiratory tract infection, which before the advent of antibiotics resulted in an increased mortality rate for this group of people.

The body of an adult with Down syndrome is usually small and broad in stature (usually not exceeding 1.5 m in height). Umbilical hernias are common. There is a tendency to hypotonia (reduced muscle tension), with the joints having an abnormal range of movement.

Hands and feet are distinctive, with the hands having a square palm with palmar crease, and a wide gap between the thumb and second finger. Fingers are short and stubby. Toes are shorter than normal and there may be a wide gap between the great toe and the second toe.

Genitalia in the male may be underdeveloped and there may be reduced fertility; however, males should not be assumed to be sterile. It is estimated that about one-third of women with Down syndrome ovulate, one-third have no evidence of ovulation, and that in the remaining third evidence of ovulation is intermediate (Newton 1992).

Edwards syndrome

Edwards syndrome was first described by Edwards and associates in 1960. It is caused by the presence of an extra chromosome on pair 18 (trisomy 18). The incidence has been calculated as 1 in 3000 and increases with advanced maternal age (Mueller & Young 1995).

Characteristics

There is an elongation of the skull, with a receding chin. The face is characterized by hypertelorism (abnormal distance) of the eyes, with underdeveloped supraorbital ridges, eyebrows and eyelashes. The ears are low set and small, and abnormal in shape. The neck is short with redundant skin folds, or webbing. The fingers are flexed and have a tendency to overlap, with distally placed thumbs. The feet are described as 'rocker bottomed', with dorsiflexed great toes. Limited abduction of the hip may be evident and the individual may have some degree of spasticity. The frontal lobes of the cerebral hemispheres may not separate normally. The degree of learning disability is severe, with associated physical handicaps, including congenital abnormalities of the heart, nervous system, abdominal organs, kidneys and ears.

The prognosis for affected individuals is poor, with most dying during the first few weeks of life.

Cri-du-chat syndrome

Cri-du-chat (or cry-of-the-cat syndrome) was first described by Lejeune and his colleagues in 1963. It is caused by a deletion of the short arm of chromosome 5. The condition is rare, with an estimated incidence of approximately 1 in 50 000

(Mueller & Young 1995). The condition is characterized by a distinctive high-pitched wailing cry, believed to be caused by a laryngeal defect. It is not until the child begins to develop that the characteristics become more striking.

Characteristics

Affected individuals tend to be small in stature, with microcephaly being common. The face is characterized by hypertelorism and downward slant of the eyes. The chin is small and the ears are low set. The nose is broad at its base and has been described as beaklike. Birthweight is low, and in the early months there is a failure to thrive and a poor sucking reflex.

Prognosis is variable, with some individuals surviving into adulthood. The degree of learning disabilities is normally severe and the development of speech is limited.

MANIFESTATIONS OF SEX CHROMOSOME ABNORMALITIES
Turner (OX) syndrome

This condition was first described in 1938. It is characterized by diminished secondary sexual characteristics: the affected individual presents as female, but lacks ovarian tissue and sex hormones, is sterile and shows primary amenorrhoea. Short stature (average adult height of 145 cm), which becomes apparent by mid-childhood, webbing of the neck, a low hairline at the back of the neck and widely spaced nipples are also features. The incidence of Turner syndrome is low, with estimates ranging from 1 in 5000 to 1 in 10 000 (Mueller & Young 1995). Affected individuals who have learning disabilities are usually described as having a very low intellect. Oestrogen therapy may be initiated at adolescence to promote the development of secondary sexual characteristics and to prevent osteoporosis during later life.

Triple X (XXX) syndrome

Birth surveys have shown that approximately

0.1% of all females have a XXX karyotype (Mueller & Young 1995). These women usually have no physical abnormalities, but can show varying degrees of reduction in intellectual functioning. Women with more than three X chromosomes show a high incidence of decreased intellectual functioning. Skeletal and neurological problems have been identified in XXX women and psychotic disorders are thought to be more frequent than in the normal population.

Klinefelter (XXY) syndrome

This condition was first described in 1942, but it was not until 1959 that the presence of the additional X chromosome was identified. This is a relatively common condition with an incidence equal to 1 in 1000 male live births (Mueller & Young 1995).

Development until puberty appears normal; the syndrome then becomes apparent when the secondary sexual characteristics fail to develop: testes are small or undescended, body hair is sparse and approximately 30% of males show moderately severe gynaecomastia (enlargement of the breasts). Adults with Klinefelter syndrome tend to have long lower limbs and are slightly taller than average. There is an increased risk of leg ulcers, osteoporosis and carcinoma of the breast in adult life. Psychotic and personality problems have also been described. The development of secondary sexual characteristics and the prevention of osteoporosis can be encouraged with the use of testosterone from puberty onwards. Many people with Klinefelter syndrome are of normal intelligence; those with learning disabilities are mainly described as mildly affected.

XYY syndrome

XYY syndrome has a reported incidence of 1 in 1000 newborn males (Mueller & Young 1995). It must be noted, however, that most XYY males do not suffer from intellectual impairment or psychopathic and criminal behaviours, as was once thought. Physical appearance is normal, with an above-average stature. Learning disabilities, if present, are usually described as mild.

GENE ABNORMALITIES

It may be helpful to group abnormalities of the genes as autosomal dominant (Fig. 2.3), autosomal recessive (Fig. 2.4), sex-linked (Fig 2.5) and polygenetic.

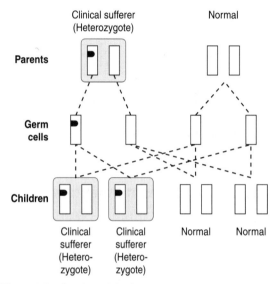

Figure 2.3 Dominant inheritance.

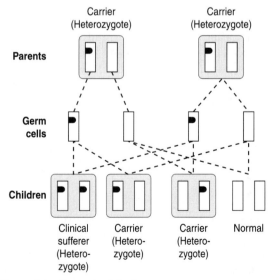

Figure 2.4 Recessive inheritance.

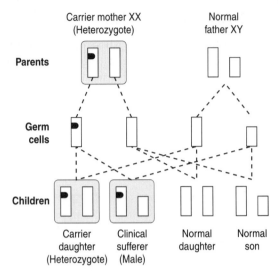

Figure 2.5 Sex-linked inheritance.

Autosomal dominant inheritance

There are at least 1000 human traits that are known to have their genetic basis in dominant genes located on autosomes (Singer 1985). Dimples and freckles are two examples of traits known to be dictated by dominant alleles.

Genetic disorders caused by dominant genes are fairly uncommon as lethal dominant genes are almost always expressed, resulting in the death of the developing embryo, fetus or child. There are, however, some conditions that are less severe, allowing the affected individual enough time to reproduce and pass on the affected gene. Achondroplasia, a rare form of dwarfism resulting from the inability of the fetus to form cartilage bone, is one example.

Autosomal recessive inheritance

There are at least 600 human traits that are known to have an autosomal recessive pattern of inheritance (Singer 1985). Many genetic disorders are inherited as simple recessive traits for example phenylketonuria and Tay–Sachs disease. To be affected, individuals must receive the gene for a particular condition from both parents. Carriers of disorders do not express the dis-

ease themselves, but can pass it on to their offspring. Offspring from consanguineous marriages (marriages between close relatives, such as siblings and first cousins) have a greater chance of inheriting two identical recessive genes and thus expressing the disease. Advice from a genetic counselling service may be of use for relatives of affected persons, enabling them to discuss the chances of their being a carrier, or of having an affected child.

Sex-linked inheritance

The Y chromosome, which contains the genes for determining maleness, is only one-third the size of the X chromosome and lacks many of the genes present on the X that code for non-sexual characteristics. For example, the gene involved in the production of certain blood clotting factors is only found on the X chromosome. Genes found only on the X chromosome are described as being X-linked. Haemophilia is a classic example of a sex-linked disorder. If a male inherits an X-linked recessive allele (from his mother) its expression is not masked because there is no corresponding allele on his Y chromosome (inherited from his father), which results in the recessive gene being expressed. In contrast, a female must have two X-linked recessive alleles to express the disease.

An example of X-linked recessive inheritance is Hunter syndrome, a form of gargoylism.

Polygenetic inheritance

Polygenetic inheritance occurs when a number of genes act together, causing complex traits. The estimated risk of inheritance is much less than in single gene inheritance, but the risk does increase with the number of first-degree relatives who suffer from the condition. Examples of congenital

Activity 2.1

If you have time, you may find it useful to find the details of your regional genetic counselling service.

conditions that are multifactorially determined are spina bifida and cleft lip.

MANIFESTATIONS OF ABNORMAL GENES

Autosomal dominant genes

Tuberous sclerosis

Tuberous sclerosis, or epiloia as it is also known, was first clearly described by Bournville in 1880. It is a rare condition caused by a gene of poor penetrance, in that it varies in manifestation both physically and intellectually. The condition has a wide range of severity, with approximately 60% of affected individuals having some degree of learning disability.

Characteristics The distinctive features of the condition are skin lesions (adenoma sebaceum, achromic naevi and fibrotic plaques), learning disabilities of varying severity, and epilepsy.

In adults and older children there is a characteristic facial rash with a superficial resemblance to acne, caused by an overgrowth of the sebaceous glands. It appears over the bridge of the nose and the cheeks and is described as a butterfly rash. In childhood the rash first appears like grains of rice under the skin, but in later life red papules appear that slowly multiply and enlarge. Treatment with an argon laser can reduce the impact for the affected individual.

'Shagreen patches' – raised areas of skin – are sometimes present in the lumbosacral region. Tumours are often found in the muscle wall of the heart and in the kidneys, lungs and brain, and can become calcified.

Children who have tuberous sclerosis may be slow in reaching developmental milestones. Mental and physical deterioration may occur, resulting in loss or worsening of skills and abilities. Life expectancy for those severely affected is considerably reduced.

Neurofibromatosis

There are several forms of neurofibromatosis, the most common being type 1 Von Recklinghausen's disease. The presence of six of more pigmented spots over 1.5 cm in diameter, and the characteristic *café-au-lait* appearance, is usually an indicator that the gene is present. Lisch nodules (harmless hamartomatous lesions) in the iris are a confirmatory clinical sign of the disease. About one-third of sufferers have one or more serious problems, including optic glioma, cerebral and spinal tumours, and mild or moderate learning disabilities, in comparison with two-thirds who are only mildly affected (Harper 1993).

Prader–Willi syndrome

Prader–Willi syndrome is the result of specific disordered function of a gene during development. It is thought that most of the syndromes described within this group are dominantly affected (Harper 1993). Prader–Willi syndrome more specifically is associated with the absence of a paternal contribution to a defined area of chromosome 15. The syndrome was first described by Prader and colleagues in 1956. It is associated with a variety of temperamental and behavioural characteristics, including extreme food-seeking behaviours, self-injury through skin picking, temper tantrums or rage reactions, lability of mood, a variety of sleep abnormalities, and stubbornness (Clarke et al 1995).

The degree of learning disability is described as mild, but more severe impairments do occur.

Autosomal recessive genes

There are a number of autosomal recessive disorders, many of which are associated with learning disabilities, for example, phenylketonuria, maple syrup disease, galactosaemia, Tay–Sachs disease, Hurler syndrome, hepatolenticular disease, Laurence–Moon–Biedl syndrome, true microcephaly, and Niemann–Pick disease.

Phenylketonuria

Phenylketonuria was first described by Asbjorn Folling, a Norwegian paediatrician, in 1934. It is probably one of the best-known genetic conditions, and, if untreated, can result in learning disabilities and a number of associated conditions.

Phenylketonuria is a disorder of protein metabolism that can be detected by a blood test. The autosomal recessive gene causes a deficiency of the enzyme normally present in the liver which converts phenylalanine to tyrosine. This results in raised blood levels of phenylalanine which are toxic to the developing brain. A blood test, or Guthrie test as it is known, is routinely carried out on all babies around the 5th or 6th day of life, provided that milk has been ingested. A child diagnosed as being phenylketonuric must be placed immediately on a phenylalanine-reduced diet. The effectiveness of the diet is monitored by regular urine tests for phenylketones and blood tests to ensure appropriate levels of phenylalanine.

Characteristics Affected children may have an increased incidence of vomiting, appear irritable, and are slow to reach developmental milestones. Hyperactivity and brain damage become evident in the second half of the first year of life. Autistic features, self-mutilation and a resistance to cuddling may be evident. Epilepsy is also characteristic in a number of children. Lack of pigmentation of the eyes, hair and skin is a result of the inability to convert phenylalanine to tyrosine, a precursor for melanin.

The degree of learning disability is dependent upon treatment, with untreated individuals being severely affected.

Galactosaemia

Galactosaemia is an autosomal recessive condition in which there is an abnormality of galactose metabolism. The condition is caused by a deficiency of the enzyme galactose-1-phosphate uridyl transferase, which is essential for the metabolism of galactose (galactose is one of the sugars of milk and is contained in nearly all naturally occurring milks). When the enzyme is deficient galactose and galactose-1-phosphate accumulate in the blood and other tissues. This is thought to be responsible for the symptoms of the disease, which is usually evident during the first few weeks of life. Affected children present with jaundice, vomiting and failure to thrive. If the condition remains untreated liver failure

occurs, and if the child survives learning disability is evident. Treatment must be started as early as possible to compromise the removal of dietary galactose.

Tay–Sachs disease

Tay–Sachs disease is an autosomal recessive disorder of the lipid metabolism that was first described by Tay in 1881 and by Sachs in 1887. The disease develops early in life, usually in the first year, and there is no treatment available that will prevent progressive mental deterioration.

With early onset of the condition death occurs in the 3rd or 4th year of life. With delayed onset, occurring in the 6th or 7th year of life, death is likely to occur in the mid-teens. The late-onset type is called Batten's disease.

Characteristics With early onset, deterioration is accompanied by spastic paralysis, blindness and convulsions. A characteristic 'cherry red' spot can be found on the macula of the retina.

Hurler syndrome

Hurler syndrome is an autosomal recessive condition in which there is abnormal storage of mucopolysaccharides in the connective tissue. It is often referred to as gargoylism because of the physical appearance of those affected. The condition is not apparent at birth but becomes evident during the first year, with its distinctive features.

Characteristics The individual is short in stature, with limited extension of the shortened limbs. The head is large with frontal bossing, the supraorbital ridges are prominent and the bridge of the nose is depressed. The eyebrows are coarse and hairy, and the eyes are low set with corneal clouding in the majority of cases. Teeth are irregular and late in appearing. The neck is short and thick. Kyphosis develops owing to abnormal vertebral deposits. Death usually occurs in adolescence, as a result of physical and mental deterioration.

X-linked recessive genes

There are a number of genetically determined

conditions associated with learning disabilities that are inherited in an X-linked manner. Females may be carriers of the conditions, with males being affected.

X-linked hydrocephalus

This is a rare form of hydrocephalus in which the aqueduct of Sylvius fails to develop fully. Without surgical intervention the cerebrospinal fluid accumulates in the ventricles and brain damage may occur.

Hunter syndrome

Hunter syndrome is a form of mucopolysaccharidosis (gargoylism). It is similar to Hurler syndrome except that it affects only males, no corneal clouding is evident and there is a much slower rate of physical and mental deterioration. Affected individuals usually survive into adulthood.

Fragile X syndrome

Fragile X syndrome was first described by Herbert Lubs in 1969. The term derives from the unusual appearance of the distal portion of the long arm of the X chromosome, which shows a fragile site. The condition causes a non-specific form of learning disability without major dysmorphic features or severe neurological abnormalities.

Fragile X syndrome has the unique and dubious distinction of being the most commonly inherited cause of learning disabilities, with an incidence of approximately 1 in 2000 males, and it accounts for 4–8% of all males with learning disabilities (Mueller & Young 1995).

Characteristics The clinical characteristics of this syndrome include a large forehead, ears and jaw, and following the onset of puberty macro-orchidism (enlarged testicles) develops. Individuals may exhibit hyperactivity, autism and self-mutilating behaviour. The degree of learning disability is said to be moderate, with a few individuals described as profoundly disabled.

Polygenic inheritance

There are a large number of conditions, some of which are rare, that are considered to be of polygenetic origin.

Sturge–Weber syndrome

Sturge–Weber syndrome, or naevoid amentia as it is also known, is a rare condition of unknown cause characterized by a facial naevus, often referred to as a 'port wine stain'. Part or all of the trigeminal nerve is affected on one side of the face. On the same side as the naevus can be found a meningeal angioma. In some cases there may be calcification in the meningeal angioma and the cerebral cortex. Epilepsy and spasticity are common features. Hemiplegia occurs on the opposite side of the body to the facial naevus. The degree of learning disability encountered can be severe.

Cornelia de Lange syndrome

Cornelia de Lange syndrome was first described by the Dutch paediatrician Cornelia de Lange in 1933. It has also become known as Amsterdam dwarfism. The incidence is approximately 1 in 40 000.

Characteristics The affected individual is dwarfed, with limb abnormalities, small hands and feet and underdeveloped genitalia. Microcephaly, facial hair, confluent eyebrows, downward-slanting eyes, small palate and irregular teeth are all characteristics.

All affected individuals have some degree of learning disability, which is often severe.

Hydrocephalus

Hydrocephalus is associated with an excessive amount of fluid in the brain. The rate of formation of cerebrospinal fluid (CSF) is often elevated, but more frequently the condition is caused by an obstruction to its flow. Hydrocephalus is often not recognized until the child is a few months old, and a considerable increase in head size can occur without evidence of significant brain damage. Severe damage to the brain substance occurs when the condition is untreated and the ventricles reach a critical point in their dilation. Surgical intervention may be required in a number of cases. The insertion of a ventriculoatrial shunt should allow the excess fluid to be drained off. Early intervention should ensure a positive outcome, but untreated cases could result in grossly distended skulls and severe learning disabilities. Strabismus, nystagmus, paralysis and epilepsy may also be evident. The reported prevalence of hydrocephalus averages 2 per 1000, but there is a higher incidence with increased parental age (Burns 1994).

Hypothyroidism

Hypothyroidism or cretinism is the name given to a group of conditions caused by a deficiency of thyroxine, which is secreted by the thyroid gland. A number of different metabolic errors result in a similar clinical picture. Although the precise cause is unknown the condition is treatable with thyroxine, usually given orally. Treatment should commence as early as possible, within the first few months of life.

The untreated individual frequently presents as apathetic, poor at feeding and sucking, a noisy breather owing to an enlarged tongue which protrudes, and also with delayed growth.

Characteristics The individual is small in stature, with severe learning disabilities, and speech acquisition is delayed until 7 or 8 years of age. The skin appears yellow in colour and is loose and wrinkled. There is thickening of the eyelids, nostrils, lips, hands and feet. Hair is usually scanty. Puberty is delayed and the external genitalia fail to develop.

ENVIRONMENT

Characteristics such as intelligence, health and body size are inextricably influenced by the environment. The individual who is deprived of food and vitamins is less likely to thrive than one who has an adequate supply. Similarly, the individual who is deprived of stimulation and education would appear to be at a disadvantage when developing intellectually, whatever their gene status. But what do we mean by environment? Like the term learning disabilities, the environment could be considered an umbrella term. Figure 2.1 shows the range of environmental factors that are considered important when studying the causes of learning disability.

ENVIRONMENTAL AND GENETIC CAUSES OF LEARNING DISABILITY BY TIME

The genetic causes of learning disability, although already identified, have been included here to demonstrate their relationship with the environmental causes of learning disabilities as identified in Figure 2.1 (p. 22).

Preconceptual

Preconceptual care and planning is for the most part a fairly new phenomenon, with the availability of valid research being limited. Good health prior to conception may not be an absolute guarantee of a healthy child, but there is statistical evidence (HC 1980, 1984; Sweet 1988) to show that unplanned pregnancies and perinatal mortality occur more frequently in the lower socioeconomic groups, in young unsupported women and in women with pre-existing medical disorders and previous obstetric complications. It would therefore seem reasonable to consider the genetic and environmental factors that may be operating during the preconceptual stage, which may assist in detecting the possibility of learning disabilities and perhaps preventing them. The organization Foresight produces information including *Guidelines for Future Parents* (Dickerson 1980) and *Planning for a Healthy Baby* (Barnes & Bradley 1990).

Heredity

Genetic counselling, which will include obtaining a detailed family history or pedigree, may be necessary for some couples, where there is a known or potential risk of abnormality (Box 2.3).

Box 2.3 Genetic counselling

Genetic counselling is a service offered to patients or relatives who may be at risk from a disorder that may be hereditary in nature. During the process patients or relatives are advised of the consequences of the disorder, the probability of developing or transmitting it, and ways in which it may be prevented, avoided or ameliorated.

The Hospital for Sick Children in Great Ormond Street, London, was the first in the UK to develop a genetic counselling service in 1946. There are now a number of regionally based centres offering this service.

Environment

Nutrition is important at any stage in the lifecycle, and any nutritional deficiencies may take many months to correct. Prospective parents should be encouraged to maintain a healthy balanced diet, not only during pregnancy but also in preparation for conception. Children conceived during periods of poor nutrition, such as in Holland in the 'Hunger Winter' (October 1944 to May 1945), were found to have a high perinatal mortality rate. In those infants who survived there was found to be an increased incidence of congenital malformation. Neural tube defects and the incidence of cleft lip and palate have been reported as having a reduced incidence (Smithells et al 1980) when mothers were given periconceptual vitamin supplements, including folic acid. Further research is currently being conducted into the implications of these findings.

Pre-existing medical disorders may have an adverse effect upon the mother and fetus: for example, a woman who was treated for phenylketonuria as a child but has now ceased taking her special diet, would have high levels of phenylalanine during pregnancy. These high levels of phenylalanine are associated with abortion, intrauterine growth retardation, congenital heart defects, microcephaly and learning disabilities (Davidson et al 1981).

Prenatal

Heredity

As previously mentioned, there are a number of known conditions caused by genetic factors operating during the developmental cycle. Mothers falling into high-risk categories by virtue of age or known family incidence, who have not considered or received preconceptual care and advice, should be offered support, counselling and access to appropriate diagnostic tests, such as amniocentesis and chorionic villus sampling, should they require it.

Environment

There are numerous environmental influences that may affect the mother and the unborn child. Appropriate health education and antenatal care may go a long way in ensuring a greater understanding of the potential risk factors, and their effects upon the mother and child.

Several factors operate during this developmental period that may have an effect upon the fetus.

Infections Maternal infections that may result in learning disabilities can be grouped under three main headings: viral, bacterial, and protozoal.

Viral

1. *Rubella* (or German measles) is probably the best-known maternal viral infection which can cause learning disability. The degree of intellectual impairment, which can range from mild to profound, can be linked to the time of contraction of the virus: the earlier the exposure to the virus during the pregnancy, especially during the first trimester, the more affected the child will be, both physically and intellectually. It has been estimated that approximately 70% of children whose mothers had rubella in the first 10 weeks of pregnancy will have some degree of handicap (Peckham 1988).

Because congenital rubella may occur in the absence of overt maternal infection it may go undetected. The principal malformations seen in congenital rubella include cataracts, deafness, congenital heart defects and microcephaly (Box 2.4) with learning disability (Harper 1993).

2. *Cytomegalovirus* means 'large cell virus'. It

Box 2.4 Microcephaly

Microcephaly (abnormal smallness of the head) may result from a variety of intrauterine causes, including congenital infection, teratogens and maternal phenylketonuria. It may also be evident as part of a genetic syndrome, such as *Cri-du-chat* syndrome. True microcephaly is the result of autosomal recessive inheritance.

---

belongs to the herpes family, along with the viruses that cause chicken pox (varicella zoster), cold sores and glandular fever. It is a common infection that usually has brief flu-like, or no symptoms. Without realizing it, by the time they are middle-aged most people will have been infected. The most frequent times for contracting the virus are in early childhood and between 20 and 35 years. It is estimated that four out of every 1000 women who are pregnant become infected, and approximately half pass on the virus to the fetus, resulting in 10% of the infected babies having a handicap (Peckham 1988).

The principal malformations seen in cytomegalovirus are deafness, blindness, cerebral palsy and learning disabilities.

3. *Varicella zoster*, or chickenpox, poses a risk to the fetus if acquired during the first 5 months of pregnancy. The principal malformations include cataract, microcephaly and learning disabilities (Harper 1993).

Bacterial Congenital syphilis is fortunately less common today than it was in the past. Improvements in general health education, antenatal care and the use of antibiotics have reduced the number of cases.

In the affected individual there is a general failure to thrive and growth is stunted. Physical manifestations include saddleback nose, peg-shaped teeth, opacities of the cornea, strabismus and nystagmus. The central nervous system is affected to various degrees and epilepsy may be present.

Protozoal When acute infection with *Toxoplasma gondii* occurs during pregnancy the parasite can cross the placenta and infect the fetus. As with the previously described infections, the earlier

this occurs in the pregnancy the more severe are the effects. Maternal infection is often asymptomatic and can result from contact with animal excrement (in particular cats), undercooked meat and unwashed vegetables. Only a small proportion of affected children would have severe manifestations, but learning disabilities and hearing defects do occur.

Maternal health Maternal nutrition and health are known to be linked to fetal development. The supply of essential nutrients and oxygen to the fetus is totally dependent upon the mother, and any interruption of this process will affect the fetus. Good health for the pregnant mother should be thought of in the widest possible context, both on a physical and a psychological level, to maximize the development of a healthy pregnancy.

Toxic agents There are a number of known toxic agents that can injure the developing fetus in some way. Smoking, alcohol, drugs and environmental pollutants have all been identified as associated factors in the causation of learning disabilities.

Smoking in itself may not be a direct cause of learning disabilities, but it does pose a preventable hazard to both the mother and the fetus. There is a wealth of evidence linking smoking during pregnancy with low birthweight, spontaneous abortion and perinatal death, as well as prenatal complications leading to handicapping conditions and deformity in the neonate (Alexander et al 1990).

Alcohol consumption has been linked with spontaneous abortion, low birthweight and fetal alcohol syndrome. This latter is characterized by low birthweight, failure to thrive, reduced motor development and microcephaly. It is unclear how much alcohol needs to be consumed to have a detrimental effect upon the fetus, but there is a view that alcohol should not be consumed in large quantities (no more than one or two units once or twice a week) and that women should not get 'drunk' during pregnancy (Plant 1987). Discussion still continues as to whether or not abstinence during pregnancy and before becoming pregnant is appropriate (Little et al 1982).

Drugs taken during pregnancy may have a teratogenic effect upon the developing fetus. The abnormality may, however, be the result of drug interaction with a nutrient, and not as a direct result of the drug action alone. The effects of the drug thalidomide have been well documented and reported. It has been suggested (Dickerson 1980) that the drug may have interacted with riboflavin (one of the heat-stable factors of the vitamin B complex), as similar effects have been recorded in riboflavin-deficient animals. Women taking anticonvulsant medication for the control of epilepsy have also been found to be at risk of producing children with malformations.

Environmental pollutants such as lead and mercury, and chemical agents such as solvents, pesticides, anaesthetic gases and ionizing radiation, have all been identified as hazardous to the developing fetus. Lead pollution in the atmosphere is known to cause stillbirth and congenital damage to the brain and central nervous system, resulting in learning disabilities (Bryce Smith 1980).

Physical factors Radiation in the form of excessive use of X-rays has been found to cause damage to the developing fetus, especially if exposure occurs during the first 3 months of pregnancy. Some pregnant women in Japan who survived the atomic bomb blasts were found to give birth to microcephalic children. Further studies of this group also identified chromosomal abnormalities and gene mutations. Ultrasound screening (a non-invasive technique that uses sound waves to visualize the position and size of the fetus and placenta) is a suitably safe alternative for examinations during pregnancy.

Maternal–fetal incompatibility (kernicterus) Rhesus factor incompatibility occurs when a rhesus-negative mother is carrying a fetus that is rhesus positive (inherited from the father). The first child is usually unaffected, but in subsequent pregnancies the number of maternal antibodies increases. The antibodies then pass through the placental barrier and destroy the rhesus-positive blood of the fetus. An exchange transfusion can be given in utero if the blood is being destroyed, or immediately following the birth. At birth an affected child will be jaundiced, and if no action is taken brain damage will occur. Anti-D gammaglobulin, if administered by injection to the rhesus-negative woman within 48 hours of the delivery of the first child, will prevent the formation of the dangerous antibodies.

Direct violence to the fetus may result in stillbirth, abortion or brain damage. The severity of the condition will depend upon the stage of gestation and the severity and nature of the violent act.

Anoxia, if allowed to continue, triggers irreversible changes in the brain. This is especially true for the developing fetus, which can only withstand very brief periods without oxygen before permanent damage occurs. Oxygen deprivation may be caused by a number of factors:

- Maternal illness, resulting in poorly oxygenated blood
- Reduction in respiration owing to maternal sedation
- Abnormal or premature detachment of the placenta.

Perinatal

Perinatal causes of learning disability occur at or about the time of birth. They include conditions such as prematurity, birth injury and/or abnormal labour.

Premature infants are those born prior to 37 weeks' gestation. Although prematurity is not in itself a cause of learning disabilities, premature and low birthweight babies experience a significantly greater number of problems during labour and the birth process, including breathing difficulties and intraventricular haemorrhage, than do full-term infants, which places them at risk for subsequent developmental problems (Kitchen & Murton 1985).

Asphyxia is the primary cause of central nervous system damage before and after birth. Asphyxiation results in hypoxia, or decreased levels of oxygen and diminished cerebral blood flow. When the cerebral blood flow is diminished the self-regulation of the brain's blood supply is impaired, leading in turn to brain swelling and haemorrhage (Wyly 1995).

Birth is a traumatic event under any circumstances, for both mother and baby, and full-term babies are also at risk from a number of factors operating during labour that can cause birth trauma or injury, including:

- Asphyxia: due to a prolonged second stage of labour, or the coiling of the umbilical cord round the child's neck
- Trauma: caused by instrumented delivery, i.e. forceps delivery. Excessive moulding of the head and breech presentation are also possible causes.

Damage or trauma to the brain may result in cerebral palsy, epilepsy or learning disabilities, depending upon the severity of the damage and the location within the brain.

Fetal monitoring, i.e. determining fetal size and presentation prior to and during labour with ultrasound and other monitoring equipment, can alert the attending professional to the signs of fetal distress and reduce the potential danger.

During the period immediately following birth, untreated hypocalcaemia, hypernatraemia and hypoglycaemia in the child can result in brain damage (Soothill et al 1987).

Postnatal

There are a number of factors that operate during the postnatal period that may result in learning disabilities, for example untreated genetic conditions, childhood infection, trauma, accidents, toxic agents, poor nutrition, and sensory and social isolation.

With appropriate health education and health promotion messages, increased awareness of these causative factors may help to reduce the incidence or promote early intervention to limit the severity of the learning disability.

Heredity

Many of the inherited conditions only become apparent in the postnatal period, for example phenylketonuria. As stated earlier, if this condition is not treated the child will become affected

---

Box 2.5   Encephalitis

Encephalitis, or inflammation of the brain, can result from a viral infection, such as rubella, mumps or chickenpox. Encephalitis following vaccination (for example whooping cough) is rare but does occur. The overall incidence of encephalitis is very low, but the effects and the degree of learning disability can be severe.

Meningitis, or inflammation of the membranes of the brain or spinal cord, can lead to brain damage and result in learning disability. Improvements in healthcare and early detection have reduced the number of recorded infections and associated complications.

Gastroenteritis, or inflammation of the mucous membrane of both stomach and intestine, can be especially dangerous in the very young. Dehydration, which may occur very rapidly, leads to brain haemorrhage, which can cause brain damage.

---

when the phenylalananine concentration rises above the critical level.

Environmental

Infection A number of childhood infections carry the risk of brain damage as a complication, which may result in the affected individual having learning disabilities and/or an associated physical handicap. Encephalitis, meningitis and gastroenteritis are three examples of infections which, if untreated, can lead to intellectual impairment (Box 2.5).

Trauma Trauma to the head can be the result of accidental or non-accidental injury.

Accidental injuries may be sustained as a result of road traffic or general household accidents, or as a result of oxygen deprivation; or they may be the result of capillary haemorrhage caused by prolonged and severe coughing during whooping cough infection.

Non-accidental injury, or battered baby syndrome, is usually caused by the main carer. Injuries include depressed fractures of the skull, haematomas and blood vessel damage. The severity of the injury will determine the degree of intellectual impairment sustained. Children who are suspected as being at risk are placed on an at-risk register and will be closely monitored (Working Together Under the Children Act 1989).

Toxic agents As in the prenatal period toxic

agents can damage the developing brain. Lead intoxication was once commonly known as a causative factor, but increased awareness of the potential problem has reduced the use of this damaging substance. Environmental pollutants are another cause for concern, and continued investigation to identify potential harmful substances is required. Mercury, copper, manganese and strontium are all seen as detrimental in the developmental period.

Nutrition Appropriate nutrition is a central element of health and wellbeing. The developing child who is malnourished may experience both physical and mental developmental delay.

Sensory and social deprivation Children learn and develop by interacting with their surroundings and environmental stimuli. Deprivation caused by impairment to any of the special senses (sight, hearing, touch, taste and smell) or social isolation may have an effect upon the child's physical and intellectual development. Therefore, in order to prevent a secondary handicap professionals should have an understanding of the holistic needs of the developing individual and be able to educate and advise those who are not so well informed or require assistance.

CONCLUSION

There is no easy or wholly satisfactory method of identifying and categorizing the numerous causes of learning disabilities. Overlaps and anomalies exist that confirm or confound the known aetiologies. However, an understanding of the known causes and manifestations of learning disabilities may enhance the quality of professionals' practice in a number of ways:

- In the provision of an appropriate package of holistic care for the individual concerned
- As a means of improving the quality of life for the individual, rather than inhibiting or artificially limiting it
- By advising parents or carers as to the nature and potential effects of the individual's condition
- By answering questions or giving information to potential parents

Summary

There are a number of known factors that contribute toward or result in learning disabilities. When looking at causation there are four quite distinct periods when learning disabilities may occur: preconceptually, pre-natally, perinatally and postnatally. The causative factors operating during these periods can be roughly divided into two areas, those of heredity and environmental factors. Each area can then be further subdivided to concentrate on the more specific causal agents.

The manifestations of the various conditions have been identified, but it must be re-emphasized that clinical features and the prognosis of a particular condition should only be used as an aid to planning appropriate care that is flexible and individualistic in approach.

- By recognizing threats to the health of people with learning disabilities caused by a known disorder.

GLOSSARY OF TERMS

Allele   Alternative form of a gene that may occupy the same site on homologous chromosomes

Autosome   Chromosome other than the sex chromosome

Centromere   A specialized region of a chromosome seen as a constriction under the microscope. This region is important in the activities of the chromosomes during cellular division.

Chromosome   Chromophilic body within the cell nucleus, visible as homologous pairs in dividing cells

Dominant trait   One which is determined by the presence of a gene in heterozygous form

Gene   The unit of inheritance, occupying a specific locus on a chromosome

Genotype   An individual's genetic makeup

Heterozygous   Having different alleles at a gene locus on each of a pair of homologous chromosomes

Homozygous   Having the same allele at a gene locus on each of a pair of homologous chromosomes

Karyotype   The chromosome characteristics of an individual arranged in pairs in descending order of size and according to the position of the centromere

Mosaicism   The presence of more than one cell type in a single individual

Mutation   A spontaneous or induced change in a gene or chromosome

Phenotype   The way in which the genotype is expressed in the body

Recessive trait   One which is determined by the presence of a gene in homozygous form

Sex chromosomes   The pair of chromosomes responsible for sex determination

Sex-linked trait   One determined by the presence of a gene on the sex chromosomes (usually X linked)

Translocation   The transfer of a segment of a chromosome to a site on a different chromosome

Trisomy   The presence of one chromosome additional to the normal homologous pair

---

REFERENCES

Alexander J, Levy V, Roach S (eds) 1990 Antenatal care: a research based approach. Macmillan Press, London

Barnes B, Bradley S G 1990 Planning for a healthy baby. Foresight, Godalming

Bryce Smith D 1980 Lead and brain functioning. In: Birch G C, Parker K J (eds) Food and health. Applied Sciences Publishing, London.

Burns J K 1994 Birth defects and their causes. Stress Books, Ireland

Clarke A M, Clarke A D B (eds) 1974 Mental deficiency, 3rd edn. Methuen, London

Clarke D J, Boer H, Webb T 1995 Genetic and behavioural aspects of Prader–Willi syndrome: a review with a translation of the original paper. Mental Handicap Research 8: 38–47

Davidson D C, Isherwood D M, Ireland J T, Page P G 1981 Outcome of pregnancy in a phenylketonuric mother after low phenylalanine diet introduced from the ninth week of pregnancy. European Journal of Paediatrics 137: 45–48

Dickerson J W T 1980 Guidelines for future parents: environmental factors and foetal health. Foresight, Godalming

Dutton G 1975 Mental handicap. Butterworths, London

Harper P S 1993 Practical genetic counselling, 4th edn. Butterworth-Heinemann, Oxford

Health of the Nation 1995 A strategy for people with learning disabilities. HMSO, London

House of Commons Social Services Committee (HC) 1980 Report on perinatal and neonatal mortality (Short Report). HMSO, London

House of Commons Social Services Committee (HC) (1984)

Follow-up report on perinatal and neonatal mortality. HMSO, London

Kitchen W, Murton L J 1985 Survival rates of infants with birth weight between 501 and 1000 g. American Journal of Diseases of Children 139: 470–471

Little R E, Graham J M, Samson H H 1982 Fetal alcohol effects in humans and animals. In: Stimmel B (ed) The effects of maternal alcohol and drug abuse on the newborn. Hawthorne Press, New York

Mueller R F, Young I D 1995 Emery's Elements of medical genetics, 9th edn. Churchill Livingstone, Edinburgh

Newton R 1992 Down's syndrome. Optima, London

Peckham C S 1988 Infection and the fetus. Medicine International 51: 2107–2110

Plant M L 1987 Women, drinking and pregnancy. Tavistock Publications, London

Singer S 1985 Human genetics, 2nd edn. WH Freeman, New York

Smithells R W, Sheppard S, Schorah C J et al 1980 Possible prevention of neural tube defects by periconceptual vitamin supplementation. Lancet i: 339–340

Soothill P W, Nicolaides K H, Campbell S 1987 Prenatal asphyxia. British Medical Journal 294: 1051–1053

Sweet B R 1988 Mayes midwifery, 11th edn.: 571–572. Baillière Tindall, London

Working Together Under the Children Act 1989 1991 A guide for inter-agency co-operation for the protection of children from abuse. HMSO, London

Wyly M V 1995 Premature infants and their families developmental interventions. Singular Publishing Group Inc., London

Development of services

C. Swann

INTRODUCTION

This chapter outlines the changes in social policy, philosophical ideals and government legislation that have taken place since the 1960s and that have subsequently influenced the development of services for people with learning disabilities in the United Kingdom. In order to understand current service provision, it is important to have a knowledge of the historical perspectives and the origins of services for people with learning disabilities. Figure 3.1 identifies the different models of care delivery over the centuries: these are put into context by a visual display in the form of a 'time line', which provides 'snapshots' from a temporal dimension from the 1400s through to the final years of the 20th century.

The time line shows that the pace of change has not always been constant. At times there appear to have been periods of stagnation, and at other times periods of great change, with considerable developments being made in a relatively short space of time. However, when an overview is taken it is clear that the developments have been far ranging and extremely effective in improving the quality of life for people with learning disabilities.

As pointed out by Bannerman and Lindsay (1993) in the previous edition of this book, there is a persistent myth that each of these successive generations views itself as the instigator of the 'Golden Age'. The danger in such a belief is the possibility of becoming complacent with a view that no new developments can be made. However, the likelihood is that there will always

Time line

1400s	1500s	... ...	1700s	1800s	1900s
'Lunatics' admitted to hospitals. Treatment consists of chaining and whipping	Borde (1542) recommends that the insane should 'be kept in a closed chamber and should have a keeper whom he fears' Witchcraft considered to have an undeniable link with madness		1736 Laws against witchcraft abolished Act of 1744 separates lunatics from vagrants and paupers Treatments include bleeding, emetics, digitalis and electricity 1763 Bill for the Regulation of Madhouses	1828 Lunatic Asylum Regulation Act Care relies on family, social networks and religious organizations Theory of deterioration of the intelligence of the general population (Darwin's Theory 1859) Lunacy Act 1890 Still no distinction between the 'mentally ill' and the 'mentally retarded'	1930s Compulsory sterilization considered in UK Nazi Germany exterminates individuals with undesirable characteristics, which include 'mental handicap' 1913 Mental Deficiency Bill classifies 'idiots', 'imbeciles' and 'feeble minded'. Introduction of guardianship and licence from institutional care, making living in the community an option for some 1959 Mental Health Act 1983 Mental Health Act Many people discharged from hospital to be cared for in the community

Figure 3.1

be change, that development will be progressive, and that probably the only thing we can be certain of is continuing change.

SOCIAL CONTEXT IN THE 1960S AND 1970S

At the time when Harold Macmillan was saying 'You've never had it so good' and when Martin Luther King gave his dramatic speech (1963) 'I have a dream ... that all men are created equal', people with learning disabilities were incarcerated in large 'mental subnormality' hospitals. While the young people of this decade were taking their fashion very seriously, undertaking regular pilgrimages to Carnaby Street, London, the then centre of world fashion, people with learning disabilities were still to achieve the luxury of owning their own clothes. They lived in substandard conditions without personal space or possessions, with routines regimented to suit the care staff and the organization rather than the needs of the patient. At the same time as Neil Armstrong was setting foot on the moon (20 July 1969), making 'a small step for man and a giant leap for mankind', deliverers of services for people with learning disabilities were dealing with more down to earth issues.

In an attempt to put life for people with learning disabilities in the early 1970s into context, a 'pen picture' of a fictitious character has been composed (Case study 3.1). It is a composite created from published authorities and anecdotal evidence supplied from people who were involved in care delivery during this time. At that time, 'institutional neurosis' was a particularly current issue. It was defined by Barton (1960) as 'a disease characterized by apathy, lack of initiative, loss of interest more marked in things and events not immediately personal or present, submissiveness, and sometimes no expression of feelings of resentment at harsh or unfair orders. There is also a lack of interest in the future and an apparent inability to make practical plans for it, a deterioration in personal habits, toilet, and standards generally, a loss of individuality, and a resigned acceptance that things will go on as they are – unchangingly, inevitably, and indefinitely.'

Case study 3.1

Pen picture of Marjorie in 1970
*It should be noted by the reader that this case study
uses terminology in use at the time depicted.*

In 1970 Marjorie was 56 years old and had lived
most of her life in a local mental handicap hospital.
Marjorie did not know if her family were still alive, as
she had not had contact with them for the last 30
years. She was first admitted to the hospital nearly 40
years ago, when it was clear that she would not be
able to find employment. Her notes on admission to
the hospital described her as 'feeble minded' and in
need of a protective environment because of the risk of
pregnancy following a number of suspected incidents
with local inhabitants. The cause of Marjorie's mental
handicap was congenital syphilis, resulting from
maternal infection. She had a typical facial appearance, which included a saddleback nose, opacities of
the cornea and nystagmus.

Marjorie lived on Primrose ward, along with 45 other
women with varying degrees of mental and physical
handicap. Primrose ward had an unpleasant smell – a
mixture of urine and faeces.

A typical day in Marjorie's life would have started at
around 7 am, when she would be wakened by the day
staff starting their duty. She would be told to go and
wash and dress. Because she was more capable than
some of the others, Marjorie was able to jump the
queue of naked bodies waiting to be bathed or
washed. Marjorie had no personal belongings, and so
washed with whatever toiletries were available. No-
one seemed to bother much about cleaning teeth.
Sometimes it was difficult for Marjorie to find a dress
which would fit from the central supply of clothes in the
cupboard. Occasionally, particularly after the weekend,
when the laundry staff had been away, it would be
difficult, if not impossible, to find any underwear at all.
Marjorie's help was often enlisted by staff to look after
some of the low-grade patients with whom she lived.
She would help them to wash and dress in the morning, help feed them at meal times and 'tuck them in' at
night. During the day, having helped to get everyone
bathed, dressed and fed, Marjorie stood outside the
front door to watch and chat with passers by. These
usually consisted of nurses and doctors going to meal
breaks or starting and finishing shifts at the hospital.

Referred to as 'teabelly' by staff and high-grade
patients alike, it was one of Marjorie's jobs to make a
drink of tea at meal times. This was made exactly the
same for all the patients: the tea was mixed with the
milk and sugar in a big teapot to save time. Meal times
were particularly noisy, with staff constantly shouting at
patients to sit down and shut up. Some of the patients
used to take Marjorie's food, which made her very agi-
tated and upset. After Marjorie had helped to clear the
pots away she would wait by the door until the staff
unlocked it, and then she would quickly go back to her
usual place outside. She only ventured back indoors at
meal times, cup of tea times and bed time.

Case study 3.1 *(cont'd)*

Bed time was at 7 pm, and everyone was in bed just
in time for the night staff to arrive on duty. Marjorie
slept in a large dormitory with the other 45 women.
Sometimes it was difficult to sleep because of the
incessant screaming and shouting of the patient who
occupied the next bed, but for Marjorie, as for many
other patients during this time, this was a way of life.

Barton identified the symptoms described
above as being a separate disorder from the one
which originally brought the individual into hospital, and suggested that it was produced by the
contemporary methods of looking after people in
mental hospitals.

It is important to recognize that people like
'Marjorie' were also suffering from institutional
neurosis, in addition to learning disability. As
Barton pointed out, the signs of institutional neurosis may vary in severity, from the mute stu-
porose 'patient' through to the 'ward worker'
(people like Marjorie), who have without protest
surrendered their existence to the institution.
Barton identified a range of characteristics commonly found in the environment which, taken
together, influence the onset of institutional neurosis. These factors include loss of contact with
the outside world, enforced idleness, bossiness
of medical and nursing staff, loss of personal
friends, possessions and personal events, drugs,
ward atmosphere and loss of prospects outside
the institution.

During the late 1960s and early 1970s there
were prolonged debates regarding the relative
merits of hospital and community-based care. By
the beginning of the 1970s the balance of advantage was shifting towards the latter. This was
perhaps fuelled not only by the belief that community care was a cheaper option, but also by the
public exposure of ill treatment of patients in
large hospitals. During this period a significant
number of reports surfaced, a notable example
being the 'Report of the Committee of Enquiry
into Ely Hospital' (1969), which identified general circumstances of low morale, impoverished

Activity 3.1

Talk to someone you know who has spent a number of years in a large 'mental handicap' hospital. Find out how their life has changed over the years.

Table 3.1 Places in local authority, private and voluntary sector services (Derived from Jay Report 1979)

	1970	1977
Local authority homes	5221	10 158
Local authority unstaffed homes	85	653
Adult training centres	26 649	40 369
Adult training centre special care	None	1672
Voluntary and private homes	1814	3404

and squalid living conditions, lack of privacy for residents, lack of activities, custodial attitudes towards patient care, a primary focus on physical care, professional isolation and administrative inertia. Public exposures such as this led to a series of moves designed to accelerate the policy of community care and improve conditions for those people remaining in hospital. The 1971 White Paper, *Better Services for the Mentally Handicapped*, was published by the Department of Health and Social Security and the Welsh Office. The report acknowledged that little or no progress had been made towards community care during the previous decade, and that hospitals still supported generally poor conditions. It gave clear targets for moving the emphasis in residential care away from hospital to community settings. The targets included a 50% reduction in hospital places by 1991 and a corresponding increase in local authority funded care, in terms of hostels, residential and day care provision. The report advocated an end to old custodial methods and attitudes and encouraged the re-education and training of hospital staff, emphasizing that the changes would require close interagency working: 'The mentally handicapped and their families need help from professions working in services administered by a variety of authorities and departments. It is important that the resources of the health services, personal social services and education services should be deployed in close and effective collaboration. Only if this is done can the relevant professional skills be most effectively used to provide complete and coordinated services' (DHSS 1971).

Initially the report was seen as innovative, but it was later criticized for failing to address the financial implications of its proposals and giving no clear guidelines on the task of transferring patients from hospitals to the community. Following the publication of the White Paper there was a steady but significant growth in local authority, private and voluntary sector services for people with learning disabilities, as shown in Table 3.1.

The transition to community care was given further impetus following the publication of the Jay Report in 1979. The recommendations of the Jay Committee were presented to Parliament by the Secretaries of State for Social Services and the Secretaries of State for Wales and Scotland in March 1979. The Committee pointed to a vision of a radically different service and non-medical caring profession which would provide care for people with learning disabilities in the future. Within its recommendations, the Jay Committee proposed a new model of care based on the principles shown in Box 3.1.

The Jay Committee recommended the end of the dual system of hospital and local authority care and a transfer to local authority care provision, and social work rather than nurse training for staff of all residential care units. The Jay proposals reflected a major change of attitude within learning disabilities care at this time; however, the report was 'quietly buried and with it the heated controversy and commitment to extra expenditure that the government was too anxious to avoid' (Ryan and Thomas 1987).

In spite of this, the report had considerable influence in that following its publication, the then General Nursing Council (GNC) revised its syllabus of mental handicap nurse training (GNC 1982), shifting the emphasis of training from hospital to the community. One of the effects of this was an increase in interagency

Box 3.1 **Jay recommendations**

- People with learning disabilities have a right to enjoy normal patterns of life within the community
- People with learning disabilities have a right to be treated as individuals
- People with learning disabilities will require additional help from the community in which they live and from professional services if they are to develop to their maximum potential as individuals

Community requirements

- People with learning disabilities should be able to live in a mixed-sex environment
- People with learning disabilities should be able to develop a daily routine just like other people
- There should be a proper separation of home, work and recreation

Individuality

- The right of the individual to live, learn and work in the least restrictive environment appropriate to that particular person
- The right to make or be involved in decisions that affect oneself
- Acceptance that individual needs differ not only between handicapped individuals but within the same individual over time
- The right of parents to be involved in decisions about their children

Service principles

- People with learning disabilities should use normal services wherever possible
- Existing networks of community support should be strengthened by professional services rather than supplanted by them
- 'Specialized' services or organizations for people with learning disabilities should be provided only to the extent that they demonstrably meet or are likely to meet additional needs that cannot be met by general services
- If the many and diverse needs of people with learning disabilities are to be met, maximum coordination of services is needed both within and between agencies at all levels. The concept of a life plan seems essential if coordination and continuity of care is to be achieved
- If high-quality services are to be established and maintained for those who cannot easily articulate and press their just claims, someone is needed to intercede on behalf of people with learning disabilities in obtaining services (Adapted from Jay Report 1979)

working, as student nurses increasingly worked alongside social workers and workers in the private and voluntary sectors.

The key to successful interagency working has always been seen as joint planning and joint financial strategy (Rose 1993). Recognizing this,

and also being aware that the delivery of care in the community was fragmented and spread between a range of statutory and non-statutory agencies, in 1976 the Government introduced joint finance arrangements. These arrangements were, however, fraught with difficulties – they were cumbersome, bureaucratic, and failed to make the anticipated impact on facilitating a move from hospital care to care in the community.

AN ORDINARY LIFE

Although the move to community care was slow during the 1970s, it became evident that informed opinion had moved steadily towards a belief that people with learning disabilities should live ordinary lives in ordinary houses and cease to be incarcerated in large hospitals. It is not surprising that this shift had been relatively slow to develop, as throughout history people with learning disabilities had been thought of as ill, and hence requiring treatment in hospital. This new approach represented a tremendous philosophical shift for both planners and deliverers of services, with a corresponding shift towards greater acceptance by society. With this new approach emerged a view that people with learning disabilities had special needs, and that with the right services they were capable of fulfilling their maximum potential. The debate about community care was stimulated by a growing acceptance of the rights of people with learning disabilities. In 1972 the first self-advocacy conference was held in Great Britain, and 'People First', an organization run by people with learning disabilities, had their first conference in 1973.

Another significant development that contributed to the notion that people with learning disabilities should live ordinary lives, was the impact of the developing concept of normalization. This was developed in Denmark in 1959 by Bank-Mikkleson, and enlarged upon by Bengt Nirje of Sweden in 1969. The principles of normalization have been an influential concept in debates concerning the shape and development of service provision to the present day.

Normalization grew out of concern for 'mentally retarded' and institutionalized people who were living in an atmosphere of unvarying stereo-typed routines. The theory has been elaborated over the years and was defined by Wolfensberger (1972) as the 'utilization of means which are as culturally normative as possible'. Normalization is a complex system which seeks to value positively previously devalued individuals and groups. In essence, normalization proposes that people with learning disabilities will only be valued by the rest of society when they are seen to be living in ways which are regarded not only as 'normal' but which are also positively socially valued. On a practical level, this means that people with a learning disability are entitled to the same rights and opportunities as all other citizens. They should be able to live near their families (if they so wish), be in everyday contact with their peers and take part in the 'normal' activities of their communities. They should have access to and make use of the same range of opportunities and services in life that the rest of the population take for granted. Normalization is not about making people with learning disabilities 'normal' – it focuses on the challenge to provide services for such people that 'ordinary' members of the community would find acceptable.

Since the concept of normalization originated in 1959 it has undergone significant change, both in response to the way in which devalued people are portrayed or perceived by society (Wolfensberger 1983) and by the recognition of the aims of normalization in terms of socially valued roles as opposed to culturally normative practices; hence the renaming of the concept as 'social role valorization'. This moved beyond an acknowledgment that people with learning disabilities have the same rights and obligations as the rest of society and began to concentrate on the ways in which society and services cast people with disabilities into particular roles, further reinforcing those roles by the way in which they respond to the needs of this minority group. The principle of normalization has seven core themes (Box 3.2).

The principles of normalization and social role valorization reflected a significant shift from the

Activity 3.2

Think about a situation in your adult life where you have been denied choice. What similarities do you see between your experience and that of someone you know with learning disabilities?

Box 3.2 Normalization

- The conservatism corollary to the principles of normalization
- The relevance of role expectancy and role circularity to deviance making and deviance unmaking
- The role of consciousness and unconsciousness in human services
- The developmental model and personal competency enhancement
- The power of imitation
- The dynamics and relevance of social imagery
- The importance of social integration and valued social participation (Wolfensberger & Tullman 1989)

---

model of care provision of previous decades – a move towards independence, choice, autonomy and the opportunity for people with learning disabilities to exercise rights and take responsibility for themselves.

SOCIAL CONTEXT IN THE 1980S

The hallmark of the 1980s was undoubtedly that of 'Thatcherism', a political revolution in British politics led by the then Prime Minister, Margaret Thatcher. This was an era that reshaped British political, economic and social life, mainly through the encouragement and support of private enterprise. It was a time of relative affluence for a significant section of society, with associated improvements in living standards for many. The era was personified by the young, 'upwardly mobile' entrepreneur complete with mobile phone. It is debatable, however, to what extent people with learning disabilities benefited from these 'boom' years.

Although the concept of normalization appeared in the literature in the late 1970s, its influence on service provision was most marked in the 1980s, when it began to significantly influence people's thinking, working practices and the organization and delivery of services (Whitehead 1993). Although there was some recognition at this time that the concept of normalization left room for damaging misinterpretations, it was on the whole accepted that normalization and social role valorization were likely to remain influential in determining the most effective ways to organize services for people with learning disabilities.

Normalization was not the only movement that focused on making the client an individual and the centre of service provision. The concept of 'accomplishments' as a standard on which to base services developed in the mid 1980s. O'Brien's interpretation of normalization made explicit that which services should try to achieve or accomplish for service users (Box 3.3).

Despite appearing relatively simple, these five major accomplishments had a profound effect on

service delivery during the late 1980s, and their subsequent effect on current service provision should not be underestimated.

In addition, the development and growth of self-advocacy groups and advocacy projects in the 1980s moved on apace. The emergence of the consumers' movement 'People First' was a significant development, and the importance of consulting service users received greater emphasis during the mid 1980s (Brechin & Swain 1988).

Despite these advances, it remained clear that limited progress was being made towards achieving the transition from hospital care to community care (Table 3.2). It was confirmed by various independent reports and by the Audit Commission (1986) that, although there had been some advances in community care, the overall rate of service development was disappointingly slow. In 1986 the Audit Commission Report *Making a Reality of Community Care* suggested that:

Box 3.3 O'Brien's interpretation of normalization

- **Community presence** is the sharing of ordinary places that define community life. Before people can participate in the social activities of a natural community, they must be physically present and involved in it. Valued activities will increase the number and variety of ordinary places that a person knows and can have access to.
- **Choice** is the experience of autonomy both in small, everyday matters (e.g. what to wear or what to eat) and in large, life-defining matters (e.g. with whom to live or what sort of work to do). Valued activities will increase the variety and significance of the choices a person makes.
- **Competence** is the opportunity to perform functional and meaningful activities with whatever level or type of assistance that is required. Valued activities will increase a person's power to define and pursue objectives that are personally and socially important.
- **Respect** is having a valued place among a network of people and valued roles in community life. Valued activities will challenge limiting, negative stereotypes about a person and provide access to valued social roles.
- **Community participation** is the experience of being part of a growing network of personal relationships that includes close friends. Valued activities will provide opportunities for a person to meet and develop a variety of types of relationships with an increasing number of people (adapted from O'Brien 1987).

- There are serious grounds for concern about the lack of progress in shifting the balance of services towards community care. Progress has been slow and uneven across the country and the near-term prospects are not promising. In short, the community care policy is failing to achieve its potential.
- Fundamental underlying problems need to be tackled if community care is to be translated from an attractive policy to reality throughout England and Wales.
- The pattern of distribution of finance is out of step with community care policies. Local authorities cannot be expected to play their full part given the loss of grant incurred for expanding services under current arrangements.
- There is considerable organizational fragmentation and confusion, with responsibility for the introduction of community care divided between a variety of separately funded organizations, who often fail to work together effectively.
- There are inadequate arrangements for training and providing opportunities in community services for existing staff in long-

Table 3.2   Progress to White Paper targets for mentally handicapped people in England and Wales (Audit Commission 1986)

	1969	1984	Target by 1991	Progress to target (%)
Hospitals (available beds, adult)	52 100	42 500	27 300	39
Residential places (local authority)	4300	18 500	29 800	56
Local authority ATC places	24 600	50 500	74 500	52

stay hospitals, and for training sufficient numbers in community-based staff.

It was clear from the report that 'a rationalization of funding policies must be undertaken' and 'adequate short-term funding must be provided to avoid the long-term waste of two inadequate services struggling in parallel indefinitely' (Audit Commission 1986).

In order to create an environment where locally integrated community care could flourish, the Audit Commission suggested that local authorities could be made responsible for the long-term needs of 'mentally and physically handicapped people', except for those who required medical supervision. The Commission suggested that the resources necessary to do this should be identified and, where appropriate, transferred from the National Health Service to local authorities, who could then 'buy in' specialized care from the NHS and the private sector. The report concluded that radical changes of this kind must occur if community care were to be effective. It seems that this change was slow to arrive, as 3 years later the Audit Commission published a further paper, *Developing Community Care for Adults with a Mental Handicap*. This paper identified that almost two-thirds of local authorities had still not yet reached an agreement with their local health authorities on the financial and practical arrangements required for resettling people into the community.

Despite the previously outlined criticism, it is fair to say that between 1980 and 1990 a 'mixed economy' of care was slowly emerging (Table 3.3). In 1988, Sir Roy Griffiths was asked to undertake a review of community care policy. His terms of reference were 'to review the way in which pub-

Table 3.3   Places available in hospitals and residential care in England 1980–1990 (DHSS 1984, DOH 1991)

	1980	1990
Beds in NHS hospitals	51 500	32 700
Places in LA residential homes	12 062	16 886
Places in voluntary homes	2129	7894
Places in private homes	1298	8383
Total	66 989	65 862

lic funds were used to support community care policy and to advise on the options for action that would improve the use of these funds as a contribution to more effective community care' (DOH 1988).

Among the main recommendations of the report was that the primary responsibility for community care should lie with local authorities. It would be their responsibility to ensure that the needs of individuals within specified groups were identified and packages of care devised, making sure that services were provided within appropriate budgets by the public and private sectors. Griffiths acknowledged the central importance of local authorities assuming the key 'brokerage' role in developing community care services, and the role of the public sector in ensuring that proper care is provided.

In 1989 the Government set out its plans for care in the community in the 21st century. The White Paper *Caring For People* (DOH 1989) endorsed many of Griffiths' recommendations. It set out six key objectives for service delivery in the community:

- To promote the development of domiciliary and respite services to enable people to live in their own homes wherever feasible and sensible

- To ensure that service providers make practical support for carers a high priority
- To make proper assessment of need and good case management the cornerstone of high-quality care. Packages of care should then be designed in line with individual needs and preferences
- To promote the development of a flourishing independent sector alongside good-quality public services
- To clarify the responsibilities of agencies and so make it easier to hold them to account for their performance
- To secure better value for taxpayers' money by introducing a new funding structure for social care (DOH 1989).

The fundamental objective of *Caring for People* was to achieve an improvement in community services by making them more sensitive to individual users and carers, and ensuring better value for money. It required the development of services with greater user involvement, services that actively sought the views of users and carers. It also required a shift towards services designed to meet people's needs, rather than attempting to fit people into existing provision. The White Paper further required a joint approach to service delivery by health authorities, local authorities and the private and voluntary sectors.

SOCIAL CONTEXT IN THE 1990S

Although the building blocks had been put into place in the form of the National Health Service and Community Care Act (1991), these developments saw the light of day in a new business-oriented environment, with the associated need to acquire funding and resources in a climate of fierce competition. In sharp contrast to the 1980s, the 1990s appear to be unfolding as a decade of economic recession, an ailing economy and endless debates in relation to economic union with other European Union States.

In 1990 *Caring for People* received parliamentary assent as part of the National Health Service and Community Care Act, providing the necessary legislative support to the proposals identified in the earlier White Paper. Within the Act the Government outlines a number of changes in the way in which social care is to be delivered and funded:

- Local authorities are to become responsible, in collaboration with medical, nursing and other interests, for assessing individual needs, designing care arrangements and securing their delivery within available resources.
- Local authorities will be expected to produce and publish clear plans for the development of community care services.
- Local authorities will be expected to make maximum use of the independent sector.
- There will be a new funding structure for those seeking public support for residential and nursing home care from April 1991. After that date local authorities will take responsibility for the financial support of people in private and voluntary homes, over and above any general social security entitlements.
- Applicants with few or no resources of their own will be eligible for the same levels of income support and housing benefit, irrespective of whether they are living in their own homes or in independent residential nursing homes.
- Local authorities will be required to establish inspection and registration units at arm's length from management of their own services. (Derived from the NHS and Community Care Act 1990.)

The Government lacked confidence in the capacity of local authorities to carry out its reforms within reasonable financial limits, and in July 1990 put forward its decision to introduce the implementation of the National Health Service and Community Care Act in three distinct phases. This was to ensure that local authorities had a longer period of time over which to spread the cost of introducing the changes. The timetable of events was as follows:

- The establishment of inspection units
- The introduction of specific grants for people with mental health problems and for people who abuse drugs and alcohol
- The introduction of comprehensive complaints procedures

By April 1992:

- The publication of a community care plan
- Preparatory work to introduce a unified assessment procedure for people in need of community care support
- Preparatory work to introduce a case management scheme for people whose service needs are complex

By April 1993:

- A unified assessment procedure in place
- A case management scheme fully introduced
- A start to the transfer of funds from the Department of Social Security to the local authority, with the consequent need for full arrangements to be in place in order to administer the transferred funds; financially assess individuals in need of community care services; supply appropriate departmental services; and purchase appropriate services from other sectors (House of Commons Hansard, 18 July 1990).

The impact of the NHS and Community Care Act on service provision for people with learning disabilities and their carers is considerable. It has provided additional impetus to the idea that people with learning disabilities should have a say in the design, development and running of the services they use, a concept that was first discussed in the 1970s.

In order to compare the tremendous changes which have taken place during the last two and a half decades, a further pen picture in relation to how Marjorie might have fared had she been born 25 years later has been composed (Case study 3.2).

One of the most profound differences between the care delivered in the 1970s and that in the 1990s is that in the 1970s it was possible to discuss in some detail a 'typical' day. Probably one of the most significant achievements in care

Case study 3.2

Pen picture of Marjorie in 1996
It should be noted by the reader that this case study uses terminology in use at the present time.

In 1996, Marjorie was 57 years old. At the age of 17 she had been admitted to a local hospital for people with learning disabilities. She remained at the hospital until 1977 when, at the age of 38, she was resettled into a social services hostel for people with learning disabilities. The hostel was a considerable change from living in the hospital. There were 25 other people living at the hostel, and Marjorie shared a bedroom with six other women of a similar age. She had her own locker for her clothes and no-one else ever wore them, as Marjorie's name was printed on the inside of each garment. Marjorie still had jobs to do during the day, largely domestic tasks such as cleaning and making beds. Meal times were much more civilized than at the hospital, although there were occasions when one of the other residents would lose their temper and start to shout and swear. There was a day centre attached to the hostel, which Marjorie had to attend. She did not enjoy going to the day centre, as all they did each day was to put coloured cocktail sticks into a wooden board and empty them out again. When the staff could acquire a driver for the minibus, Marjorie would be taken out into town for a special treat. On one occasion the staff took everyone at the hostel to Blackpool for the day.

After 12 years at the hostel Marjorie was asked if she would like to be considered for a place with three other women in a small group home close to the centre of town. The next few months consisted of numerous visits from a variety of people employed by the social services, the housing association, health service and befriending agencies. After some months of preparation, Marjorie moved out into her new home. During the next few years Marjorie was able to learn a number of daily living skills, such as how to take a bus to a given destination, to choose her own clothes and cook a simple snack. She now attends the local college of further education twice weekly, where she is learning to improve her reading and writing skills. Marjorie also attends a cookery and housekeeping class at the resource centre and has a part time job in a local hairdresser's, where she makes tea and undertakes general cleaning duties.

At present, Marjorie is looking forward to a holiday which she has been involved in planning, she has a close friend and a busy social calendar. She keeps in touch with some of the people who still live in the hostel, and particularly enjoys the freedom she now has to choose how she will spend the rest of her life.

development is that it is not now so easy to discuss a typical day, as each day varies in response to the needs and wishes of the individual. The extent of opportunities and choices for Marjorie has vastly increased, she has regular holidays, has sampled other cultures and is a long way towards full integration within her own society. Marjorie has many decisions to make with respect to the clothes she wears, how she spends her time, who she spends it with, and major decisions related to her future and the shape her life will take.

THE FUTURE FOR LOCAL AUTHORITIES

Local authorities have become the 'gatekeepers' to and for community care, with the responsibility for coordinating needs assessment and the production of community care plans. Although the responsibility for assessment rests with the local authority, there is a clear remit to include all agencies involved with the client in the assessment process. Once a package of care has been determined it is the role of the local authority to ensure that the agreed services are in place, and that wherever possible cost-effective services from the voluntary, not-for-profit and private sectors are used. The role of local authorities has been endorsed by government as arrangers and purchasers of care services, rather than monopolistic providers of care.

THE FUTURE FOR HEALTH AUTHORITIES

The responsibilities of the health service remain essentially unaltered: it will continue to adopt a community-based focus, replacing the reliance on long-stay institutions with the services of general practitioners and community health services such as community nurses, speech and language therapists, occupational therapists, physiotherapists, doctors and psychologists. It is still the responsibility of health authorities to meet the healthcare needs of the population they serve. In situations where it is difficult to make a clear distinction between health and social care, it is essential that the responsible authorities work together. Health authorities will be involved in the development of community care policies and the provisions they intend to make for community care. Close integration between the work of primary healthcare teams, community teams for people with learning disabilities, local authorities and other agencies involved in the delivery of care is vital if they are to enable people with learning disabilities to remain in the community.

THE FUTURE FOR THE INDEPENDENT SECTOR

Voluntary-sector and not-for-profit agencies have grown considerably over recent years, and are continuing to flourish in response to the increased demand for individualized care packages. *Caring for People* (DOH 1989) identifies that, although domiciliary and day services are available and provided by local authorities to enable people to live in the community, the provision of such services is uneven and poorly coordinated. This creates considerable scope for the independent sector to develop more flexible and intensive health and social care services for people who would otherwise need institutional care.

MEMBER COUNTRIES OF THE UNITED KINGDOM

It has to be acknowledged that there is considerable variation in service provision across the United Kingdom, and although the general principles previously discussed apply equally there are differing approaches within each of the member countries. The main thrust of each is outlined within this section.

Northern Ireland

Northern Ireland has its own distinctive structure for the management of health and social ser-

Activity 3.3

List the different roles and responsibilities of the main care providers for people with learning disabilities.

vices, and although the recommendations in *Caring For People* (DOH 1989) are equally applicable to Northern Ireland, the Government has published a separate policy paper that takes this uniqueness into account.

In 1973, services for people with learning disabilities in Northern Ireland were reorganized and integrated into the general health and personal social service structures. The majority of people with learning disabilities in Northern Ireland have been cared for at home, with varying degrees of support. In 1978 there were 1337 patients in learning disability hospitals and 362 patients with learning disabilities in psychiatric hospitals. By December 1986 the numbers of people with a learning disability in hospital care provision had fallen to 1289 and 216 respectively. By 1992 they had fallen from 1289 to 926, and from 216 to 121. The relatively small decline between 1978 and 1986 has been attributed to slow growth in alternative community residential and day care facilities (DHSS 1995); however, the shift in government policy has created a significant growth in the development of private and voluntary sector care provision in Northern Ireland. In 1993, of 1544 places available 30% were provided by the statutory sector, 20% by the voluntary sector and 42% by the private sector. Nursing homes provided 27% of the total number of places available.

Partnerships between statutory and non-statutory organizations are continuing to develop, along with an extensive range of home-based supports for people with learning disabilities and their families.

Wales

The Welsh Mental Handicap Strategy was launched in 1983. One of its aims was to develop community-based support for individuals with a mental handicap and to improve the quality of care. The strategy was based on three guiding principles:

- The right to ordinary patterns of life within the community
- The right to be treated as individuals
- The right to additional help from community professionals (Welsh Office 1983).

The Secretary of State has reaffirmed the principles of this strategy, extending them to the year 2003. The provision of the mental handicap service in Wales is based on a shared philosophy between health and social service departments, and there is a recognition that in order to achieve their stated objectives there must be partnership and commitment between all agencies involved in the delivery of care to people with learning disabilities. The guidance document issued by the Welsh Office in 1994 highlighted the significant progress made between 1983 and 1993 (Table 3.4). One of the keys to the success of the strategy was the political commitment given to the development of services by the Secretary of State for Wales at the time of its launch in 1983, and his agreement to a 10-year funding programme of £1.5 million per annum on a cumulative basis. This has resulted, with inflation, in an extra £50 million per annum now being available for those specific services.

Although there is still a reliance on long-stay hospitals, it can be seen that the number of people living in hospital care provision dropped by almost half between 1983 and 1993, and the development of residential provision in ordinary housing increased dramatically. The overall objectives of the strategy have been identified as:

Table 3.4 (Welsh Mental Handicap Strategy. Guidance 1994)		
	1983	*1993*
Adults living in their own home in the community	166	1427
Families receiving support in their own homes	41	4691
Individuals with especially difficult behaviour receiving support	16	610
Individuals receiving new patterns of care	0	3665
Residing in long-stay hospitals	2089	1058

- An 'individual plan' for everyone who wants one, coordinating care throughout their life and properly reflecting their needs and preferences
- A range of care and support which meets the needs of children and their families
- Help and support for most children to attend local schools, and for adults to attend local colleges and evening classes
- Help to obtain a real job for most adults, and support to help them keep it
- Help to become part of the community and to take part in leisure activities alongside other local people
- A range of accommodation which meets the needs and preferences of individuals and their carers, including the resettlement of everyone living inappropriately in a hospital
- Support for those living in the community, whether by themselves or with carers, that helps them to continue living in the community
- Access to the same healthcare as others living in the community, with additional support to meet their special needs (Welsh Office 1994).

Caring for People (DOH 1989) confirms that the strategy has made possible an unprecedented expansion of community services, and in turn a reduction in the numbers of people living in long-stay institutional facilities in Wales. In 1992 the Welsh Health Planning Forum devised a 'Protocol for Investment in Health gain' specifically for people with learning disabilities. The Forum was established in 1988 by the Secretary of State for Wales, as an advisory subgroup of the Executive Committee of the Health Policy Board of the National Health Service. Its role was to give advice on the planning of health services, its aim 'to add years to life and life to years'. The strategic intent was outlined as follows: 'Working with others the National Health Service aims to take the people of Wales into the 21st century with a level of health on course to compare with the best in Europe' (Welsh Office 1992).

The protocol complements the principles of the strategy and considers where further investment in care provision could bring worthwhile gain, and identifies where current practices are 'questionable and reinvestment might be considered'. The overall strategic intent of the protocol is based on 'health gain' and, taken into account with the All Wales Strategy, enables a complementary approach to the development of future services in Wales.

Scotland

In Scotland, the development of health and social care is a well established policy objective, with increasing efforts aimed at enabling people to stay longer in their own homes. The Scottish local authorities and health boards have developed, both separately and jointly, a range of services and facilities that have helped to progress the shifting emphasis from hospital to community-based services. Between 1979 and 1987, the number of people with learning disabilities in long-stay hospitals fell by 21%, and day care provision rose by 39%. Places in residential homes for people with learning disabilities during this period of time have risen by 73%. One of the recommendations of the Working Group which was constituted to examine the contribution of the hospital services to care for people with learning disabilities in Scotland (Scottish Office 1992) was as follows: 'In the future it should be the norm that people with a mental handicap who are unable to be looked after in their own home, should be cared for in small, locally based residential facilities. These facilities should be developed by the NHS, local authorities and voluntary and private organizations.'

Although the report went on to point out that the 'potential for placement of people with learning disabilities in the community in Scotland has not been adequately developed', there has been a

Activity 3.4

Consider the home of a person with learning disabilities. Is it a home or a residential facility? Is there a difference?

Activity 3.5

List the range of services currently available to people with learning disabilities in your area.

marked escalation in the development of small, locally based living units and a significant move to provide people with learning disabilities with the opportunity to join in the life of the community to its full extent.

CONCLUSION

Over the past 35 years there have been significant changes in the ideologies and concepts underpinning service provision for people with learning disabilities (Figure 3.2). A move can be traced from segregation to integration, from incarceration to socialization, and from a medical to a social model of care. These changes, although

generally beneficial to people with learning disabilities, have provided a number of challenges: hospital closures have created a clear need for the development of a whole range of residential options, not least the development of residential and day care facilities that cater for people with a combination of complex and special needs.

There have been significant changes to the way in which services are funded. Local authorities now have the remit to plan appropriate packages of care, subsequently purchasing services from a variety of providers. The distinction between health and social care means that local authorities and health authorities will need to collaborate and determine locally how they share objectives, responsibilities and funding. In essence, it is suggested that the introduction of care management will result in care agencies accepting responsibility for meeting the needs of consumers; integral to this will be the requirement of care agencies to provide appropriate information to consumers in relation to service delivery. It should be acknowledged, however,

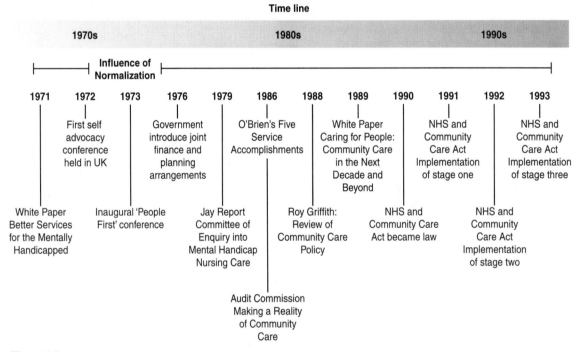

Figure 3.2

that care management and the extent of its implementation is variable across the country, as Waddington (1995) points out: 'It is beyond question that the delivery of anything like the full promise of *Care in the Community* over the next decade and beyond will require more effective collaboration between agencies everywhere. Without that, progress will not be possible much beyond a culture of collaboration characterized by "fine words and wish lists", as in traditional joint planning and community care plans.'

He goes on to acknowledge that some areas have travelled down the joint commissioning road in a relatively short period of time, and that factors supporting successful implementation include 'learning by doing', realism, incrementalism, time, good relationships, managerial support, clarity of joint objectives and a willingness to commit joint finance.

Central to the reforms proposed in *Caring For People* (DOH 1989) was the principle of a needs-led approach to assessment; a tailoring of services to meet individuals' requirements; and consideration of the resources available from both statutory and non-statutory services, ensuring that they are more responsive as a result of linking assessment, purchasing and commissioning. Although it is clearly still the responsibility of health authorities to meet healthcare needs, it is essential that, where there is overlap between health and social care, or where the distinction between the two is unclear, the responsible authorities work together to achieve the desired objective; it should be a 'seamless' service which removes the possibility of consumers falling into the 'health and social care gap' which may be created as a result of this division of care. Henwood (1992) warned that the health and social care divide was always going to be the 'Achilles heel' of the community care reforms, in that some needs can clearly be identified as health or social, and there is a 'grey' area where health and social care merge. This need not be a problem, provided that one or both agencies meets such needs.

As we approach the next millennium and consider those factors essential in the provision of successful health and social care for people with learning disabilities, it is clear that the future lies with interagency working, close collaboration and liaison with professionals sharing a common set of values and a willingness to work together. Such cooperation can only succeed if the views and opinions of people with learning disabilities and their carers are an active and integral part of the process.

REFERENCES

Audit Commission 1986 Making a reality of community care. HMSO, London

Audit Commission for Local Authorities in England and Wales 1989 Developing community care for adults with a mental handicap. Occasional Paper 9, HMSO, London

Bannerman M, Lindsay M 1993 Evolution of services. In: Shanley E, Starrs T A (eds) Learning disabilities handbook of care, 2nd edn. Churchill Livingtone, London

Barton R 1960 Institutional neurosis. Stonebridge Press, Bristol

Brechin A, Swain J 1988 Professional and client relationships: creating a 'working alliance' with people with learning difficulties. Disability, Handicap and Society 3: 213–226

DHSS 1971 Better services for the mentally handicapped. Cmnd 4683, HMSO, London

DOH 1988 Community care: agenda for action (Griffiths Report). HMSO, London

DOH 1989 Caring for people: community care in the next decade and beyond. Cm849, HMSO, London

DHSS 1995 Review of policy for people with a learning disability. HMSO, Northern Ireland

Ely Report 1969 Report of the Committee of Enquiry into Allegations of Ill Treatment of Patients and other Irregularities at the Ely Hospital, Cardiff. Cmnd 3975 HMSO, London

General Nursing Council 1982 Training Syllabus for Registered Nurses for Mental Subnormality Nursing. General Nursing Council for England and Wales, London

Henwood M 1992 Twilight zone. Health Service Journal 102: 28–30

House of Commons Hansard, 18 July 1990, cols 999–1014. HMSO, London

O'Brien J 1987 A guide to life-style planning. In: Bellamy G T, Wilcox B (eds) The activities catalog. Paul H Brookes Publishing Co, London

Report of the Committee of Enquiry into Mental Handicap Nursing Care 1979 (Jay Report) Cmnd. 74681 (I) and (II), HMSO, London

Rose S 1993 Social policy: a perspective on service developments and interagency working. In: Brigden P, Todd M (eds) Concepts in community care for people with learning difficulty. Macmillan, London

Ryan J, Thomas F 1987 The politics of mental handicap. Free Associated Press, London

Scottish Office Home and Health Department Scottish Health Service Advisory Council 1992 The future of mental handicap hospital services in Scotland. HMSO, Edinburgh

Waddington P 1995 Joint commissioning of services for people with learning disabilities: a review of the principles and the practice. British Journal of Learning Disabilities 23: 2–10

Welsh Office 1983 All Wales strategy for the development of services for mentally handicapped people. Welsh Office, Cardiff

Welsh Office 1992 Protocol for investment in health gain. Mental handicap (learning disabilities). Welsh Health Planning Forum, Cardiff

Welsh Mental Handicap Strategy: Guidance, 1994 Guidance, Cardiff (p 3)

Whitehead S 1993 The social origins of normalisation. In: Brown H, Smith S (eds) Normalisation – a reader for the nineties. Routledge, London

Wolfensberger W 1972 Normalisation: the principle of normalisation in human services. National Institute of Mental Retardation, Toronto

Wolfensberger W 1983 Social role valorization. A proposed new term for the principle of normalization. Mental Retardation 21: 234–239

Wolfensberger W, Tullman S 1989 A brief outline of the principle of normalization. In: Brechin A, Walmsley J 1989 Making connections. Hodder & Stoughton, London, p 215–217

4

Providing quality care

J. Pougher

INTRODUCTION

Providing quality care for people with learning disabilities poses challenges for nurses and service providers at a time of significant changes in underlying belief systems and the nature of service provision. Among recent key changes have been a growing emphasis on individual rights, the promotion of service user involvement in planning and evaluating services and a move from institutional care to provision in the community. Service providers have also had to demonstrate a commitment to improving quality standards in response to government initiatives and the growing expectations of service users and their carers.

This chapter reviews some of the key processes that nurses and other professionals working in organizations providing healthcare need to adopt in order to provide high-quality care. These processes are equally valid for organizations whatever their size and whether they are in the statutory or non-statutory sector. For an organization to deliver a quality service and care to people there are three basic requirements:

1. A value base
2. A framework for delivering services
3. An appropriate range of quality tools and systems.

Before examining these requirements it is important to define the concept of quality, briefly review its history in health provision, and consider why it is important to have a programme to address the promotion of quality in an organization.

What is a quality service?

Service providers constantly highlight their commitment to providing a quality service, yet what is meant by the term quality is not always clear. Generally, if something is referred to as being of good quality it is because it has some positive attribute. The first question that must be asked, however, is who decides whether a service has a positive benefit – those providing the service or those receiving it. The views of both are important, but traditionally the professionals' view of what constituted a quality service was predominant and was rarely questioned by those receiving it. However, during recent years increasing attention has focused on the service user's perspective. Defining what constitutes a quality health service has also involved a range of different groups, including patient representatives, professional staff, managers, carers, the Government, pressure groups, health commissioners and community health councils. Despite the involvement of so many groups, any attempt to define the nature of quality must first and foremost be viewed from the perspective of the user.

It is not sufficient to leave the definition of a quality service at this point, because what constitutes a quality service differs between one service user and another. Indeed, it is often said that quality, like beauty, is in the eye of the beholder. Take, for example, a visit to a service user's home by a community learning disability nurse. For most people the outcome of such a visit will be the key quality indicator. Other people might consider the key quality indicator to be how quickly the nurse responded to the request for a visit, or flexibility in visiting hours. For other individuals these matters may be of relatively little importance, and they will be more concerned with how smartly dressed the nurse is or the degree of courtesy exhibited by the nurse. The fact is that people have different expectations and different needs. Therefore, when we talk about a quality service we are talking about one that identifies and meets people's individual needs.

It must also be remembered that an individual's views and expectations can change over time, and that what was found to be satisfactory a few years ago may now be considered inadequate. Also, it must be appreciated that occasionally service users may be unsure or unaware of what services they may need, or may request inappropriate interventions. Providing a quality service, therefore, also involves working in partnership with service users to identify their individual needs, delivering the appropriate and agreed care, and constantly monitoring its relevance and effectiveness with them.

Providing a quality service also means ensuring that people's individual needs are met efficiently and that resources are used effectively and not wasted. No organization has unlimited resources, and it is important that they are well managed to deliver the best possible care. For example, in an outpatients' department staff should arrive on time and clinics should run to schedule, as well as providing the correct treatment. Money that is wasted in an organization by any department could have gone to helping more people or providing better-quality care.

Finally, if an organization aims to provide quality care it must ensure that all those who need a service receive it. It is not sufficient to provide a good service to a small number of people while a large number of people's needs remain unmet or even unidentified. Providing a quality service is about ensuring that the needs of all customers are being met.

Given the above considerations, a definition of a quality health service that will be used in this chapter is: a service that has identified all its customers and consistently meets their agreed needs in a cost-effective manner.

A background to quality: the nursing perspective

For nurses, providing a quality service is not a new concept. As far back as 1854 Florence Nightingale was establishing standards and reducing the costs of poor-quality nursing care. Recent years, however, have seen a growing interest in and focus on what constitutes a quality service, with an increasing willingness to involve service users in defining standards.

There has also been a significant change in opinion regarding a role in society for people with learning disabilities, the key change being the rejection of the 19th century approach which saw the rise of institutions to ensure that people with learning disabilities were kept segregated from the rest of society.

Legislation and social policy has played a significant role in promoting changes in patterns of care for people with learning disabilities. The White Paper *Better Services for the Mentally Handicapped* (DOH 1971) promoted the principle that people with learning disabilities should be treated as ordinary citizens and enjoy the right to live a normal life in the community. The move to promote community provision for people with learning disabilities was reinforced with the publication of the White Paper *Caring for People: Community Care in the Next Decade and Beyond* (DOH 1989).

Changes in service philosophy and patterns of care have also been championed and challenged by a number of agencies. The King's Fund, the Independent Developmental Council, People First, and the Joseph Rowntree Foundation for Research and Development, among other groups, have been instrumental in defining and improving standards for people with learning disabilities.

A key landmark in defining quality standards in the field of learning disabilities came with the publication of *Pursuing Quality: How Good are Your Services for People with a Mental Handicap?* (Independent Development Council 1986). This booklet drew on quality management theory and supported user involvement and the values of *An Ordinary Life* (King's Fund 1980). It also laid down clear guidelines as to how services could be organized to establish and improve the quality of care.

Nurses, along with other healthcare professionals, have also been at the forefront of helping to improve services. Nurses have responded positively to the challenges raised by changing expectations and advances in the delivery of healthcare. The Code of Professional Conduct (UKCC 1994), changes in nurse training and a focus on continuing professional development

have all contributed to improved nursing care. On a formal level nurses have also worked on setting explicit written standards of care. An important milestone was the establishment of RCN Standard of Care Project in 1965. This is now a major national programme, with current activity focused on the Dynamic Standard Setting System (RCN 1990).

Why is it necessary to establish a system to manage quality?

Although most people agree that providing a quality service is important, many question the need to set up a formal system to manage quality. Faced with an additional workload, a substantial investment of resources and an uncertain outcome, many staff are reluctant to advocate change. Some might respond by simply indicating that they are just too busy, others that they have seen things like it before and they did not change anything. It is therefore important that staff are made aware of the advantages to formally managing quality. Some of these are as follows:

- A quality management system reduces costs, helps eliminate wasteful practices and enables scarce resources to be targeted where they are most needed.
- It makes the work of staff easier. They spend less time dealing with problems and more time focusing on their work.
- Staff can respond more effectively to the needs of individual service users, and thereby enhance user satisfaction with the service.
- An organization that has a good reputation for delivering quality care will attract good staff, which will further help enhance the quality of services provided.
- Finally, an effective quality management system will give the organization a competitive edge: people will want to use the services you provide.

The three requirements necessary for providing quality care – a value base, a framework and quality tools and systems – will now be explained in some detail.

THE VALUE BASE

The foundation for any organization committed to providing quality care is an agreed explicit set of values that clearly set out what the service is seeking to achieve. Values are critical because they define what services should be like, and thus provide a basis for setting explicit service outcomes.

An organization's values should:

- Clearly state the organization's basic beliefs regarding the role of people with learning disabilities in society
- Identify how the organization will establish and review its goals
- Indicate how the organization will work with people with learning disabilities.

Only when an organization has determined its values can it establish the scope of its business plan. This will outline what services it will offer, to whom and where. Having done this, the organization can then identify the nature and skills of its workforce and the extent of resources required to deliver that plan.

As values are so important it is essential that an organization clearly sets out how they will be determined. It is also important that the organization regularly reviews its values and the objectives derived from them to ensure they continue to reflect the needs and aspirations of service users and staff. Both staff and users need to set and monitor the organization's values. This should not involve just professional staff or managers – everybody, at all levels, in all departments of the organization, should be consulted. People need to believe in and support the values of the organization they work for if they are to champion them. If they have not been involved in deciding upon them or reviewing them they may at best be half-hearted in their support for what the organization does. Changes in values can also result in resistance from some staff: new values can take time to gain acceptance. Values also need to be written in a language people can understand and relate to: they should not contain jargon or buzzwords.

In determining its values or in reviewing them

an organization should listen to and value the views of local service users. These may be obtained on a one-to-one basis, or user groups can be established. The important point is that users and their advocates should have a genuine ability to influence the outcomes of debate. Organizations should also consult with carers, voluntary bodies and other agencies, such as social services, to ensure that the views of other provider agencies and the wider local community are taken into account.

The values espoused by an organization should also be influenced by the prevailing values in society. Occasionally a new set of values appears that have a significant effect on the way people think and act. One such set of values in the field of learning disabilities has been that of normalization.

Normalization

Normalization may be seen as part of a larger change in the way people with learning disabilities are perceived, i.e. away from their being seen as a threat to society and requiring to be segregated. It is part of a wider belief that services should fit the needs of the individual, rather than the individual being made to fit into what the service provides. There is insufficient scope within this chapter to examine the principle of normalization in depth, but it is useful to consider some of its key concepts.

The concept of normalization originated in Denmark, where the Mental Retardation Act (1959) sought to develop services for people with learning disabilities as close as possible to normal living conditions (Bank-Mikkelsen 1980). This concept was refined in Scandinavia during the 1960s, and had an increasing influence on service provision in Scandinavia. Its popularization owes much of its success to Wolfensberger, who developed the concept further in America during the late 1960s (Wolfensberger 1980).

The central value of normalization is that people with learning disabilities have the same human value as anyone else in society. It does not argue that everybody should be normal: rather, it states that people with learning disabilities should be able to engage in socially valued activities. Normalization acknowledges that people with learning disabilities are generally devalued by the rest of society, and argues that they need positive help and support to establish them in socially valued roles. Unfortunately, the services set up to care for people with learning disabilities reflect the opinions of society, and often do little to support the individual development of service users. Normalization argues that service providers need to be aware of what they are doing, and to work alongside service users to create positive expectations for people with learning disabilities. Until such people are able to engage in socially valued activities they will continue to be devalued.

Putting values into action

The values of normalization are of little use if they are not put into practice. The principles of normalization have found expression in evaluation materials that determine the extent to which they are implemented. Perhaps the best known of these is the 'program analysis of service systems implementation of normalization goals', more commonly called PASSING (Wolfensberger & Thomas 1983).

Another popular approach to interpreting the principles of normalization within the United Kingdom has been O'Brien's five service accomplishments (O'Brien 1987a). Basically, these are ways in which the service can enhance the quality of an individual's life. In effect, O'Brien's accomplishments take the principles of normalization into the field of service provision, and an organization can use them to monitor its activities from the perspective of the user. The accomplishments are outlined in Box 4.1

Having an explicit set of values alone does not of course provide all the answers, yet they are an essential starting point to ensuring a quality service. Once a set of values has been agreed, the next step is for the organization to develop a framework to ensure that the values and the objectives derived from them can be achieved.

Box 4.1   Service accomplishments of O'Brien (1987)

Respect
Service providers should create opportunities for people with learning disabilities to engage in activities and develop behaviours that project a positive image. In doing so, however, the service should be careful that in the provision of specialist services people do not become even more stigmatized.

Community presence
People with learning disabilities have a right to live in the community, in ordinary homes that are indistinguishable from those around them. They should also be able to shop, work and spend their recreational time with fellow citizens in their local community. They should not have to use different facilities, or the same facilities at different times of the day.

Relationships
People with learning disabilities have the right to socialize with people whom they choose. It is not sufficient that they just live in the community: as with everybody else, they should have the opportunity to be able to form lasting, meaningful relationships with both handicapped and non-handicapped people.

Choice
People with learning disabilities have the right to make choices concerning their life. These may range from small decisions, such as choice of meal, to larger ones like where to live, and occupation. People with learning disabilities may need support in making some decisions.

Competence
This principle recognizes that people with learning disabilities may need to develop skills and attributes that enable them to fully enjoy the facilities within the community. A range of specialist help may need to be made available. Ultimately, the goal is for each individual to live as independently as possible.

Activity 4.1

Consider your own values and beliefs regarding people with learning disabilities.

Have they changed over time? Have your views been shared by colleagues you have worked with?

Finally, consider how your values might influence the way you interact with people who have learning disabilities.

A FRAMEWORK FOR QUALITY

A framework is basically a set of working principles that define how an organization will conduct its activities and evaluate the effectiveness of what it does. A framework provides structure and coordination, and forms the basis of the organization's business strategy. A business strategy should indicate what services will be delivered to whom and how. Without a properly formulated business strategy an organization may find it is delivering a potentially wonderful service, but not to those most in need of it. An organizational framework should enable staff to operate in a supportive and coordinated environment that enhances learning. One organizational framework that has received an increasing amount of support in recent years is total quality management (TQM).

TQM basically comprises of a set of principles that guide staff in how they should work and focus their activities. Developed in the commercial sector, initially in Japan, the model has become increasingly popular in the west, in both private and public sectors. The introduction of TQM in the NHS can be dated to 1989–1990, with the Department of Health funding 17 demonstration sites. There is nothing revolutionary in the principles of TQM – indeed, most of them are common sense ideas that many successful organizations have employed for a long time. The key feature that makes TQM different is that these principles have to be applied to the whole organization in a systematic and coordinated way. Senior managers have a key role to play in applying the principles of TQM, but all staff are involved. Although there are several different models of TQM in existence there are certain common principles.

Whatever framework is adopted by an organization it will need to be adapted and developed to ensure that it meets the needs of local service users and reflects the skills, history and aspirations of staff. Outlined below are the key principles that make up the TQM framework.

Focus on customers

Central to the TQM philosophy is the importance of the customer. To ensure success an organization must identify their individual requirements and meet them consistently. Indeed, some organizations who adopt a TQM approach express an intention not only to meet needs, but even to delight customers and exceed their expectations.

To provide quality healthcare an organization must be in constant touch with the needs, opinions and aspirations of service users. Needs can be assessed on an individual basis through assessments undertaken by staff as part of an individualized plan of care for each service user. How well services continue to meet individual needs can also be monitored via care plan reviews. For the organization to be truly in touch with opinions and aspirations, however, the users should also be involved in planning, running and evaluating service provision. This involvement should not be token participation but genuine informed involvement. It might, for instance, involve users in a residential home choosing the staff who will help care for them, or being involved in staff training and development activities.

As not all service users will necessarily be involved in running, planning and evaluating services, it is important that there are also opportunities, both formal and informal, for them to express their opinions. Feedback is necessary so that providers can plan services and direct resources where they are needed. One very important means of obtaining feedback is through complaints, which should be viewed positively and indeed encouraged as a key means of improving services. Complaints should be dealt with as soon as possible – often all the complainant requires is an apology or a simple explanation, and people should have the opportunity to comment upon services at the earliest possible moment. Although the analysis of complaints is important, an organization should also pay equal attention to expressions of commendation. It is important to develop complaint systems that are accessible to service users who have difficulty in understanding the written word. For example, a complaints procedure has been developed by the Hull and Holderness Community Health NHS Trust (1996) that uses Makaton and simplified text to enable users to directly access the complaints system. Views and opinions can also be obtained through the use of patient satisfaction surveys. These can involve questionnaires or interviews, and it is important that they are carried out by trained and experienced individuals. Care should also be taken to avoid bias, and to ensure that the information obtained is meaningful. The results must also be incorporated into the organization's decision-making process.

It is also important to remember that if a service starts receiving more complaints it does not necessarily mean that it is becoming worse: it may indicate that the organization is more open, and service users feel that it is likely to deal with the issues they have raised. It is also important to appreciate that if user expectations are low, they may be reasonably happy with whatever quality care they receive, or see little point in complaining as they do not believe anything will be done. Yet as expectations grow, users may only be satisfied with continually improving levels of service provision.

Reducing waste

No organization does everything right first time, every time, and never makes a mistake or wastes money. TQM requires an organization to strive to eliminate all mistakes and wasteful practices. In a typical organization large sums of money are wasted in putting mistakes right, duplicating effort, or just by spending on the wrong things or the right things at the wrong time. TQM defines such waste as the cost of quality. There is of course a cost associated with ensuring that no mistakes happen, but most organizations spend

considerably more to put mistakes right than they are likely to spend in eliminating wasteful practices.

Identifying the costs of making mistakes is not always straightforward. In practice there are two main ways of doing this: the PAF method and the process cost method.

The PAF Method

The PAF method breaks down costs into one of three categories: prevention, appraisal and failure. Prevention is basically ensuring that mistakes do not happen. Appraisal means checking how well the organization is performing against its agreed standards. Appraisal costs will therefore include money spent on clinical audit and routine inspection of equipment. Failure costs are those associated with putting things right once they have gone wrong. The only legitimate costs an organization should really incur concern prevention activities, although it is likely that a small amount will always be spent on appraisal. Ultimately no money should be spent in relation to the failure category. This method has been criticized because health organizations can find it difficult to assign certain costs to the given headings.

The process cost method

The process cost method basically requires an organization to identify its key processes and determine what the cost would be if everything went right for each one. For instance, the organization could examine the cost associated with running an outpatients clinic if all the patients turned up on time, all the staff were present, all the case notes were up to date and accessible, and all appointments ran to schedule. The organization could then conduct a survey to find out what really happens and attach a cost to the activities that go wrong, for example the cost of staff time wasted in trying to find notes, or because people do not turn up, or because the right equipment is not available. This method is generally more useful for healthcare providers.

Once quality costs have been identified an

Activity 4.2

Consider an organization or an area that you have worked in, preferably recently, and then answer the following questions:
- How much time was spent in putting mistakes right?
- What were the most common problems, and what could have been done to solve them?
- If everything had been done right and no money wasted, what could have been done with the money saved?

organization must be in a position to tackle them; this requires commitment and technical skill. Whatever system is used, it is essential that all levels of staff are involved in identifying the costs. It is also important that the initiative is not seen as a cost-cutting exercise: staff need to be informed of the purpose of the exercise. An appropriate training programme will also need to be conducted to enable staff to undertake the exercise effectively.

Empowerment

It is important that all staff in an organization are given the authority to do their jobs effectively. The contributions of staff, particularly those at the most junior level, need to be explicitly recognized. Staff are an organization's most valuable asset, and their expertise and experience need to be fully used. To this end many organizations reward significant or exceptional work through either a certificate scheme or a financial reward scheme to help buy equipment or aid developmental work. The ultimate objective is to develop a culture where all staff feel valued.

In order to promote staff involvement many organizations have established staff groups based on working environments. A group could, therefore, be based around the members of a community learning disability team, or staff in a residential home. In the past these groups were often called quality circles, but are now more likely to be called quality implementation teams or quality action groups. Typically, group members brainstorm ideas on how they can improve services in their area, and come up with their own solutions to problems that affect them. Such groups will only prove effective, however, if they have support from managers and the team members have been appropriately trained.

Staff training and development

The nature of service provision for people with learning disabilities is subject to constant change and review. In order for an organization to deliver good-quality care it is therefore important that all staff are trained and competent in the latest advances in practice and research findings. Training must be coordinated – it is too important to be left to chance.

The first step is to identify staff training needs: these should be agreed between staff and their line managers. The range of training required will be determined via the identified needs of service users and the objectives of the organization as outlined in the business plan. Once identified, there needs to be a system to evaluate the effectiveness of the training. The key question to ask is whether the training has improved practice.

Given the nature of the work undertaken by nurses it is important that they have the opportunity to take part in multidisciplinary and multiagency learning forums. The opportunity to attend training events with service users should also be encouraged.

Individual staff members should have their own training plan which records their progress and identifies future needs. These plans should be drawn up during meetings with line managers and reviewed on a regular basis. Qualified nursing staff, of course, have a duty to update their nursing knowledge in line with post-registration and education requirements (PREPP; UKCC 1994), but all staff should ensure that they work in accordance with accepted best practice.

If an organization is committed to TQM staff also need to be trained in its key principles. As with all training, individual needs must be identified and outcomes made explicit. The content of a typical training programme would be:

- The organization's approach to quality
- The organization's philosophy
- Team building
- Problem-solving techniques
- Customer care
- Clinical audit
- Evaluation and monitoring techniques
- Identification of internal customers and suppliers
- Managing change
- Process improvement
- Benchmarking
- Effective communication.

Team work

Running an organization is a complex task. Although the insight of individual members of staff is very important to the success of an organization, TQM argues that the ability of staff to work effectively as a team is very important. Several advantages for teamwork over individual effort have been claimed:

- Teamworking is an effective means of promoting organizational change. Staff are more likely to support change if they have been involved in it.
- Working in teams supports cooperation within an organization rather than competition. It should improve communications between departments and help build trust and develop interdependence.
- People can bring into a team a wide range of skills and experience that can be shared. Thus, a greater number of problems can be solved than could be tackled by one individual.
- The standard of decision making in teams tends to be high, and recommendations from teams are therefore more likely to be implemented.

Staff need to understand and appreciate the skills and ideas that colleagues from different professions can bring to the delivery of services. Promoting good teamwork, however, is not always an easy matter: good teams do not just happen. Many teams do not operate at maximum efficiency and individual members can come into conflict. Staff need to work at becoming effective team members and to appreciate that different people will bring different skills into the team. There is also the danger that promoting teams can result in rivalry between teams in the same organization. This is not appropriate for TQM, as teams are supposed to work in a complementary way.

Internal customers

TQM does not just recognize the importance of meeting the needs of external customers (service users), it also promotes the concept of internal customers. Essentially within any organization there exists for each team or department a series of suppliers and customers. For example, the finance department may be seen as a supplier to operational managers. In a community home, the people preparing a meal rely on those who ordered or purchased the food: if they do not have the right ingredients they cannot make the meal. Each supplier should know exactly what their customers want. If operational managers want timely, accurate and easily understood financial information, that is what they should receive. The quality of work of one department affects the quality of output from another, and ultimately affects the service delivered to the external customer. Any organization hoping to deliver a quality service must ensure that staff work together effectively.

The problem is that many organizations have poorly developed internal customer chains. If teams or departments are not receiving the appropriate service and support, it is not sufficient to complain: there must be a commitment to do something about it. It is important that different departments or professions understand each other's roles and make a commitment to support each other, rather than put their department's interests first.

Different teams/departments within an organization need to communicate their requirements effectively. A series of supplier/customer workshops can be established where staff are brought together to discuss problem areas and identify solutions. If internal customer requirements are not clearly understood, then problems can arise, including unrealistic targets being set, ill-defined requirements and departments blaming each other for mistakes.

Effective communication

The quality vision, i.e. what the organization is seeking to achieve, needs to be effectively disseminated. Every member of staff must have the same understanding, and so messages must be carefully worded and jargon avoided.

Good communication between members of the same team, between teams and between the organization and other organizations is essential. For any organization to work effectively, staff must be in possession of relevant, timely and accurate information. Good-quality information is essential for tackling problems and being able to monitor performance.

The organization also needs to keep up-to-date information on its activities, and this should be accessible to all relevant staff. This should help prevent situations where, for example, one group of staff wastes time researching and developing an idea that has, unbeknown to them, already been successfully implemented in another part of the organization. Effective use should be made of newsletters and information boards. A newsletter is a useful tool to publicize and celebrate successes. It could include interviews with staff, staff suggestions, and highlight future events. Many organizations also have a briefing system to ensure that communications are transmitted to all staff within a given time frame.

Continuous improvement

The organization should commit itself to a programme of continuous improvement in all departments. In reality, no organization can claim that it has reached its ultimate quality goal: new research will come along that will dictate a change in working patterns; new technology will solve problems but pose new challenges; service user expectations will change; there will be calls to deliver greater output but with the same or diminished resources. Within such a challenging, complex, changing world an organization needs to constantly review its targets and methods, and keep closely in touch with the needs and aspirations of its users.

Management structure for the delivery of quality

Most organizations establish some structure to ensure that quality is effectively managed. Some programmes rely entirely on existing management structures, where quality issues and initiatives are a part of the normal activities. Others set up a full shadow structure for quality, establish-

ing separate committees and team meetings specifically to examine quality matters. Often these shadow structures are time limited and cease to function when the drive for quality becomes integrated into the normal business activities.

Where an organization establishes a structure to manage quality, there is typically a steering committee to direct activities and support the activities of work-based quality implementation teams. The respective roles and tasks of these bodies are outlined in Table 4.1.

It is also important for the head of the organization to make a visible commitment to the quality programme (Oakland 1993). Quality management is essentially a management change process and therefore a managerial responsibility. Senior managers must:

- become the catalysts of change
- act as teachers and role models
- encourage staff to put forward ideas
- support skill development and, in conjunction with staff, set key targets
- act as champions of change by demonstrating visible commitment.

Most organizations appoint a TQM specialist or specialist team when embarking on a TQM programme. However, care must be taken to ensure that staff do not believe that quality is the responsibility only of the quality department.

To ensure successful implementation all staff must be clear on how the organization's commitment to quality will be conducted. There should be a written strategy that clearly outlines how the organization will manage quality, detailing principles, responsibilities and objectives. This document should be used by staff to guide them in their day-to-day work and help ensure that they are all working towards common goals.

The quality culture

TQM often requires a fundamental shift in the way people think and work. It requires people and processes to work in harmony; a commitment to preventing mistakes from happening, rather than spending resources and time in

Table 4.1 The roles of quality structures	
Role of the steering committee	Role of the quality implementation teams
Determine the success criteria for the total quality management programme	Identify local priorities for action
Ensure, with the support of staff, the ongoing development of the quality philosophy, purpose and guiding principles	Provide ongoing support for staff
Ensure sufficient resources, training and support for staff are available	Identify cost improvement activities
Monitor the progress of the organization in achieving its quality goals	Monitor local performance
Resolve issues between departments and functions within the organization	Make recommendations to managers
Support quality implementation teams throughout the organization	Help ensure the views of staff are represented at all levels of the organization
Review the quality strategy in light of time and changing circumstances	Offer developmental opportunities for staff
Give visible commitment to the quality strategy	

putting things right; a culture where all staff are committed to delivering a high quality of care focused on meeting their customers' needs; a culture where departments work cooperatively and not in competition with each other. This means breaking down barriers between professionals and departments. TQM means a commitment to viewing mistakes as learning opportunities. It means establishing an open learning environment where staff learn from each other, and everybody sees it as part of their business to deliver quality. Finally, TQM demands a commitment to continuous quality improvement.

It should not be expected that an organization's culture will change overnight: it may take many years, but this is not to say that significant progress cannot be made in the short term.

DELIVERING A QUALITY SERVICE

Once the organization has a structured framework such as TQM it will still need to use a range of tools or systems to help meet the needs of its service users effectively. The tools and systems used will depend largely upon the nature of the organization's activities. This section will examine some of those commonly used in health settings. They may also of course be used in an organization that does not have a structured approach to development, but to make the best use of them the organization should be committed to continuous quality improvement.

Quality assurance

Quality assurance is basically a system which ensures that an organization consistently adheres to a certain standard that its customers can rely upon. Quality assurance involves setting standards, monitoring them and feeding back the results in order to improve practice. Quality assurance systems focus on the delivery of services and seek to prevent errors. There is sometimes confusion as to the relationship between TQM and quality assurance. Quality assurance is not the same as TQM: TQM is a wider-based initiative involving strategic planning, changing values to build a new culture, promoting teamwork and integrating quality into the organization's business. Quality assurance does, however, often play a key part in a TQM strategy. Indeed, many organizations start with a quality assurance strategy and then develop a wider approach to quality such as TQM.

One of the best-known quality assurance systems is the internationally accepted ISO 9000 series, formerly known as BS5750 in the UK (British Standards Institution 1987). This system involves an organization determining its critical functions for success, setting up a comprehensive range of standards in predefined areas around these functions, and then auditing these standards. Other quality assurance systems may be relatively small scale and developed locally. Many will involve the use of other tools that will be considered in this section.

Clinical audit

Clinical audit ensures that practice is developed in a coordinated and effective manner. The Department of Health has stated that 'Clinical audit involves systematically looking at the procedures used for diagnosis, care and treatment, examining how associated resources are used and investigating the effect care has on the outcome and quality of life for the patient' (DOH 1994). Clinical audit may be seen as a quality assurance system applied to the activities of a group of healthcare professionals.

Clinical audit done well can provide a number of benefits:

- A reduction in the number of clinical mistakes made
- Improving the general quality of care
- The promotion of more consistent care
- A reduction in the amount of money wasted.

Whereas clinical audit obviously focuses on clinical care, there are other audits that focus on how organizations plan their activities and manage resources. One of the best-known of these is the King's Fund Organizational Audit. Some audits may also, of course, examine both clinical delivery and organizational issues. Audit should not be confined to clinical staff but should be used across all aspects of an organization's activities.

In introducing audit, it is best to let staff decide upon priorities for action and agree upon what the relevant standards should be. Audit should not be imposed by managers. It is also important that service users should be involved in the audit process.

Staff will need support and training to conduct audit effectively. Sufficient time and resources should be set aside, and staff also need to be open and honest if audit is to be successful. Although many audits are still fairly simple and small scale, larger, more complex audits will require the use of computers.

A range of different methods are used in collecting information for clinical audit. These include questionnaires, review of records, interviews, and physical observation.

It is not sufficient to merely audit the services that one provides, or just to find out what is happening: audit should be a continuing process aimed at improving services. This is known as the audit cycle (Figure 4.1). For this to succeed, it is important that there is a commitment from managers and staff to actioning the results of audit. Finally, audit should also form part of continuing professional development.

Standard setting

As can be seen from Figure 4.1, standard setting is essentially the first phase of the clinical audit process. An organization needs to set standards before taking steps to measure performance against them and then take action as appropriate. A standard is an expectation of performance. Standards define the quality of service that users

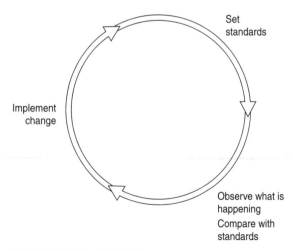

Figure 4.1   The audit cycle.

can expect. It is important that standards should not be seen as just a bureaucratic exercise or as a means of inspection from above.

Nurses and healthcare staff can find themselves working to a wide range of standards. For instance, nurses work in line with professional standards established by the United Kingdom Central Council. There are also standards set by purchasers of services through contracting arrangements, and by the Government through initiatives such as the Patient's Charter. Finally, and just as important, there are standards set by staff themselves. Standards can also cover a wide area, including professional conduct, written records, communication and clinical practice.

Where to start setting standards and at what level can pose an interesting challenge for staff. Where possible, standards should be underpinned by research evidence and involve service users. It is also useful to involve the multidisciplinary team, as all staff can then sign up to and work to a consistent standard, although there still remains a place for unidisciplinary standards.

Imposing a detailed range of standards that have been developed elsewhere can often be counterproductive. It is usually better for staff to work on developing their own standards, using what has been done elsewhere for guidance and developing this to meet their own particular circumstances. One common mistake is to set a standard for everything an organization does: this can result in a lot of time and resources being spent on setting standards that are of little importance. It is better to prioritize the work that needs to be done.

A very popular approach to setting professional standards has been the Donebedian method. This breaks a standard into three parts: structure, process and outcome. The structure part contains all the elements that are necessary to achieve the standard; the process part outlines the actions that are necessary to achieve the standard; and the outcome part outlines what should happen when the standard is achieved.

Whatever format is used, standards should detail specific outcomes and be achievable within given resources. They may be difficult for a team to achieve, presenting a significant challenge and taking time to accomplish, but ultimately they must be achievable, as staff will become discouraged if they can never reach the required grade in spite of their best efforts. There is also little point in setting standards below the level that is currently being provided. Standards should also be written in a way that people can easily understand. Also, most importantly, standards should be measurable: it is a waste of time and resources to set standards that cannot be readily and simply evaluated. Finally, standards should not be set in stone but be open to critical challenge and regular review.

Benchmarking

A benchmark is a reference point against which to compare oneself. Benchmarking is a structured process whereby an organization evaluates its performance, services and practice against another organization with the aim of achieving and maintaining enhanced performance. Benchmarking is effectively about trying to achieve best practice.

Although benchmarking obviously involves setting standards, it is not just another name for standard setting. In benchmarking the ultimate aim is to explicitly compare one's own standards against those of an outside organization (often a competitor), and then to set up a system to ensure a continuing platform for enhancing performance up to and beyond the level of that organization. The other organization need not be in the same field or even in the same country: you could, for instance, measure your performance against the best in the world. Benchmarking is often broken down into four types (Bell et al 1994).

1. **Internal benchmarking** This is where an organization compares performance only between its own departments. Internal benchmarking is relatively straightforward and does not require a great deal of time and resources. Its value may be fairly limited, but

it is often a useful first step towards the other forms of benchmarking.

2. **Competitive benchmarking** This is where an organization compares its performance in certain functions against other organizations (competitors) within the same industry.
3. **Functional benchmarking** Here an organization seeks to compare specific functions against the very best of any organizations' performance worldwide, irrespective of the nature of the business being conducted.
4. **Generic benchmarking** Here the organization seeks to compare all its functions with those of other organizations worldwide, regardless of the business being conducted.

The organization must decide upon an appropriate data collection method and identify the areas to be benchmarked first. When engaging in external or competitive benchmarking it is useful to visit the target organization to see how they conduct their activities. Benchmarking does not just involve collecting and comparing data: the organization must understand how the target organization achieves its performance. Having set performance targets, the organization must then determine how it will achieve its improvements. The targets should not be set in isolation, but integrated into the business planning process. The benefits of benchmarking are that it:

- promotes and demonstrates the organization's commitment to value for money
- helps promote a culture focused on continuous improvement
- enables organizations to become leaders in service provision
- gives an organization an insight into how other organizations have tackled problems, and thereby access to proven solutions
- establishes credible standards of best practice.

To be successful managers need to ensure that findings are understood and acted upon. Finally, benchmarking should be promoted as a method of working more efficiently, not as more work to be undertaken.

Research-based practice

It is generally acknowledged that much work is conducted upon the basis of custom and experience, yet ideally, nursing, along with other professions, should move towards evidence-based practice. As with other professions, nurses need to know what interventions and treatments work. Research-based practice is in effect the foundation for good practice (Culyer 1994). There are several advantages in operating research-based practice:

- Research can develop new knowledge that leads to improvements in practice, benefiting service users, their families and the community.
- The relevance and effectiveness of established approaches to delivering healthcare can be evaluated via research.
- Research can result in the more effective use of resources by eliminating inefficient practices.

Although it is important to undertake research to improve the delivery of care, it is equally important that research findings are effectively disseminated to staff. There is little point in undertaking research if the findings and benefits are not put into practice. It is therefore essential that the organization not only supports research, but also ensures that findings are acted upon, incorporated into standards, and inform the development of practice.

It is not vital that all staff be skilled researchers, but all should be able to evaluate research findings objectively and determine their usefulness in their work. Research is not an elitist activity, nor is it relevant only for clinical staff – it is important for all staff. It is important, for instance, that the human resources department uses the most effective training strategy, or that the IT department has the most effective equipment for its needs.

Clinical supervision

In *A Vision for the Future* (NHSME 1993) clinical supervision is highlighted as a means of supporting nurses in maintaining and developing high standards of practice and developing credible new means of delivering care. Managed effectively, clinical supervision protects standards, enhances competence and enables nurses to extend their abilities.

Clinical supervision is a process of regular contact between a member of staff and their supervisor. The role of clinical supervisor has often been likened to that of a professional guide, with the expert guiding and teaching the novice. Discussions at clinical supervision sessions can be very wide ranging, and may include giving feedback on performance, reviewing professional developments, and advising on caseload management. The relationship between the staff member and the supervisor enhances the ability of the nurse to put professional knowledge into practice. Supervision may be on a one-to-one basis, within a group or team, or on a peer review basis (Hawkins & Shoney 1989).

To be effective, staff should be trained in communication and counselling skills. The effective supervisor must also be skilled in promoting trust and confidentiality, and be reliable and open. An appropriate agreed amount of time should be set aside for the sessions. There also needs to be agreement and a clear understanding of the aims of the sessions. Clinical supervision may also play a part in more formal appraisal and review.

Individual Programme Plans (IPPs)

It is important that, whatever tools or systems are used, the potential benefits must be translated into actual practice. The individual programme approach to service delivery has been widely accepted as providing a structured and effective means of determining and meeting an individual's needs. It is also an important means of enabling the organization to determine how well it is meeting the individual planned and agreed needs of service users. Central to and underpinning an individual programme approach to meeting needs are several key principles:

• The individual owns the system with regard

to the service they receive: their wishes are central and overriding.
• The individual is viewed as a person in their own right.
• The individual should be encouraged to reach his or her full potential.
• Individual needs should define the nature of service provision. The needs of the individual should not be made to fit into the current pattern of service provision.

All individual plans should contain a comprehensive assessment. As the plan should focus on the needs of the individual, the service user needs to be involved in the assessment planning and evaluation. The individualized care plan should also identify a strategy in order to meet the set goals. It should clearly set out the commitment other individuals make to the user's care. Finally, individualized plans should identify service deficiencies and indicate what action needs to be taken. For individual care planning to be carried out effectively, staff require certain key skills. These include knowledge of the individual, insight into the assessment technique to be used, and observational and time management skills.

EVALUATION OF SERVICES

Having established a framework for developing services and adopted an appropriate range of quality tools and systems, it is important that an organization constantly and critically monitors how well it is functioning. If an organization does not know how effectively it is achieving its objectives, it cannot take the appropriate action to correct the problems and improve services. Before embarking on any programme to improve services it is essential that an organization establishes explicit guidelines on what should be evaluated, who should be involved, and the method to be used.

What to evaluate

There are several indicators an organization can use to evaluate how well it is doing. First, it

Activity 4.3

- Consider a service (or an aspect of a service) that you have worked in.
- How would you evaluate whether it was successful or not?
- On what criteria did you base your evaluation? Who did you involve in your evaluation?

should of course monitor how well it is doing against the objectives derived from its value base and made explicit in its business plan. An organization might evaluate its performance against business objectives and financial targets. It might also evaluate the level of service interventions delivered. Another aspect of an evaluation might be whether the services provided are available to the whole community or just a selected few. Whatever indicators are used, however, it is essential that service user satisfaction is monitored.

One popular model to evaluate the performance of an organization is the European Model for Quality Management (Hakes 1995). This focuses attention on nine key components of an organization's activities: leadership; people management; policy and strategy; resources; processes; people satisfaction; customer satisfaction; impact on society; and business results.

Who should be involved?

Given that user satisfaction is the most important means of evaluating the performance of an organization, it is important that service users be involved. To do this effectively requires a genuine commitment to listening to, and valuing the views of users. Self-advocacy – speaking up on your own behalf – should be supported by health providers (for an overview of advocacy see Gates 1994). Evaluation of service performance must first and foremost be through the perspective of the user. The organization should also obtain feedback from carers and other organizations that provide services, such as social services and the voluntary sector.

Method of evaluation

One of the first decisions that must be taken is whether the evaluation should be internal or external.

Internal

Internal evaluation could be by means of a senior management review, whereby senior managers review the performance of staff/departments against agreed criteria, or it could be by a peer review process, where nurses working in a community team might evaluate the performance of each other. To be successful there does need to be clear guidelines, and the process should have the support of the staff involved. Although not usually as threatening as an external evaluation care still needs to be taken to reassure staff, who often feel very vulnerable during any evaluation process. Sufficient time needs to be set aside for the process and staff need to be appropriately trained. An appropriate location should be chosen that allows staff to meet without interruption.

Involving staff in reviewing and evaluating their services has several advantages. It can promote greater understanding among staff of their respective roles. It also develops a degree of expertise among staff in the areas of service monitoring and evaluation. Finally, it helps staff appreciate the importance of promoting quality, and that it is as much their responsibility as anybody else's.

External

An external evaluation could be by a group of service users, or possibly a consultancy firm. An external evaluation may often give a more objective view of the performance of the organization. External evaluations are, however, often seen as threatening, and time must be taken to reassure staff and explain the purpose and extent of the evaluation.

Evaluations can also focus at various levels within an organization: on individual staff, a team or a department. Whatever means is used it is important that evaluation is done in a sensitive and understanding manner. Staff need to feel at ease and be free and open with the process. Finally, there is no point in undertaking an evaluation if there is no commitment to acting upon the results.

CONCLUSION

For an organization to deliver quality care on a consistent basis it must have three key features in place. First, the organization must have a clear set of values from which it derives its objectives. Secondly, it must have a framework for delivering these objectives. Thirdly, it must employ a range of relevant tools and quality systems in a coordinated and systematic way to consistently enhance service provision.

The whole focus of activity for the organization must be the service user, to identify and meet his or her individual needs. To achieve this the organization must not only communicate regularly with its users, but also genuinely involve them in the planning, delivery and evaluation of services.

There must be an explicit commitment to managing the issue of quality and a clear understanding by all staff on how objectives will be achieved. A quality strategy should detail the criteria against which the success of the organization will be evaluated. The organization's approach to delivering services must also be open to constructive criticism, and regularly reviewed. The strategy must also detail how the organization will reduce waste and achieve continuous improvements in the quality of its services.

All staff must be able to work in a supportive environment that recognizes their needs and promotes integrated training and development. All staff must also have the opportunity to contribute positively to the way the organization conducts its business. It is not only the organization that has a key role to play: individual staff must also acknowledge a personal responsibility to deliver best practice. Finally, it is important that the drive to deliver quality is seen as an integral part of the business of the organization, and not as an add-on. The promotion of quality is not the reserve of managers or a quality assurance department: the responsibility for delivering quality care is the everyday business of everybody.

REFERENCES

Bank-Mikkelsen N 1980 Denmark. In: Flynn, R J Nitsch K E (eds) Normalisation, social integration and community services. Pro-Ed, Austin, Texas

Bell D, McBride P, Wilson G 1994 Managing quality. Butterworth-Heinemann, Oxford

British Standards Institution 1987 BS 5750/ISO 9000 Quality management systems. BSI, London

Culyer Report 1994 Supporting research and development in the NHS. HMSO, London

DOH 1971 Better services for the mentally handicapped. Cmnd 4683, HMSO, London

DOH 1989 Caring for people: community care in the next decade and beyond. Cmnd 848, HMSO, London

DOH 1994 The evolution of clinical audit. Department of Health, London

Gates B 1994 Advocacy: a nurse's guide. Scutari Press, Middlesex

Hakes C 1995 The corporate self assessment handbook for measuring business excellence. Chapman & Hall, London

Hawkins P, Shoney R 1989 Supervision in the helping professions. Open University Press, Milton Keynes

Hull and Holderness Community Health NHS Trust 1996 Complaints procedure in Makaton. Hull and Holderness Community Health NHS Trust, Hull

IDC 1986 Pursuing quality: how good are your local services for people with mental handicap? Independent Development Council, London

King's Fund Centre 1980 An ordinary life: comprehensive locally based residential services for mentally handicapped people. King Edward's Hospital Fund, London

NHSME 1993 A vision for the future: the nursing, midwifery and health visiting contribution to health and health care. Department of Health, London

Oakland J S 1993 Total quality management. Heinemann Professional Publishing, Oxford

O'Brien J 1987a A guide to life planning: using the activities catalogue to integrate services and natural support systems. In Wilcox B W, Bellamy G T (eds) The activities catalogue: an alternative curriculum for youth and adults with severe disabilities. Brookes, Baltimore

O'Brien J 1987b A guide to personal futures planning. In: Bellamy E T, Wilcox B (eds) A comprehensive guide to the activities catalogue: an alternative curriculum for youth and adults with severe disabilities. Paul H. Brookes, Baltimore

R C N 1990 Dynamic standard setting system. Royal College of Nursing, London

United Kingdom Central Council for Nurses, Midwives and
    Health Visitors 1994 Future of professional practice – the
    Council's standards for education and practice following
    registration. UKCC, London
Wolfensberger W 1980 The definition of normalisation:
    update, problems, disagreements and misunderstandings.
In Flynn R J, Nitsch K E (eds) Normalisation, social
    integration and community services. University Park
    Press, Baltimore
Wolfensberger W, Thomas S 1983 PASSING: Programme
    analysis of service systems implementation of normalisation
    goals. National Institute on Mental Retardation, Toronto

FURTHER READING

Brown H, Smith H 1992 Normalisation: a reader for the
    nineties. Tavistock/Routledge, London
A comprehensive account and appraisal of the philosophy of
    normalization. The theoretical underpinning of
    normalization and its potential to bring about positive
    change, as well as the problematic issues it raises, are
    discussed in detail.
Ellis R, Whittington D 1993 Quality assurance in health care:
    a handbook. Edward Arnold, London
An informative guide to quality assurance and its
    application in healthcare. A detailed account is given of
    the historical development of quality assurance, methods
    of application and its management. The book also
    contains a comprehensive reference section and a useful
    glossary.
Koch H 1992 Total quality management in health care.
    Longman, Harlow
A guide that specifically examines the application of TQM in
    healthcare. There are particularly useful sections on
    preparing organizations for the introduction of TQM and
    the management of TQM projects. This book is useful both
    as an introductory text and as a reference guide for those
    responsible for implementing quality systems.
Joss R, Kogan M 1995 Advancing total quality management in
    the National Health Service, Open University, Buckingham.
A wide-ranging review of TQM initiatives within the
    National Health Service. There are sections on the key
    concepts of TQM, case studies from the commercial sector
    and recommendations as to how TQM can be more
    successfully applied within the health service. This guide
    is essential reading for health organizations about to
    embark on a total quality management programme.
Oakland J S 1989 Total quality management. Heinemann
    Professional Publishing, Oxford
Deservedly recognized as one of the standard works on
    TQM, the book covers a comprehensive range of topics,
    including understanding and planning for quality, training
    for quality, team work and culture change. Although both
    the public and private sectors are considered, there is more
    emphasis on the private sector.
Robertson L 1992 Quality assurance for nurses: a guide to
    understanding and implementing ISO 9000/BS5750.
    Longman, Harlow
An accessible account of how ISO9000 can be applied to
    clinical and community nursing. Key principles of the
    system are explained and interpreted from the nurse's
    perspective. The relationship of the ISO9000 to TQM and
    standard setting is also clearly identified. A useful
    reference book for nurses wanting to develop a quality
    assurance system.

Ethics

R. Billington

INTRODUCTION

In this chapter a variety of ethical issues are addressed which the learning disabilities nurse, carer or relative may face at some time in the care or supervision of a person with learning disabilities. It would be difficult to provide answers to all of the issues raised, and indeed would not be right to do so, as readers will have their own views and will have formed their own opinions. The intention here is to provide the reader with the opportunity to provoke thought and discussion and to put into some perspective the range of issues with which an individual may be confronted during their nursing career or caring experience.

WHAT IS AN ETHICAL ISSUE?

In our everyday language we tend to talk about moral and ethical issues and use these words almost interchangeably. 'Morals', however, tends to refer to the standards of behaviour actually held or followed by individuals or groups within society. 'Ethics', on the other hand, refers to the science or study of those morals. Because of this, 'ethical' and 'moral' tend to be used as terms of approval, as opposed to 'unethical' or 'immoral' to convey our feelings of disapproval, whether that be a personal perspective or one held on behalf of a group within society.

Ethical problems and dilemmas confront us with choices that involve our beliefs and feelings about what we regard as fundamentally 'good' or 'right' in our opinion, i.e. what we regard as our own moral standards and principles. It is when these values and principles are challenged by some external force or situation that difficulties or conflicts may arise within us, causing our beliefs to be challenged or forcing us to re-examine our opinions.

The words 'problem' and 'dilemma' are often used almost interchangeably in situations such as these, but again there are subtle differences. If we refer to a 'problem', this tends to give the impression that there is a solution to the situation. If, on the other hand, we use the word 'dilemma', this gives the impression that there is no solution, or no single solution, to that particular situation. Ethical issues do not remain static for a variety of reasons. Technology is now available that enables improved care and treatment, which themselves are not static, but dynamic and ever changing. Not many years ago it would have been inconceivable to be able to keep someone alive, almost indefinitely, on a life support system in order to allow time for the body to begin recovery, or for treatments to be carried out over a longer period of time. Who would have thought it possible that people who had been immersed in extremely cold water for considerable lengths of time could possibly be resuscitated, when once they would have been presumed to have drowned?

DIFFERENT ISSUES FOR DIFFERENT PEOPLE

An ethical issue or dilemma for one person may or may not be the same as for another person, for a variety of reasons. There may be many contributing factors to this, such as a person's religious beliefs or lack of them, their upbringing, the influence of peers, sexual orientation or sexual preference, their personal life experiences so far, their nursing (or other caring) experiences, their education or the information that they may or may not have had access to. There may of course be a variety of cultural issues which could have a bearing on the establishment of an individual's belief system, behaviours or opinions, and these may not necessarily be the opinions of the individual concerned, but may be those of the society or culture to which the individual must be seen to be conforming. As we will see later in this chapter, religious or cultural beliefs may have some bearing on the nursing and caring professions, particularly if individuals wish to 'opt out' of some situations in which they do not feel able to participate because of their own beliefs.

It is also possible that the law can have an influence on the way we act as individuals, in spite of the way in which we might prefer to behave, and may be beyond our control and enforce constraints upon us. An example of this could be in the use of the Mental Health Act (1983), of which learning disability and mental health nurses in particular are likely to have experience at some time in their career. The law can also have a great influence on the way in which we work, which can sometimes conflict with our own beliefs. Such an example would be in the case of euthanasia, which is illegal in Great Britain but in which a great many people believe. According to an opinion poll carried out in April 1993 by National Opinion Poll on behalf of the Voluntary Euthanasia Society (VES 1993), it would seem that about 79% of the general population in Britain – 4% more than in 1989 – would be in favour of voluntary euthanasia in some instances if it were to become legal. Although the nurse must conform not only to the laws of the land but also to various codes of conduct (for example UKCC 1992), it would be naive to assume that nurses are any different from other people, and many believe that voluntary euthanasia should be available to people under certain circumstances and in a professionally legislated and strictly controlled manner. There are also those who would see that to hold such beliefs must contravene certain codes of conduct or codes of ethics (ICN 1973, UKCC 1992) and so could not be compatible within a nursing career. Conflicts such as these could undermine the trust that is put in people as guardians or advocates for people with learning disabilities.

CHANGING ISSUES

Life-prolonging treatments and life-sustaining

equipment are frequently used throughout all branches of nursing and midwifery across the age spectrum of patients in our care, whether they be people with learning disabilities or not. Many ethical issues are not confined solely to learning disability, but they may have a different perspective or focus if the people in our care are not able to speak for themselves, or are at times regarded by others as being less worthwhile or less deserving than those who do not have learning disabilities. Several dilemmas may arise in relation to this treatment and care:

- Who decides who does and who does not receive such treatment and care?
- Should this treatment and care be available to anyone, regardless of the cost?
- Do we consider what the expected outcome is for the patient by giving or withholding treatment and care with regard to what we judge is going to be their standard or quality of life in the future?
- How soon after the birth of a child with gross physical defects, which could assume concurrent learning disability, are treatment and future care choices made, and does this have any influence on the choices made or the 'rationing' of treatment in favour of someone else's perceived need?
- Who should be involved in such treatment decisions?

The scenario in Case study 5.1 may be useful as a means of discussion with your peers or fellow students.

EUGENICS

Situations such as the one illustrated in Case study 5.1, some would argue, could possibly be seen to be entering into the realms of the eugenic movement. The word 'eugenic' is Greek, meaning 'of good stock' (Chambers 1955), also defined in this same dictionary as 'pertaining to race improvement by judicious mating', and 'eugenics' is therefore the science of such. The eugenics movement was founded by Sir Francis Galton (1822–1911), a British anthropologist and the cousin of Charles Darwin. He advocated selec-

Case study 5.1

A Down syndrome baby is born with gross cardiac defects. He requires immediate surgery within the next 24–48 hours to give him any reasonable chance of survival. The family and the professionals involved are at great variance as to what should be done. The parents want no active intervention – they wish their child to be christened, kept comfortable and free from any physical distress and allowed to pass away peacefully.

The junior doctor believes this is the wrong course of action and wants to arrange for the necessary operation immediately, in case the baby deteriorates any further. He instructs the ward sister to prepare the baby for theatre. The sister is torn between respecting the wishes of the parents and carrying out the doctor's instructions. Some less experienced members of staff (who may be student nurses, nursing assistants or other qualified staff) cannot understand why the sister is agreeing with the parents. Surely this conflicts with training, personal philosophy or the whole ethos of nursing and medical care – i.e. to preserve life and promote wellbeing.

Activity 5.1

Who do you consider is right in the situation depicted in Box 5.1 and why?
- The doctor?
- The parents?
- The ward sister?
- The less experienced staff?
Now consider:
- How would you respect the rights of the baby and act in his best interests?
- Should rationing of healthcare enter the equation in situations such as these?
- Who do you believe should have the final power to decide the course of action for this baby?
You may find it useful to discuss some of these issues with your peers in the form of a debate and see if it is possible to reach a consensus.

tive breeding to improve the human stock and aimed at 'the improvement of the physical and mental quality of a people by agencies under social control' (Horsley 1986).

The eugenics movement at the end of the nineteenth and beginning of the twentieth centuries questioned the status of individuals with learning difficulties as persons, often advocating isolation or incarceration, formal sterilisation and in extreme cases even termination of pregnancy on the basis that such individuals were subhuman or degenerate species.

(Tschudin 1994)

Thankfully, nowadays little is heard of opinions such as these but more of the rights of the unborn child, consideration of the choice and opinions of individuals as to treatment and care options available for brain-damaged fetuses and children, and the rights of those with learning disabilities as to what they require and deserve as human beings.

CONTRACEPTION, STERILIZATION AND TERMINATION OF PREGNANCY

Although in some ways these issues should be treated entirely separately, there is much overlap in the ethical issues that surround them. At one time it was not uncommon, if not the norm, for female patients who were seen as 'promiscuous' to be prescribed some form of contraception, usually in the form of the pill, and for male patients who might be seen to be capable of 'taking advantage of the female patients' to be on such medication as benperidol (Anquil), prescribed for 'the control of deviant and antisocial sexual behaviour'. On whose judgement they were placed in this category is sometimes unclear, and the prescribing of any medication was rarely, if ever, discussed with junior ward staff or the patients themselves.

Nursing and social care of people with learning disabilities has come a long way in 20 years. Such people are now given information regarding their treatment and care, and offered a choice in what is done to and for them and by whom. It is of course acknowledged that in some cases this cannot be done because of the severity of the individual's condition, but there is no reason why relatives, advocates or carers cannot be given this information. Consider the situation described in Case study 5.2.

There are no easy solutions to these ethical issues, and situations will vary from relationship to relationship. There can be no hard and fast rules which will suit all situations and be acceptable to all parties involved.

Case study 5.2

Two people in their 20s, with a moderate learning disability, have formed a strong friendship at the community home in which they live as permanent residents. They now want to get married. Some of the staff working in the home do not agree that this couple should be allowed to marry. A variety of concerns have been raised, such as whether or not contraception would be an issue, the sexual health of the people concerned, the possible exploitation of one person with a learning disability by another. On the other hand, some staff are very much in favour of this and wish to assist the couple in any way they can, with issues such as sex education and the promotion of positive sexual health, advice about contraception and its availability, and support in order that they can maintain a good relationship with as much privacy as is possible within a care environment.

Activity 5.2

Again it may be useful to split into groups to discuss some of the issues raised by the situation described in Case study 5.2. You will probably find that again there are no easy solutions in these situations if you want to respect the rights of people with a learning disability, allow for choice in whether they need or even want contraception or not, and whether you should consider if relationships such as these should ever be allowed to develop in the first place.

- Is the choice their own in this situation, or do they have to have the permission of their relatives?
- Would the situation be any different if the couple concerned were of the same gender?
- Are there any different considerations if one of the couple is much older than the other?
- What if one of the couple has a more severe learning disability than the other?
- Are there any special issues if one of the couple is far more physically disabled than the other?
- If the situation were slightly different, in that one of the couple lived independently, away from a care environment and wished that they could live together after the marriage without the support of the community home, could this pose any new difficulties?

Sterilization is another issue which poses difficulties and arouses much heated debate among professionals and relatives. In the past sterilization was often more or less automatic following the birth of a child to a woman with a learning disability, the child being taken into care and offered for fostering or adoption. Sterilization was also sometimes used as a form of contraception, and indeed in extreme cases with no other satisfactory alternative, may still be considered the only option. There are two things at issue here: whether the sterilization is being performed as a means of contraception or whether it is being done for medical reasons to prevent deterioration in or improve the health of the woman. In either case it may be difficult in some instances to obtain informed consent from an individual with a learning disability. In this country there are no legal grounds for compulsory sterilization, but some people may argue that there should be such legislation to prevent the transmission of certain genetically inherited disorders. At present genetic counselling and support could be offered, but decisions concerning contraception and sterilization should remain with the individual(s) concerned.

Termination of pregnancy is perhaps an even more difficult situation to address. Even if it has not been considered before, we have another dimension to the proposal of pregnancy termination: religious or cultural beliefs and rules, not just those of the individual but also of the people who care for that person in residential accommodation.

Some people may suggest that people with learning difficulties do not have religious beliefs because they do not have the cognitive or conceptual ability to understand the tenets of any religion, and consequently the nurse's obligation to respect their religious wishes does not apply.

(Tschudin 1994)

It may be somewhat easier to accommodate the religious views and beliefs of nurses and other carers within large institutions by ensuring that they only work in areas where these situations are unlikely to arise, for example if caring for elderly people or those with profound physical or learning disabilities. Dilemmas are more likely to arise now that the vast majority of care takes place within much smaller, family-sized units in the community, where staff have probably less or even no freedom of movement to work in another home if these types of situation arise.

Activity 5.3

Consider the following dilemmas.
- If a pregnant woman has been brought up as a Roman Catholic and has some understanding of her religion, should anyone else have the right, legally or morally, to advocate a termination of pregnancy solely because the woman has a learning disability, even if she wishes to continue with the pregnancy?
- If the pregnant woman has been brought up as a Roman Catholic but has little or no understanding of the meaning of this, or the implications that it may have on her life, can she make the decision to have her pregnancy terminated without the intervention of her next of kin?
- What might be the issues raised for those people caring for this woman? Are their religious and moral beliefs to be taken into consideration?

WITHHOLDING OR RATIONING OF TREATMENT AND CARE

Difficulties often arise for nurses faced with treatment decisions for people in their care with which they do not always feel entirely comfortable. Most nurses at some point in their career will be faced with problems regarding financial constraints within healthcare. To most people it would seem to be morally wrong that the choice and availability of treatment and care could ever be governed by financial constraints, staffing problems or bed availability, but this is unfortunately the situation with which we are now often faced. This has implications for treatments available to people with a learning disability as opposed to people who, in the opinion of some, are seen to be more deserving of limited resources. The scenario in Case study 5.3 may help to illustrate some of these points.

Decisions such as these may be seen to be in conflict with some parts of the UKCC Code of Professional Conduct (1992), which states:

Each registered nurse, midwife and health visitor shall act, at all times, in such a manner as to:

Safeguard and promote the interests of individual patients and clients.

As a registered nurse, midwife or health visitor, you are personally accountable for your practice and, in the exercise of your professional accountability, must:

1. act always in such a manner as to promote and safeguard the interests and well-being of patients and clients;
2. ensure that no act or omission on your part, or within your sphere of responsibility, is detrimental to the interests, condition or safety of patients and clients;
5. work in an open and co-operative manner with patients, clients and their families, foster their independence and recognise and respect their involvement in the planning and delivery of care;
8. report to an appropriate person or authority, at the earliest possible time, any conscientious objection which may be relevant to your professional practice.

Case study 5.3

An 82-year-old woman with severe learning disability is living in a residential home. She develops a chest infection. The decision is taken by the doctor who is called in that no antibiotics should be prescribed in this situation – 'let nature take its course'. The manager in charge of the home agrees, but some of the other staff are not so sure. They feel that this woman has a right to the best treatment and care available, as would a relative of their own who did not have a learning disability. The relatives of the elderly woman have not been consulted, but they have been contacted to inform them of her deteriorating condition and the expected outcome. When her younger brother and sister-in-law arrive, they enquire as to what medication has been prescribed and are horrified when they find out that this has not been done. They demand to know the reason why, and ask to see the doctor immediately. On his arrival he explains that 'after all, she is 82, has a severe learning disability, no understanding of her current situation, a very poor prognosis and no real quality of life'.

Activity 5.4

- Who do you consider should make decisions in situations such as the one in Case study 5.3, and should they be made only by the doctor or be a team decision?
- Should the relatives be involved in such decisions, or merely informed of the outcome in this case?
- Is a nurse truly able to advocate for the elderly woman in this instance if she strongly believes that treatment should be prescribed?
- Would your decisions be any easier or a lot more difficult if the person were only in their 30s but had no known relatives?

Activity 5.5

Using the excerpts from the UKCC Code of Professional Conduct, discuss how they may conflict with or assist you in your role as a nurse involved in the care of someone such as the elderly woman described in Case study 5.3.

THE QUALITY VERSUS QUANTITY OF LIFE DEBATE

Discussion continues as to whether or not it is possible to balance the quality of a person's life against the quantity, in order to find a solution to some complex problems. There are two fundamental points at issue here:

- The quality of the individual's life (in the opinion of others) and whether that perceived quality can be measured.
- The expected lifespan of the individual, whether that be with medical intervention or not.

The beginning of the debate on quality of life rather than just being alive, and whether one person has the right to decide what another person's quality of life is or will be has been put forward by a number of people (Oosthuizen 1978, Humphry 1986, Scally 1995). Oosthuizen stated that: 'Life and the quality of life are concepts that can never be divorced, but increasing emphasis is put on the quality of life as a dominant consideration.' Rachels (1986) also suggests that there may be a difference between 'having a life' and 'being alive', i.e. the quality versus quantity of life debate.

The question in Activity 5.6 was highlighted most recently by a case near Hull where the parents of a severely brain-damaged little boy

Activity 5.6

- Discuss whether artificial feeding is a treatment that can be withdrawn or withheld to allow a person to die.

wished to have the abdominal tube through which he was being fed removed, in order to allow him to die. This was to prove something of a test case, and may even have led ultimately to changes in the laws on euthanasia in the UK.

The following is an extract from the *Hull Daily Mail* (Foulkes & Makel 1996) that outlines the case.

September 24 1993 should have been a joyful day for the Creedons with the birth of baby Thomas, but it became clear very quickly that their son had suffered horrendous brain damage during pregnancy. Within seven hours of coming into the world he had started suffering fits. A brain scan four days later showed that Thomas had suffered global brain damage and the doctors inferred from that, that he would have little or no quality of life. Thomas was blind, deaf, could not swallow and had no control over his muscles. Parents Con and Fiona asked doctors at Hull Maternity Hospital not to start artificially feeding their baby. Their argument was that artificial feeding was as much a life support system as a ventilator. The Creedons felt even then that nature did not intend Thomas to live. The family spent many months fighting for Thomas's right to die.

Thomas finally succumbed to a chest infection and died in February 1996. The case never reached the courts.

Understandably, there are no easy answers to what the outcome would have been had the case reached the High Court, but if the Creedons had won their case it could have meant that more parents would have had some choice in allowing their brain-damaged children to die. Would this then have created further ethical dilemmas for nurses, and possibly another opportunity for nurses to 'opt out' of participating in this kind of treatment or withdrawal of treatment issue?

A similar situation arose with the case of Tony Bland, a young man who was left severely brain damaged following a football stadium disaster in Sheffield in 1989. He was caught in a crush, during which his brain was starved of oxygen, resulting in irreversible damage to the cerebral cortex. The brain stem continued to function, allowing him to breathe independently and retain many of the reflex actions that gave the appearance of consciousness, but because of the damage to the cerebral cortex – the part controlling thought and emotion – he remained in a coma, unable to express himself or to communicate in any way and had to be fed artificially. Tony eventually died in 1993, after a High Court ruling that hydration, medication and nutrition could legally be withdrawn because of the irreversible state of his condition (Williams 1996).

Cases such as Thomas Creedon and Tony Bland are not dissimilar in some ways, but of course are vastly different in legal, medical and nursing terms. Thomas Creedon was not brain dead, whereas Tony Bland was – a fundamental and very important difference in medico-legal terms. The similarity lay in the fact that in both cases the person concerned was unable to make decisions concerning their treatment options. There can never be hard and fast rules in cases such as these, and each must be judged on its own individual merits and circumstances. Ethical guidelines may be of some use in these situations, and the law must also always play a part so that control is maintained. From the standpoint of the nurses involved though, there are many decisions that must be made on an individual basis.

Obviously these two cases are individual in their own right, and much depends upon consideration being given to the wishes of family and friends as well as medical and nursing opinion. Wilkinson (1996) has emphasized the need for

Activity 5.7

It may be useful to discuss some of the following points with your peers.
- Is there any fundamental difference between the cases of Thomas Creedon and Tony Bland?
- If Thomas Creedon had survived the chest infection, what do you think the court decision would have been?
- What do you believe should have been the outcome in this situation?
- Do you think that the right decisions were made in the case of Tony Bland?
- Have we somehow now set a precedent for the future?
- How would you have felt in the two situations described, and how easy would it have been for you to voice your opinions?

nurses to be involved in decisions concerning individual patients:

What is crucial for nurses is that they are involved in every stage of the decision making process and each individual case is dealt with from a multidisciplinary approach. Nurses have got to be included in any ultimate care decisions as they provide eighty-five per cent of direct patient care and work very closely with the families of these patients.

(Wilkinson 1996)

In situations such as these it is essential that nurses are given adequate support and supervision to enable them to discuss their concerns and have a forum in which to air their views without fear of disciplinary action being taken against them. Bailey (1996) ex-chair of the RCN ethics forum, firmly believes that all nurses need adequate preparation in order to be able to deal with decisions such as allowing patients to die, and also so that they are free to opt out of these situations if they so wish without any fear of recrimination.

ISSUES RELATED TO MEDICATION

Medication has played a vital role in the care and management of people with learning disabilities, particularly over the past 20–30 years, during which time new drugs have become available for the treatment of epilepsy in particular, and drugs have been refined and improved in order to minimize the side effects that, with some drugs, could be more debilitating than the condition being treated. Dosages have also improved so that the minimum amount of medication can be used to obtain the desired effect. Drugs have been developed to reduce behavioural difficulties but unfortunately have sometimes been used as a means of control or medical restraint, leaving the person unable to function effectively. Training and education for nurses and doctors in the use of behaviour modification techniques has greatly reduced the need, in a large proportion of cases, for the overuse of major tranquillizers in order to control patients. Improved staffing ratios and better living environments have had good effect on the behaviour of individuals with a learning disability. Staff are more able, through time and improved education, to put into use techniques such as gentle teaching, relaxation therapies, anxiety and anger management training, and the use of Snoezelen – all things which were deemed almost impossible 10–15 years ago – with inadequate staffing levels and financial constraints. In some cases, however, the use of major tranquillizers is still the only option, either on a long-term or a short-term basis, and each individual should be carefully monitored for any side effects. Provided medication is regularly reviewed in accordance with local policy, the least possible drug combination and administration will be achieved. However, in spite of rigorous training and policies being in place, mistakes do sometimes happen. Consider the scenario in Case study 5.4.

Errors such as those described in Case studies 5.4 and 5.5 should not of course happen. It is no excuse to say that you did not know the client very well, and a plea of this nature would not stand up in a disciplinary hearing if the matter were to be reported and actioned in this way. Although these are ethical dilemmas for the nurse concerned, they are also professional matters: nurses should not be placed in a position where they are performing any task for which they have not been trained or in which they are not competent.

The UKCC Code of Professional Conduct makes the situation quite clear:

As a registered nurse, midwife or health visitor, you are personally accountable for your practice

 Case study 5.4

The ward/unit manager hands you some medication for a client in your care. None of the clients are able to communicate, so confirming their names with them is impossible. You give the medication to the client for whom you believe it is intended. While returning to the drugs trolley you hear another nurse call out the name of the client to whom you have just given the medication, and see that she is walking towards a different client on the ward. You realize that you have just wrongly administered medication intended for someone else.

Activity 5.8

Discuss the implications of the error in Case study 5.4

- Do you keep quiet or own up to your mistake?
- If you own up, what is the course of action for the person in charge?
- Are they equally accountable in this situation or do you have to take the entire blame for your actions?
- What do you do about the incorrect entry on the medicine card – the person in charge has signed for medication that has been incorrectly given?
- Do you need to inform the pharmacy about the resulting discrepancies in tablet numbers?
- You realize that the medication that you have given will not have any serious side effects for the person concerned, it was just one dose of antibiotic that is highly unlikely to have any effect on the person at all. Does this make any difference to your decisions and ultimate course of action?
- The medication was a large dose of a major tranquillizer. The person for whom it was intended has been on this medication for many years and has developed a tolerance to it. The person to whom it has been given, however, has never been prescribed any major tranquillizer before, let alone a drug with a dose of this magnitude.
  Does this make any difference to your decisions and ultimate course of action?
- Do you keep quiet, observe the client and hope that their resulting drowsy condition will be attributed to tiredness?
- Do you inform the person in charge immediately, knowing that this could result in some form of disciplinary action for you?
- If the person in charge says that they will cover up your mistake, would you feel comfortable with this decision?
- Do you feel that you now owe them a favour?
- Does this situation affect how you feel about your professional status and the trust that has been placed in you?

Case study 5.5

The clients in your care have only a mild learning disability and are living in a home in the community. You have only recently come to work there and do not know them very well. The person in charge hands you some medication and you approach the person for whom you believe it is intended. The woman protests, saying that this is not her medication, she 'doesn't have any white ones', only a pink one and a blue one. You return the medication without administering it, but are told that this client always says this and are asked to go back and give it.

Activity 5.9

Consider the situation described in Case study 5.5.
- Do you administer the medication in spite of the woman protesting?
- Do you try and pacify her by telling her that the colours of the tablets have changed?
- Are you absolutely certain that you have got the right person?
- How could you double check in this instance?

and, in the exercise of your professional accountability, must:

4. acknowledge any limitations in your knowledge and competence and decline any duties or responsibilities unless able to perform them in a safe and skilled manner.

(UKCC 1992)

On the other hand, the person in charge cannot abdicate responsibility in a situation such as this and must take some of the blame for your errors.

Refusal on the part of a person with a learning disability to take their medication is sometimes a difficult situation to resolve. There may be differing courses of action if the person is a voluntary resident within an institution or community home, than for someone who is being detained under a section of the Mental Health Act (1983). Likewise, detention under a section of the Mental Health Act does not automatically allow for the administration of medication against a person's will. In some cases, enforced administration of medication could be considered an assault.

With the ever-changing treatment regimens for clients within our care, and the competition between drug companies to produce cheaper medications, we have a responsibility to update

Activity 5.10

- Discuss with your colleagues which sections of the Mental Health Act would allow the administration of medication to a person under the circumstances discussed above, and what particular conditions need to be adhered to.

and maintain our knowledge base in accordance with current practice and prescribing policies.

COMMUNITY VERSUS INSTITUTIONAL CARE

By far the greatest proportion of people with learning disabilities are cared for either within their own home or in some form of residential home within the community. Care provision in the community has expanded greatly, particularly over the last decade, with the closure of the large, long-stay institutions which were mostly of Victorian origin, when the emphasis on 'care' was seen as custodial, controlling and away from society in general. Although many of these large institutions were imposing and foreboding from the exterior, the care, some would argue, was of the highest standard, and it must not be assumed that everything that went before so-called community care was bad, and that now everything is perfect. Far from it. We can never be complacent about care provision, otherwise improvement will never take place and change will not be seen to be necessary. Any kind of institutional or community care within a residential establishment will have its drawbacks and shortcomings, but has its place for some people with learning disabilities. This must, of course, include those people who are detained for treatment under sections of the Mental Health Act (1983) within the special hospitals because they are a danger to themselves or others. Likewise, not all people living in their own homes are living in an ideal environment – they may have less access to the wider community than those living in a residential establishment because of geographical isolation, elderly carers or financial constraints on access to services.

There are seldom any easy answers to dilemmas such as those posed in Case studies 5.6 and 5.7, and, as in other situations, each one has to be examined from its own perspective and from a variety of angles, taking everyone's opinions and best interests into consideration. What must not be forgotten is that it is important for the person with the learning disability to have stability of care provision within a secure and loving envi-

Case study 5.6

A 42-year-old man with a moderate learning disability lives with his father, who is now in his 70s, in a small village with few community facilities. He attends a day centre from Monday to Friday, which he considers to be his place of work, and is very happy there. He has never spent any time away from home because his father does not want him to. The community nurse involved with his care is worried that the time will come when he has to go into some form of care because his father is no longer able to cope.

Activity 5.11

Consider the scenario in Case study 5.6.
● If the father refuses any sort of support or respite care, are you in a position to do anything about it?
● In whose best interests are you trying to advocate in this instance?

Case study 5.7

The father becomes ill very suddenly and is taken into hospital for treatment, which necessitates his remaining there for 2 weeks. Accommodation has to be found quickly for the son with the learning disability, and a place is found for him in a residential home near the day centre he attends. Many of his friends from the day centre also live here, and he soon settles and begins to enjoy this new environment, with stimulating activities as well as the company of his friends. When his father is well enough he is discharged home and wishes his son to return to live with him, even though the community nurse feels that a longer period of respite care would be in both their interests and the son is reluctant to leave the residential home.

ronment. The needs of the carers must not be forgotten, nor their right to have a say in these situations. They usually have the ultimate power of decision here, unless overruled by a court or by the use of the Mental Health Act. The nurse can often have conflicts of interest here – trying to advocate in the best interests of the client, assisting carers in maintaining the client within their own home, and a professional responsibility to balance all these to suit everyone's purposes and interests. There has been and continues to be much discussion regarding the best place for people with learning disabilities to be cared for if they are unable to support themselves or live with relatives. Many charities have set up therapeutic communities in rural or urban areas in order to try and meet the needs of these people and endeavour to give them a choice of where to live. In reality this has often meant that people were placed or offered a place whenever a vacancy arose. Organizations such as the Camphill Village Trust have striven to address this problem by opening residential facilities of varying sizes all over the world, in both rural and urban areas. Once accepted into these communities, people have the flexibility to move between establishments in order to best meet their needs. This is also true for the staff working in these places, so that if an environment is too quiet, for example, there is the ability to move and live in another Camphill community. No matter where people with learning disabilities live, there will always be criticism from some quarter, for example those favouring segregation as opposed to integration. However, integration may not

always be the key if the society into which people are placed is not willing to accept them. This could, in fact, be more isolating, and lead to more institutionalization than one would expect of a community placement. Restriction on movement and true integration becomes a barrier to the individuals concerned and detrimental in the long run.

WORK, THERAPY OR EXPLOITATION OF LABOUR?

For many years now people with learning disabilities have been encouraged to participate in some form of activity, either within the institution or home in which they lived, or at a local day centre. For these 'tasks', which are often referred to as 'work', they receive a small remuneration. (The reason for this remuneration being so small is so that any financial benefits they receive, or which their carers receive on their behalf, are not affected by this 'paid employment'.) Within the institutions it was not uncommon for patients to have specific jobs – delivering the milk, meals or newspapers to the wards and departments, working in the gardens or greenhouses, making rugs, baskets, soft toys, or doing woodwork in the occupational therapy department. All these activities were viewed as ethical, not exploiting people, and giving them valuable employment and a sense of worth and achievement as well as a degree of responsibility. They often looked upon these activities as 'their job', for which they received 'wages' at the end of the week – money to call their own, and which they could spend as they chose.

Attitudes to this kind of task orientation have changed much over the past 20 or so years. More emphasis is being placed on finding work or activities in keeping with the level of ability of each individual, and according to their own choice. Less emphasis is now placed on contract work, although there is still a place for this, and many people in society, not just those with learning disabilities, undertake very repetitious work on a daily basis for many years. The difference is in the fact that the person with the learning disability may have little or no choice in the type of

Activity 5.13

- What are the differences between a person being encouraged to work for therapeutic reasons and told that he *must* work?
- List the advantages and disadvantages of a person having a specific job, particularly if this involves work of a regular or repetitive nature.

Activity 5.14

- Define a geographical area near to where you live or work, and identify types of employment which exist within that area.
- From these types of employment, identify which may be suitable for people with a learning disability to undertake.
- What are some of the constraints to employing people with a learning disability in your identified areas of employment?
- Try and ascertain whether anyone in your chosen geographical area is employing anyone with a learning disability.

Case study 5.8

George has been attending an adult training centre for many years and has now reached 65 years of age. He is due to retire from the work that he has been doing there, but has no concept of what retirement will mean and no plans for anything to replace what he has been doing. He enjoys the company at the centre and no-one else in the home in which he lives is retired, which will mean that apart from the staff, there will be no company for him during the day.

Activity 5.15

Consider the scenario in Case study 5.8

- Is it right that George should be forced to retire from the adult training centre if he does not wish to?
- If he were allowed to stay there for some time longer, do you think that there comes a point when others would view his work as exploitative?
- What could the staff have done to better prepare George for his impending retirement?

work offered, and there is unlikely to be an option for a change to alternative employment within the area.

Many mentally handicapped people would like some form of employment, not only because it is the normal thing for most people but also for the equally normal reason that they would like to earn money. Britain has a very poor record of promoting the employment of people with disability, and much more could be done to improve matters. Many people with mental handicaps may find it very difficult to compete in a restricted labour market and this has meant that it has often been easy to assume that employment is impossible.

(Stewart 1993)

Because of the views of society about people with learning disabilities, it has rarely been easy for them to find gainful employment, if at all. Unfortunately, with the economy and the unemployment situation as it stands at the moment, this situation is unlikely to improve in the foreseeable future. Employment within sheltered sit-

uations perhaps needs to become more meaningful and less task orientated. An end product of employment is that it helps individuals to acquire a sense of accomplishment and improved self-esteem. There will always be those who, because of the severity of their disability, will not be able to undertake employment, and there will be those who do not wish to. Finding the right occupation (in the broadest sense) is essential, and careful assessment by a coordinated team of care providers must be undertaken, together with the person concerned, so that the needs of the person can best be met within the constraints of the disability and employment options.

CONCLUSION

This chapter has attempted to identify a range of ethical issues relevant to people with learning disabilities. It is impossible to address all the issues or answer all the dilemmas, and indeed it would not be correct to do this. It is important that the reader uses the references given as widely as possible and explores the issues raised, with colleagues, peers and people with learning disabilities as well, in order to try and balance arguments, encourage discussion and reach conclusions where possible. When satisfactory conclusions cannot be reached or a consensus of opinion is impossible, try to appreciate all points of view. This will help throughout your caring career by encouraging dialogue and questioning the role of nurses in these situations, so that the best possible care can be offered to people with learning disabilities.

REFERENCES

Bailey S M 1996 Cited in: Williams K 1996 Each decision is different. News analysis, Nursing Standard 10: No 27

Chambers 1955 Shorter English Dictionary. Chambers, London

Foulkes D, Makel J 1996 A blessing in disguise. Hull Daily Mail, 27 February, p6

Horsley E M 1986 Hutchinson factfinder – concise encyclopaedia. Guild Publishing, London

Humphry D 1986 The right to die. An historical and legal perspective on euthanasia. The Hemlock Society, Eugene, Oregon

International Council of Nurses 1973 Code for nurses: ethical concepts applied to nursing. ICN, Geneva. Cited in: Rumbold G 1993 Ethics in nursing practice, 2nd edn. Baillière Tindall, London

Oosthuizen G C et al (eds) 1978 Euthanasia. Human Sciences Research Council, Publication No. 65, Oxford University Press, Cape Town

Rachels J 1986 The end of life. Euthanasia and morality. Oxford University Press, Oxford

Scally J 1995 Whose death is it anyway? Euthanasia and the right to die. Basement Press, Dublin

Stewart H 1993 Cited in: Shanley E, Starrs T A (eds) 1993 Learning disabilities. A handbook of care. 2nd edn. Churchill Livingstone, Edinburgh

Tschudin V 1994 Ethics: nursing people with special needs, Part II. Scutari Press, London

UKCC 1992 Code of professional conduct. United Kingdom Central Council for Nursing, Midwifery & Health Visiting, 3rd edn. UKCC, London

Voluntary Euthanasia Society 1993 The Voluntary Euthanasia Society Newsletter April, Issue No. 48

Wilkinson R 1996 Cited in: Williams K 1996 Each decision is different. News analysis, Nursing Standard 10: No 27

Williams K 1996 Each decision is different. News analysis, Nursing Standard 10: No 27

2

Helping people towards independence

6

Health

D. Vernon

INTRODUCTION

Many people with learning disabilities have lived for many years in institutions, having minimal contact with society in general. As a result, their healthcare needs were met by the staff who worked in such institutions. During this period of institutionalization, the medical model of health, which defined people in terms of diagnosis and symptoms, prevailed. According to the medical model health is viewed in terms of disease, and on this basis it is presumed that an individual in whom no trace of illness can be detected is healthy. Within this model, care and treatment are only offered when symptoms of ill health arise. Darbyshire (1991) has made the point that 'it is perhaps an indication of just how pervasive the influence of the medical model has been ... that issues of health ... have been among the least discussed aspects of care'. Indeed, studies show that the healthcare needs of many people with learning disabilities are unmet. Beange (1986) asserted that 'developmentally disabled people are basically a population with many unmet health needs'. More recently, Rodgers (1994) stated that 'the health care needs of people with learning disabilities are in danger of being ignored'. Sadly, these claims are substantiated by a series of studies. Howells (1986) reported the results of health screening for 151 people with learning disabilities who attended an adult training centre in Wales: 75% of these adults were found to have common health problems that were not known to their general practitioners and/or were not being managed. These included problems known to be associated with Down syndrome. Seventy-five people with learning difficulties had visual or hearing problems, 20 had weight problems and 36 had circulatory and respiratory disorders. Clearly, such conditions serve to compound the difficulties that people with a learning disability face. In the same year, Cole (1986) carried out a study of 53 people with learning disabilities who attended a social education centre, 66% of whom were found to need medical attention. Once again, a number of visual defects and dental problems were identified. Conditions such as hypertension and obesity were common. Four years later, Wilson and Haire (1990) found that out of 65 people with learning disabilities who were attending another British day centre, 80% had a previously undetected health problem. In particular, 10 individuals were found to have unmanaged disorders of their circulatory and respiratory systems. At variance with good practice, 26 people were taking anticonvulsant medication by repeat prescription, without review. More recently, Meehan et al (1995) screened 191 adults with learning disabilities and found that 83% had previously undetected and treatable conditions, including abnormalities in blood pressure, weight, urine, breasts, testicles, ears, eyes and blood results. Despite the fact that many of the conditions highlighted in these studies are 'generally seen as being preventable' (Meehan et al 1995), it would appear that preventive procedures are 'not performed as frequently for people with learning difficulties' (Langan et al 1993). It is clear, therefore, that there are deficits in essential aspects of healthcare, and it appears that 'many health care professionals appear to adopt complacent attitudes towards people with learning disabilities' (Meehan et al 1995). The movement towards care in the community (see Chapter 3) underpins the need for staff to become more responsive to the changing needs of people with learning disabilities. Specialist learning disability nurses have a key role to play in ensuring that the healthcare needs of their patients are given top priority, and that such individuals are served by an appropriate range of services. In so doing, however, carers must avoid overemphasizing physical symptoms

and diagnoses. Rather, a much broader, holistic model of health should be embraced. In view of this, the following section explores the concept of health as being much more than the 'absence of disease' (WHO 1946).

WHAT IS HEALTH?

This section will first look in some detail at the topic of health. What is meant by the concept of health? What does being healthy mean? Is health just a physical condition or, as Seedhouse (1986) has asked, 'Is it a commodity? A state which enables functioning? Or is it a reserve of strength?' An examination of the relevant attributes of health provides the foundations for working with people with learning disabilities. It is only through the acquisition of such knowledge that nurses can contribute to the enhancement and maintenance of the health of this group of people.

First, health must be defined. There are no simple or obvious ways in which this can be done, as a great deal of literature over the past 20–30 years has testified. It is widely accepted, however, that health is a multidimensional, as opposed to a unidimensional, concept. Perhaps the most celebrated statement of this position is found in the constitution of the World Health Organization, which states: 'Health is a state of complete physical, mental and social well-being and not merely the absence of disease and infirmity' (WHO 1946). Such a view avoids equating health with the absence of disease and acknowledges the various arenas in life in which health operates – the physical, the mental and the social. However, this definition has its shortcomings. It portrays health as a utopian and unattainable state. Some authors (Sims 1990) have gone so far as to say that health is not so much defined as simply restated in terms of the equally elusive concept of wellbeing. As such, if learning disability nurses are to stretch their practice beyond the treatment of disease and illness to activities concerned with enhancing the health of people with learning disabilities, then further exploration of the multidimensional nature of health is necessary. A basis for discussing the relationship between health and the everyday life of people with learning disabilities will thus be provided.

Dimensions of health

A multidimensional approach to health has been described by Beck et al (1988), who consider there to be five aspects to the individual. These are illustrated in Figure 6.1. Within this model, health is defined as 'more than an absence of disease. It is a dynamic, active process of continually striving to reach one's own balances and highest potentials. Health involves working towards optimal functioning in all areas. This process varies among people and even within individuals as they move from one life stage to another.' Beck is careful to define health in terms of the individual's specific potentials throughout life. Health is thus an individualized notion whose emphasis changes from person to person. Indeed, ideas of health mean different things to different people at different points in life. How

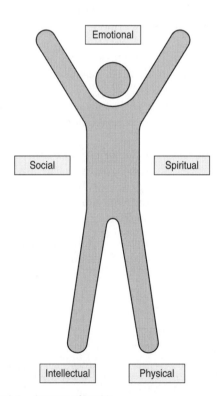

Figure 6.1   Aspects of health.

we may conceptualize health in the lives of people with a learning disability requires further examination. This may be achieved by examining what other people have said about health.

Lay health beliefs

The ways in which ordinary people think about health have been termed 'key concepts of health' or 'lay health beliefs'. Lay concepts of health have been seen as an interesting topic of research since the early 1970s. Although there have been no attempts to explicate the lay health concepts of people with learning disabilities, existing studies of lay health beliefs provide detailed information on what being healthy means. The remainder of this section concentrates on three studies that have provided information about the nature of health. Perhaps the most notable was one of the first: Herzlich's (1973) study of a sample of predominantly middle-class individuals from Paris and Normandy. Herzlich's findings confirmed that people do not think of health as the polar opposite of illness. Health, for her respondents, was identified as having three dimensions:

- Health-in-a-vacuum
- A reserve of health
- A state of equilibrium.

The first, health-in-a-vacuum, refers to the absence of illness. That is, one only knows one has health when illness strikes. The second, a 'reserve of health', is characteristic of the individual and refers to an innate or cultivated constitution that endures despite episodes of illness. Finally, Herzlich found that people spoke of health as a state of equilibrium, i.e. something that could be lost or regained. It is worth noting that Herzlich's respondents sometimes expressed several ideas together in their statements. The study also suggested that health cannot be assumed to be the condition of someone not carrying a medical diagnosis. Rather, concepts of health connect with many areas of life, giving it meaning in terms of emotions and abilities regarding activities and other people. The important idea to grasp here in relation to learning disability is that to think of oneself as healthy is to think of oneself in a particular relationship to society. That is, health is something that is exercised and proved in the person's active involvement in society. These conclusions are substantiated by the results of another qualitative study that examined the lay health concepts of a group of people, all aged over 60, in Scotland (Williams 1983, 1990). Williams (1983) identified three main conceptions of health:

- Health as the absence of disease
- Health as a continuum of strength
- Health as being fit for work.

The positive effects of continued normal living were found to relate to all three concepts of health. Williams (1990) highlighted that it was involvement in social activities, such as gardening, pensioners' clubs and discussing baking recipes, that informants believed generated good health. The importance of these findings in relation to people with learning disabilities cannot be overlooked. Clearly, social activity is 'not just an index of good health, but also a medium through which it may be generated' (Radley 1994). As such, the health of people with learning disabilities is inextricably entwined with their social world. It is, however, the health and lifestyle survey carried out by Blaxter (1990) that provides us with the most comprehensive overview of what constitutes 'health'. Some 9000 people were interviewed in their homes and extensively questioned on a variety of health matters. Beliefs about health were derived from two main questions:

1. Think of someone you know who is very healthy. Who are you thinking of? How old are they? What makes you call them healthy?
2. At times people are healthier than at other times. What is it like when you are healthy?

Blaxter (1990) identified seven broad categories in response to these questions:

1. Health as not ill – in which health is defined as not suffering any symptoms, never having anything more serious than a cold, never seeing a doctor, having no aches and pains.
2. Health as a reserve – in which being healthy is recovering quickly from illness, or innate because the individual comes from a family with strong constitutions.
3. Health as behaviour – health is defined in terms of the individual's virtuous behaviour, for example eating a well-balanced diet, taking exercise, not smoking, avoiding alcohol.
4. Health as physical fitness and as vitality – emphasis is placed upon physical fitness, for example the ability to play sport, a feeling of energy, and/or a willingness to undertake household tasks.
5. Health as social relationships – this involves defining health in terms of being actively involved in social activities, being outgoing and talkative, having good relationships with others and/or having sufficient energy to care for other people.
6. Health as a function – this is the idea of health as the ability to perform one's duties. Health is defined as being able to do what you want to when you want to, such as the ability to look after the garden, hold down a job and be self-sufficient.
7. Health as psychosocial wellbeing – Blaxter (1990) argued that the concept of health as psychosocial wellbeing is closely related to being happy and relaxed, mentally alert, content, proud and self-confident.

On the basis of these findings, Blaxter (1990) highlighted that health is not a unitary concept:

Activity 6.1

Take several minutes to consider these questions. Note down answers to each one.

Activity 6.2

Think of a person you know who has a learning disability. Do you consider them to be healthy in each of Blaxter's (1990) categories?

ideally it includes many dimensions, but the achievement of health in each of these categories is often an elusive scenario. In particular, people who have a learning disability may face a number of obstacles to the achievement of optimal health. In view of this, it is pertinent to address those challenges that prevent people with learning disabilities from achieving health.

CHALLENGES TO HEALTH

What are the obstacles to health facing people with learning disabilities? To understand this complex issue fully it is necessary to focus on the physical and psychosocial aspects of learning disability. This will allow the reader to see how particular conditions influence the health of the individual. It will also provide a basis for discussing how the attitudes of carers can influence their charges' health.

Physical aspects of health and learning disability

'People with learning disabilities experience the same health problems as the rest of the population' (Department of Health 1995), but there are some health problems that are more common among people with a learning disability. The Centre for Research and Information into Mental Disability (CRIMD) in 1990 highlighted these problems as hypertension, chronic bronchitis, epilepsy, cerebral palsy, gross obesity, spinal deformities and skin disorders. In particular, people with genetically determined causes of learning disability have unique health concerns. For example, there are some 'important features of Downs syndrome that may impinge upon the health of the individual' (Burns & Gunn 1993). The most serious of these are congenital heart defects, which have been reported in about one-third of children born with Down syndrome. If neglected, such defects may seriously reduce life expectancy. Fortunately, most defects are correctable by medical and surgical intervention. There are also a number of orthopaedic problems associated with Down syndrome that may affect

the mobility of the individual. The most severe of these is atlantoaxial instability. Tredwell et al (1990) warned that instability occurs in 9–22% of adults and children with Down syndrome. This condition can lead to dislocation of the vertebrae and subsequent damage to the spinal cord. Clearly, if left undetected severe mobility disturbances occur that have an adverse impact upon the quality of the individual's life. Other impairments associated with Down syndrome include hypothyroidism. Hypothyroidism has an effect upon levels of activity and is generally associated with sluggishness. Burns and Gunn (1993) pointed out that hypothyroidism also has a 'permanent deleterious effect on intellectual functioning'. From this brief account it can be seen that there are certain characteristics of Down syndrome that may affect the physical health of the individual. A summary of physical problems associated with other genetically determined causes of learning disability is given in Box 6.1. This list is by no means exhaustive – it merely serves to provide the impetus for nurses to acquire knowledge of those physical problems associated with learning disabilities. Without this knowledge, the ability of the nurse to enable an individual to achieve optimal health will be severely compromised.

Box 6.1 Common physical problems associated with specific conditions

Down syndrome
Congenital heart defects
Megaloblastic anaemia
Orthopaedic vulnerability
Cleft palate
Recurrent chest infection

Tuberous sclerosis
Epilepsy
Tumours
Respiratory disorders
Disorders of the central nervous system

Klinefelter syndrome
Cardiac disease
Osteoporosis
Kidney problems
Gastrointestinal bleeding

Psychosocial aspects of health and learning disability

The psychosocial aspects of health in relation to learning disability are the non-physical components of the individual that embrace thoughts, feelings, motivation and mental health status, and the parts of their life that are affected by or dependent on other people. Psychosocial health, therefore, refers to positive, valued and caring relations with others that promote feelings of self-worth and a sense of mastery over the environment. The achievement of psychosocial health is dependent upon a wide range of factors. These are illustrated in Figure 6.2. People with a learning disability, however, frequently face barriers to achieving psychosocial health. In particular, there is significant evidence that rates of mental ill health are higher among people with a learning disability than in the rest of the population (Jacobson &

Ackerman 1988). There is a lack of research findings to account for this, but theories have been put forward suggesting factors such as underlying abnormalities of brain structure and function, or the effects of increased prevalence of epilepsy (Holland & Murphy 1990). Among people with mild learning disability Russell (1991) has suggested that mental health problems might be due to social and psychological factors, such as being aware of differences between self and the rest of society, or social attitudes towards disability that can lead to isolation and segregation. Not surprisingly, people who have a learning disability are vulnerable to the full range of mental health disorders: organic psychoses, schizophrenia, paranoid states, obsessional neuroses and personality disorders are perhaps the most common. In addition, Russell (1991) has noted that substantial numbers of people with learning difficulties are vulnerable to problems such as hypersensitivity to criticism, excessive dependency and social inadequacy. Mental health problems, however, cannot be seen in isolation. Specifically, the individual cannot be separated from society. Complex societal demands that affect all people may adversely affect this group to a greater extent. Appreciation of this fact will enable nurses to consider that the mental health of people with learning disabilities is integrally linked to social factors. Sociological factors involve those variables that influence an individual's performance of social roles and their position within society. For example, nearly all people establish a social network around themselves. Social networks have the potential to fulfil important functions, including:

- closeness to others, often involving relations with others that are safe, warm and expressive
- cooperation with others, involving shared experiences among people in similar situations with common goals
- practical assistance, advice and guidance, shared problem solving
- reassurance of worth, self-esteem and self-confidence.

It is unfortunate that people take personal rela-

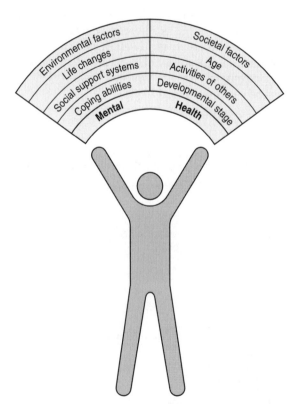

Figure 6.2   Determinants of mental health.

tionships with others for granted. It has become increasingly recognized, however, that people with learning difficulties often lack such closeness to others. Such a lack is not always evident, however, as people with learning disabilities are often surrounded by others who live or work in group homes or hostels. Despite this, 'many people with learning disabilities are, in fact, quite lonely' (Richardson & Ritchie 1991) because they face a number of barriers to establishing personal relations. These include:

- a lack of opportunities to meet new people
- an assumption among some parents and professionals that people with learning difficulties have no need for friends
- lack of self-confidence
- communication difficulties that restrict the expression of thoughts and feelings.

For all these reasons, people with learning difficulties are often unable to establish and maintain personal relationships as easily as other people. Indeed, they may often be lonely and are likely to have many unequal relationships with others. However, studies of lay health beliefs have highlighted the centrality of social relations with others to health. Clearly, a lack of close relationships can adversely affect the quality of the individual's life. It needs to be appreciated, therefore, that relationships are central to the lives of people with learning difficulties (Richardson and Ritchie 1991) and that failure to consider the social aspects of an individual's life may serve to hinder the achievement of health.

An examination of the physical and psychosocial aspects of health in relation to learning disability has highlighted a number of challenges facing such individuals. It behoves the carer, therefore, to address themselves, as a matter of priority, to the physical and psychosocial health needs of their clients. On this basis, the central aim of the learning disability nurse should be to remove obstacles to the fulfilment of a person's potential. The next section, therefore, examines how the nurse may enable people with learning disabilities to maximize their potential in relation to health.

THE ACHIEVEMENT OF HEALTH

A number of theorists subscribe to the view that the achievement of health involves maximizing human potential. The psychologist Abraham Maslow (1954) developed one of the earlier theories based upon human need. Maslow believed that certain basic fundamental needs (Figure 6.3) must be met before one can make maximal use of one's abilities and potential. Seedhouse (1986) maintained that health involves maximizing individual and environmental conditions for the fullest achievement of human potential. All individuals possess the ability to progress towards self-actualization. People with a learning disability, however, may sometimes require assistance to maximize their potential and ultimately embrace health. Nurses and other healthcare workers can assist individuals, families and communities in establishing effective plans for the achievement of health. Such plans must be flexible and tailored to specific needs, as well as being revised as needed to fit changing conditions and goals.

The process of maximizing the potential of the individual can be described as the health gain approach. The health gain approach is con-

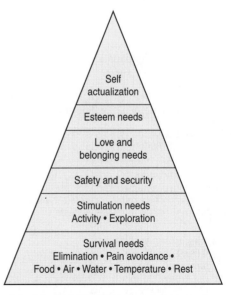

Figure 6.3 Maslow's (1954) hierarchy of needs

cerned with the removal or avoidance of challenges throughout life that prevent individuals from achieving health gains. It encompasses the physical, psychological and social aspects of health. At the same time, it acknowledges that the way in which a person achieves a health gain is highly individualized. Emphasis is placed upon prevention and health promotion. The recent report by the Department of Health (1995) entitled *The Health of the Nation – a strategy for people with learning disabilities* emphasizes that people who have a learning disability require assistance in maintaining and promoting health. Clearly, nurses have a crucial role to play in enabling individuals to achieve a health gain.

In order to maintain and promote the health of individuals it is vital that learning disability nurses are capable of functioning at three levels of prevention:

- Primary prevention: actions taken to prevent health loss before it occurs
- Secondary prevention: actions related to early detection of health loss
- Tertiary prevention: action taken to avoid needless progression of health loss.

Examples of such activities in relation to learning disability are presented in Box 6.2.

Box 6.2   Levels of prevention

Primary prevention
Protection against infectious disease
Health education, e.g. healthy eating, smoking cessation
Accident prevention
Self-care education, e.g. toothbrushing
Identification of threats to mental health, e.g. limited social network

Secondary prevention
Screening for sensory deficits
Screening for hypertension, diabetes, breast cancer, atlantoaxial instability, hypothyroidism
Identification of behavioural changes

Tertiary prevention
Management of epilepsy
Management of diabetes
Remedial therapy to minimize disability, e.g. postural drainage, passive movements

---

Primary prevention

Interventions to prevent loss of health are the most desirable form of intervention. Primary preventive efforts spare the individual the discomfort and threat to their quality of life that health loss poses. Early breakthroughs in primary prevention centred on control of acute infectious diseases, and resulted in mass immunization programmes. One of the principal primary preventive interventions is health education. This is a planned process aimed at helping individuals achieve and maintain a level of health that is appropriate for them. Efforts should be directed at assisting rather than coercing individuals to adopt a healthy lifestyle. Examples include counselling, educative efforts directed at weight control to prevent the onset of diabetes, nutritional education to maintain normal blood pressure, and the development of self-care skills such as toothbrushing to prevent the development of dental caries.

Health education must begin with assessing how much information the individual needs, wants and is able to learn. Observation of behaviour and data contained within the assessment of the individual's strengths and needs may provide some information. Sensory deficits, attention span and communication abilities will influence the degree to which the individual can become actively involved with the education process. Specific conditions also require consideration: for example, the presence of diabetes will determine the way in which a programme aimed at promoting healthy eating is developed. Equally, genetic influences need consideration. For example, individuals who have Prader–Willi syndrome commonly overeat (Murphy 1994). Clearly, such factors require careful consideration when developing a health education programme. The past experiences of the individual will also influence the education process. For example, have sweet foods previously been used to reinforce behaviour?

The way in which programmes of health education are presented also requires careful consideration. Traditional health education techniques have relied upon information-giving activities

Activity 6.3

In pairs or small groups, discuss how you would devise a preventive health programme aimed at educating an individual with a learning disability about the dangers of one of the following:
- Smoking
- Human immuno deficiency virus/acquired immuno deficiency syndrome
- Exposure to sunlight as a risk factor for skin cancer

such as making available videos and leaflets. Most information, however, is targeted at the general public and 'demands reading skills which may be far beyond the abilities of some people with learning disabilities' (Meehan et al 1995). Although time-consuming, 'the interpretation, simplification and even complete rewriting of the materials' (Lawrie 1995) is often necessary. Sociocultural factors will also affect the health education process. For example, income levels and financial awareness will determine the approach taken to the promotion of a healthy diet.

Primary prevention is also important in the area of mental health. The ability to 'recognise, avoid or deal constructively with problems or situations that may pose a threat to mental health is an important preventive measure' (Pender 1987). The provision of social support, opportunities to learn new skills, family and individual counselling and advice on managing stress are examples of how nurses may promote mental health at a primary level.

Secondary prevention

Preventive measures at a secondary level involve the early detection of symptoms of health loss. Members of the general public are encouraged to monitor their own health and report symptoms of health loss; many people with learning disabilities, however, rely upon their carers to detect early symptoms of ill health. Not all symptoms, however, are easily recognizable. For example, the onset of cervical cancer or hypertension may

not be immediately apparent. Screening programmes aimed at early detection of a health problem can reduce the effects that might otherwise result from advanced illness. Screening also serves to limit disability by identifying at an early stage problems such as hearing or visual deficits, which might otherwise compound learning disabilities 'causing communication difficulties and isolation' (Rodgers 1994). The learning disability nurse has a central role to play in relation to health screening and surveillance. The significant contribution that nurses can make may be defined in terms of monitoring, observation, education and liaison. Specifically, nurses can help clients to monitor their weight, blood sugar levels or blood pressure, for example.

The onset of symptoms of ill health, including physical and/or behavioural changes, requires astute observation on the part of the carer. Nurses may also use their knowledge and expertise to enable people with learning disabilities to monitor their own health. For example, 'teaching women to examine their own breasts is crucial' (Roth & Brown 1991). Similarly, teaching men to self-examine for testicular changes is equally important. Health screening also involves liaison with generic services. The learning disability nurse can make 'a distinctive contribution to enable people to gain access to, and use ordinary facilities' (Rose & Kay 1995). Some members of the primary healthcare team, however, may have had little or no contact with people with a learning disability. They may therefore share many of the initial anxieties and prejudices held by some members of the general public. Thornton (1994) also voiced concern about the lack of awareness of the needs of people with learning disabilities among members of the primary healthcare team. Indeed, Langan and Russell (1993) concluded that people with a learning disability were less likely than other patients to be offered cervical screening, breast examination or hypertension screening. Clearly, there is a 'need to raise people's expectations about the health of people with a learning disability' (Rose & Kay 1995). This may be partly achieved by means of a jointly formulated protocol for healthcare, for people with learning difficulties (Rodgers 1994). 'Well person' clinics for people with learning difficulties 'should also be seen as essential' (Meehan et al 1995). Enabling members of the primary healthcare team to come to know the person with a learning disability as an individual may also serve to reduce initial prejudices and anxieties as well as establishing rapport and mutual understanding. This may be achieved by arranging for the client to visit the generic healthcare facility some time before an appointment. In this way, the client can begin to become familiar with both the environment and the relevant healthcare worker in a non-threatening atmosphere. It is also vital that the learning disability nurse prepares the individual prior to the process of health screening. Efforts should be made to explain the nature and importance of the screening procedure, since 'people who have been educated about their health are more likely to cooperate with treatment regimes' (Roth & Brown 1991). Issues regarding consent to examination and treatment also require attention (see Chapter 5 for a comprehensive account of such ethical issues in relation to learning disability). Some individuals who have a learning disability may find 'waiting times at routine clinic visits difficult to cope with' (Lawrie 1995). It may be useful, therefore, to contact the clinic beforehand to find out if the appointment time is likely to be delayed. Roth and Brown (1991) have also advised that nurses should consider taking some activity to pass the time in the waiting area. During the consultation individuals may have problems articulating their general health concerns and needs. Nevertheless, they should be encouraged to answer questions independently, with assistance from the carer where necessary. When the consultation is over it is important to establish whether or not the 'client was satisfied with the way the appointment was conducted' (Roth & Brown 1991) and that 'appropriate treatment and follow-up is available' (Meehan et al 1995).

In relation to mental health, secondary preventive efforts involve the early identification of behavioural changes such as those described in Box 6.3. This list is by no means exhaustive, but

Activity 6.4

Pauline, 54, has a moderate learning disability. She has recently moved into a small group home with continual staff support, after living in a long-stay hospital ward for 38 years. As a result, Pauline has recently registered with a local general practitioner and has now been invited to attend a 'Well Woman' clinic. How would you prepare Pauline for her visit to the clinic?

Box 6.3   Behavioural changes commonly signalling the onset of a mental health problem

Aggression towards others
Self-injurious behaviour
Loss of appetite
Social withdrawal
Mood swings
Insomnia/early morning wakening
Onset of bizarre, repetitive movements
Restlessness
Inhibition
Anxiety

represents some of the most common behavioural changes that may signal the onset of mental health problems. Of course, behavioural changes may also be associated with physical factors such as toothache or headache. Moreover, specific conditions such as Fragile X syndrome and Lesch–Nyhan syndrome are particularly associated with behavioural difficulties. In all cases it is the role of the nurse to identify behavioural difficulties at an early stage, in order to devise a therapeutic plan involving any combination of physical care, education, social support or individual therapy to make the continuation of behavioural difficulties less likely.

Tertiary prevention

According to Strauss (1975), the ultimate goal of tertiary prevention is to help clients live full and productive lives. Tertiary prevention, therefore, focuses upon rehabilitation and remedial therapy. In the rehabilitative care process the nurse can gently explore and expand the potential of the individual and facilitate sensitive integration into the community. The rehabilitative care process must therefore be based on an assessment of need in consultation with the individual.

The development of skills forms a core component of rehabilitation. Skill development at a tertiary level may include, for example, teaching an individual self-administration of medication or enabling an individual to identify and participate in a leisure pursuit that they find enjoyable. Remedial therapy involves minimizing the residual effects of disability. Correct positioning to prevent deformity, passive movements to minimize spasticity and the use of aids that promote independence, such as walking frames or cutlery adaptations, are examples of care at a tertiary level. Tertiary prevention activities must also be directed at the management of physical conditions such as epilepsy or diabetes. This involves the administration of medications as well as enabling access to the appropriate mainstream services so that such conditions can be monitored.

Another aspect of tertiary prevention concerns the management of challenging, disturbed or aggressive behaviour. Chapter 9 provides a comprehensive account of the nature of, and the skills and expertise required of the learning disability nurse in relation to the management of behavioural difficulties.

A PROGRAMME FOR HEALTH EDUCATION

A consistent focus of primary, secondary and tertiary levels of prevention is health education. Health education in relation to learning disability presents the nurse with an exciting challenge. People with learning disabilities have specific needs with regard to education, that is, 'they generally learn at a slower pace' (Lawrie 1995). Therefore, any programme of health education must address this need.

The learning disability nurse as health educator

The teaching–learning process is an interactive one. Health teaching must be designed to meet the needs of the individual, and the nurse is responsible for creating the atmosphere in which learning occurs. 'Effective health teaching occurs in an environment which is supportive, non-judgmental and unhurried' (Coutts & Hardy 1991). Educative programmes should be systematic, and it is often beneficial if the teaching programme is presented in stages rather than providing the learner with large amounts of information. The nurse must also make use of the considerable opportunity for health education to take place within daily nursing care. For example, healthy food choices may be reinforced during shopping trips. The use of 'specific means of intervention, including behavioural techniques such as modelling' (Lawrie 1995) may also be utilized to reinforce the learning process. Carers who 'help individuals to control their weight are not effective models if they themselves are overweight' (Coutts & Hardy 1991). Finally, it is important that the nurse is consistent, supportive and sincere. These qualities must be balanced with a degree of flexibility, that is, health education should avoid a prescriptive approach, where learning is closely defined and controlled. Assisting a healthy lifestyle, as opposed to enforcing healthy options, is the essence of good teaching.

Some aspects of learning

- **Learner motivation** The key to learning is motivation, and one way to motivate the learner is to set realistic goals. Formal teaching sessions should 'last no longer than 30–40 minutes' (Lawrie 1995), and enable the learner to achieve a degree of satisfaction. The achievement of a goal provides encouragement, support and further motivation to learn.
- **Stage of the learner** Learning is a process of steps and stages that the nurse should gear to the abilities of the individual.
- **The language used** No-one will be able to learn if the language used is inappropriate. The person's ability to learn, therefore, will be governed to some extent by the vocabulary used. Identifying the key terms used by the learner

provides a 'familiar starting point' that 'facilitates the absorption of new material' (Coutts & Hardy 1991). The use of the individual's own vocabulary should be encouraged.

- **Learning materials** The materials used in the process of health education should be appropriate to the individual. The use of pictures, simple text, everyday living items and video equipment may be beneficial.

- **Reinforce learning** The Department of Health report (1995) entitled *The Health of the Nation – a strategy for people with learning disabilities*, acknowledges that the health message 'should be targeted, sustained into adult life and repeated'. This statement highlights the importance of reinforcing learning.

CONCLUSION

This chapter commenced by recognizing that the healthcare needs of people with a learning disability have been in danger of being ignored. It has been illustrated that people with learning disabilities frequently have specific health problems, 'but use health services less than the general population' (Department of Health 1995). The movement towards care in the community underpins the need for nurses and other healthcare professionals to become more responsive to the healthcare needs of people with a learning disability. The narrow biological view of health that emphasizes diagnosis is no longer appropriate: it is crucial that learning disability nurses embrace a much broader, holistic model of

health. By doing so, the nature of health in the everyday lives of people with learning disabilities is clarified. That is, health is inextricably entwined with the physical and psychosocial aspects of the individual. The existence of a learning disability compromises the individual's ability to achieve health independently. Hence, learning disability nurses have a central role to play in maximizing the potential of the individual to achieve health. A high standard of preventive care can minimize the occurrence of health loss and its complications. Effective preventive care is likely to produce significant health gains that have a beneficial impact upon many areas of the individual's life. Learning disability nurses also have an important role to play in health education. They can assist people to 'choose a healthy way to live' (Department of Health 1995), based upon individual needs. Of equal importance, nurses must enable people with learning disabilities to gain access to comprehensive healthcare services. This means that the learning disability nurse must establish alliances with generic health services and enable appropriate care to be developed in an atmosphere that is receptive to the individual's needs. In conclusion, health promotion, preventive interventions, the teaching of skills and enabling access to appropriate services form the core components of the health gain approach. Assistance will be needed to some degree if people with learning disabilities are to achieve a significant health gain. Surely, this principle must underpin the terms upon which learning disability nurses base their practice.

REFERENCES

Beange H 1986 The medical model revisited. Australia and New Zealand Journal of Developmental Disabilities 12(1): 3–7

Beck C M, Rawlins RP, Williams SR 1988 Mental health psychiatric nursing: a holistic life cycle approach. CV Mosby, St Louis

Blaxter M 1990 Health and lifestyles. Tavistock/Routledge, London

Burns Y, Gunn P 1993 Down syndrome – moving through life. Chapman & Hall, London

Cole O 1986 Medical screening of adults at social education centres: whose responsibility? Mental Handicap 14(6): 54–56

Coutts L C, Hardy L K 1991 Teaching for health – the nurse as health educator. Churchill Livingstone, London

CRIMD 1990 Primary health care for people with learning disability. Policy paper No. 1. Centre for Research and Information into Mental Disability, University of Birmingham

Darbyshire P 1991 (ed) In: Roth S, Brown M (authors) Advocates for health. Nursing Times 87(21): 62–64

Department of Health 1995 The health of the nation – a strategy for people with learning disabilities. HMSO, London

Herzlich C 1973 Health and illness: a social psychological analysis. Academic Press, London

Holland T, Murphy G 1990 Behavioural and psychiatric

disorder in adults with mild learning difficulties. International Review of Psychiatry 2: 117–136

Howells G 1986 Are the medical needs of mentally handicapped adults being met? Journal of the Royal College of General Practitioners 36(27): 449–453

Jacobson J W, Ackerman L J 1988 An appraisal of services for persons with mental retardation and psychiatric impairments. Mental Retardation 26(6): 377

Langan J, Russell O 1993 Community care and the general practitioner: primary health care for people with learning disabilities. Norah Fry Research Centre, Bristol

Lawrie K 1995 Better health care for people with learning disabilities. Nursing Times 91(19): 32–34

Maslow A 1954 Motivation and personality. Harper & Row, London

Meehan S, Moore G, Barr O 1995 Specialist services for people with learning disabilities. Nursing Times 91(13): 33–35

Murphy G 1994 Understanding challenging behaviour. In: Emerson E, McGill P, Mansell J (eds) Severe learning disability and challenging behaviours. Chapman & Hall, London

Pender N J 1987 Health promotion in nursing practice. Appleton & Lange, California

Radley A 1994 Making sense of illness: the social psychology of health and disease. Sage Publications, London

Richardson A, Ritchie J 1991 We all need a friend. Health Service Journal 26 September: 31.

Rodgers J 1994 Primary health care provision for people with learning difficulties. Health and Social Care 2: 11–17

Rose S, Kay B 1995 Significant skills. Nursing Times 91(36): 63–64

Roth S, Brown M 1991 Advocates for Health. Nursing Times 87(21): 62–64

Russell O 1991 Presentation of psychiatric illness in the mentally handicapped. Medicine International 95: 3975–3977

Seedhouse D 1986 Health: the foundations for achievement. John Wiley, Chichester

Sims J 1990 The concept of health. Physiotherapy 76(7): 423–428

Strauss A L 1975 Chronic illness and the quality of life. C V Mosby, St Louis

Thornton C 1994 Primary health care for adults with learning disabilities who live in the community – is a specialist required? Journal of Psychiatric and Mental Health Nursing 1(2): 125–126

Tredwell S J, Newman D E, Lockitch G 1990 Instability of the upper cervical spine in Down syndrome. Journal of Pediatric Orthopaedics 10(5): 602–606

WHO 1946 Constitution. World Health Organisation, New York

Williams R 1983 Concepts of health: an analysis of lay logic. Sociology 17: 185–205

Williams R 1990 A protestant legacy: attitudes to death and illness among older Aberdonians. Clarendon House, Oxford

Wilson D N, Haire A 1990 Health care screening for people with mental handicap living in the community. British Medical Journal 301: 1379–1381

7

Education

D. Dickinson L. Dickinson

INTRODUCTION

The provision of effective education for people with learning disabilities has been the subject of considerable debate, legislation and development. The right of access to an education that meets an individual learner's needs has placed far-reaching demands upon professional knowledge and practice.

Effective education is a complex process. Teaching is far more than the imparting of knowledge and skill: it relies upon sophisticated approaches to assessment and intervention that recognize the particular learning needs of the individual. This chapter explores how educational legislation and the development of professional practice support the process of meeting the individual and special educational needs of children with learning disabilities.

THE CONTEXT

The last quarter of the 20th century has seen significant developments in special education. There have been major changes in thinking about how to provide education for children with learning disabilities, and these changes have had far-reaching effects upon professional practice.

The concept of special educational need: Warnock and the 1981 Education Act

The Warnock Report (1978) and the 1981 Education Act marked fundamental changes in approaches to the education of children with learning disabilities. The formation of a government committee of enquiry chaired by Mary Warnock was, in large part, a response to concerns that:

- Special education had focused for many years upon children's 'handicapping' conditions, rather than individual needs. This focus often detracted attention from the children's abilities and aptitudes and served to set children with learning disabilities apart from those considered to be learning normally.
- This approach had led to the formation of statutory categories of handicap into which children with disabilities were placed. The development of special schools designed to cater for the categories of handicap led to the further separation of children with disabilities from those considered to be learning normally. This segregation of children with disabilities potentially limited their access to a broad and balanced curriculum.
- There were many more children with learning disabilities in the education system than the relatively small number attending special schools.
- The support professionals (medical, psychological, educational and social) employed to identify and categorize children's handicaps might be better deployed in the long-term support of their education.
- There was limited formal involvement of parents in the educational decisions taken for their children.

The key recommendations of the Warnock report included the following:

- Abolition of the statutory categories of handicap and an end to the distinction between handicapped and non-handicapped children.
- The introduction of the concept of special educational need, focusing attention on the individual learning needs of children rather than their handicapping condition. Special educational needs should take into account the child's existing abilities and the need for special facilities and resources in order to maximize the child's learning.

- The recognition that approximately 20% of children will experience some form of special educational need at some time in their school career.
- Wherever possible, children's special educational needs should be met in ordinary schools. There was also a recognition that approximately 2% of children may experience significant learning difficulties that would require their special needs to be met in a special school.
- Special schools should continue to play an important role in meeting the special educational needs of those children for whom the facilities and resources did not exist in ordinary schools. This role should broaden to include active collaboration with ordinary schools.
- The introduction of a staged approach to the assessment of special need, initially involving the child, parent and the teacher and moving through the stages to involve outside agencies and local education authority resources.

The 1981 Education Act responded to the Warnock Committee recommendations in a number of ways. Legislation did indeed abolish the statutory categories of handicap, and these were replaced by a formal recognition of a concept of special educational need (this will be explored in more detail later in the chapter). Furthermore, the 1981 Act instituted a process of assessment, based upon the Warnock 'stages'. Local education authorities were charged with the duty to identify the needs of children (aged 2–19) through a process of multidisciplinary assessment involving parents, teachers, educational psychologists, medical professionals and the social services. If a child was identified as having a significant level of need, then the LEA was required to make appropriate arrangements for provision. These arrangements were safeguarded by the making of a statement, a legally binding document identifying the needs of the child and stating how the LEA intended to meet those needs. Significantly, the 1981 Act also gave formal recognition to the Warnock recommendation that, wherever possible, the special educational needs of children should be met in ordinary schools.

In many senses, therefore, the Warnock Committee and the 1981 Education Act served to change the emphasis of special education away from where the child's needs should be met to how they should be met. The focus was now more upon the facilities and resources required to meet identified needs, and more attention was turned to the capacity of ordinary schools to provide for children with learning disabilities.

Integration versus segregation

The term 'integration' was coined in the Warnock Report to refer to the processes involved in meeting special needs in an ordinary school. There has been much debate (e.g. Portwood 1995) since the Warnock Report about the ways in which integration can be achieved, and the continuing purpose of segregation (i.e. the process of meeting needs in special schools etc.). Some have argued that all needs could be met in ordinary schools, given appropriate levels of resources (Dessent 1987, Sayer 1983a, b), yet segregation continues to be a feature. Although the statutory categories of handicap were abolished by the 1981 Education Act, special schools in many areas of the country continue to provide for categories of learning difficulty (e.g. severe and moderate learning difficulties, emotional and behavioural difficulties).

The capacity of ordinary schools to respond to wider ranges of special educational needs has undoubtedly increased since the 1981 Education Act. Parents are more aware of their rights to expect access to ordinary schools for their children (reinforced by the 1993 Education Act – see later in the chapter). Consequently there are more children in ordinary schools with a wider range of learning needs. This has placed considerable demands upon the processes of multidisciplinary professional support for children, their schools and parents.

In order to ensure that children receive appropriate support in an integrated setting, it is important that all professionals involved understand precisely what is meant by 'integration'. Warnock outlined three fundamental aspects of integration:

- Locational integration. This is where a special school or class is located on the same campus as an ordinary school.
- Social integration. This is where children with special learning needs may enjoy contact with children with ordinary learning needs, but there are no formal arrangements for them to learn together in the same classes.
- Functional integration. This form of integration is the most sophisticated. Children with a wide range of learning needs across the spectrum from ordinary to special learn together in the same classes. At its most sophisticated, functional integration demands the provision of differentiated approaches to the teaching of individual children. These differentiated approaches recognize the learning needs of individuals and provide the right level of access to a curriculum that all children in the class are following. This, of course, places considerable demands upon teachers' skills and approaches to learning needs.

The demands created by functional integration (mainly upon resources, teacher skills and organization in ordinary schools) have meant that for some children the most appropriate place for their education has continued to be in a segregated special school. It is important to remember, however, that there is formal and legislative recognition that, wherever possible, children should have their needs met in ordinary schools. This continues to provide an impetus to the process of enhancing the capacity of ordinary schools to meet a wider range of needs.

Multidisciplinary assessment and statements

The replacement of categories of handicap with a more sophisticated process of defining special educational need required the development of professional practices that could respond to new expectations. The 1981 Education Act outlined new responsibilities for LEAs to identify special educational needs, and to specify the provision necessary to meet those needs via a statutory process of 'multidisciplinary assessments' and 'statements'. The Warnock Report, however, recommended that the statutory identification of special need should be preceded by a less formal and staged approach to assessment, as outlined below.

- **Stage 1** Where a teacher identifies that a child may have a learning difficulty then the parents and the headteacher should be informed. Special arrangements are made for teaching the child in the mainstream classroom and for assessing their progress.
- **Stage 2** If the child continues to demonstrate special learning needs in the classroom, then the school should inform the parents and involve more specialist teaching from within existing school resources, perhaps by providing individual teaching for key skill areas.
- **Stage 3** Where the school feels that the child's needs are not adequately met by the stage 1 and 2 approaches, then the parents should be informed and advice or input should be sought from outside agencies (e.g. peripatetic specialist teachers, educational psychologists, speech therapists etc.).

The next two stages were those formally introduced by the 1981 Act.

- **Stage 4** If the child is considered to be demonstrating special learning needs that are beyond the resources deployed at stages 1–3, then a request can be made to the LEA to make a statutory multidisciplinary assessment of the child's needs. If the LEA decides that there is a case for such an assessment to be made, then, with parental consent, requests are made for reports from the school, an educational psychologist, the health authority and social services. Representations are also sought from the parents regarding the needs of their child. Once the reports are received then it is the duty of the LEA to consider the advice and to decide whether a statement is necessary. A statement is a legally binding document that lists the child's special educational needs and indicates how and where they are to be met. Parents are given 15 days to agree or disagree with its contents before it is finally issued. The LEA is then committed to the provision of the facilities and resources promised

in the statement. The statement must be reviewed annually.

- **Stage 5** The statement is now put into operation. The process of annual review should involve the parents and the professionals in consideration of the effectiveness of the provision. If there is general agreement that the child's needs have changed, then the LEA can decide to change the provision or cease to maintain the statement. All children with statements must be reassessed formally between the ages of $13\frac{1}{2}$ and $14\frac{1}{2}$.

These latter two stages have come to be known commonly as 'statementing'. However, it is important to draw a distinction between stages 4 and 5 and to recognize that 'statementing' should refer only to stage 5. The stage 4 multidisciplinary assessment is, by law, a non-prejudicial process where no assumption should be made that a statement will be issued at the end.

Over the decade following the introduction of the 1981 Education Act there were many problems encountered in the operation of the staged approach to assessment. The 1993 Education Act attempted to address many of these. Before detailed consideration of the 1993 Act, however, it is important to examine another development in educational legislation that had significant effects upon the education of children with learning disabilities – the 1988 Education Act and the National Curriculum.

The 1988 Education Act and the National Curriculum

The introduction of the National Curriculum by the 1988 Education Act provided a structure for the education of all children throughout their school careers (ages 5–16) and a set of expectations for what a child should be able to achieve within core and foundation subject areas. These expectations were based upon a detailed breakdown of the skills and knowledge (statements of attainment) that the child should learn within four key stages of learning development (key stage 1 being up to age 7, key stage 2 up to age 11, key stage 3 up to age 14 and key stage 4 up to age 16). Across the 5–16 age range there are 10 detailed levels of attainment in each of the core and foundation subjects.

The introduction of national testing of children (standard assessment tests) was intended to provide a picture of a child's attainments against the expectations of the National Curriculum. At each key stage there are expected levels of attainment, and these are intended to give an indication of how a child is performing at the end of that stage. To illustrate: at key stage 1 (up to age 7) if children are performing at level 2 then they are considered to be attaining at the expected level within the National Curriculum. Performance at level 1 (or lower) or level 3 (or higher) gives some idea of variation either side of the expectation.

The National Curriculum has important implications for the education of children with learning disabilities. Some of these implications can be seen as advantageous, others not so.

Advantages:

- A clear structure of expectations exists against which to gauge a child's learning development.
- An outline is provided for the teaching of skills and knowledge.
- The National Curriculum provides a basic assessment tool for parents, teachers and other professionals to help identify children's learning needs.

Disadvantages:

- The National Curriculum expectations may be too broad to cater for the specific needs of many children with learning disabilities.
- This may reinforce a picture of 'failure' against national expectations.
- The statements of attainment may be too broad or too steeply graded to cater for the more finely graded achievements of children with learning disabilities.
- There are no guidelines on how to break down the statements of attainment into finer steps.

Many children with learning disabilities will, throughout their school career, perform well below the National Curriculum expectations, and the lack of finely graded steps might call into question the relevance of the Curriculum for

such children. In recognition of this, the 1988 Education Act provided for children with special educational needs to be exempted from following the National Curriculum. This exemption can be provided for all or part of the Curriculum, and must be confirmed by a statement of special educational need.

In many cases nationally, however, this path has not been followed. There appear to be three main reasons for this:

- In a context of integration the child has an entitlement to the same curricular access as all children.
- If a child is exempted from the National Curriculum, then the school and LEA must formally outline an alternative. If the child is not exempted then the concept of 'working towards' a level of attainment can replace the need for a formally rewritten curriculum. In this case it is up to the teacher to identify the more finely graded steps required for a child to be taught effectively.
- In an integrated classroom the teacher can provide the same curriculum for all children, but differentiate the ways in which information is presented, in recognition of individual learning needs. Assessment of progress can similarly be differentiated.

Since the introduction of the National Curriculum approaches to assessment have continued to develop, in recognition of the complex processes involved in defining the special needs of children with learning disability. A significant step forward in this latter respect was marked by the provisions of the 1993 Education Act and the introduction of the 'code of practice on the identification and assessment of special educational needs'.

The 1993 Education Act and the code of practice

In the years following the passing of the 1981 Education Act there were many criticisms of the ways in which LEAs and schools carried out the new statutory expectations. These criticisms centred on:

- a lack of national consistency in the ways in which the processes of identification, assessment and meeting of special educational needs developed. This was highlighted by a survey carried out by the Audit Commission and Her Majesty's Inspectorate of Schools (Audit Commission 1992), where 13 LEAs were investigated in terms of their implementation of the 1981 Act
- delays in the processing of multidisciplinary assessments and the issuing of statements
- a lack of guidance from the Department for Education regarding effective implementation of the 1981 Act
- a lack of rigour in the implementation of the five-stage Warnock model of assessment.

In late 1992 the Audit Commission and Her Majesty's Inspectorate of Schools published their recommendations, based upon the preceding survey, of how LEAs might improve their processes of assessment and identification of special educational needs (Audit Commission 1993). Many of these were embodied in the 1993 Education Act, which introduced the requirement for a national code of practice on the identification and assessment of special educational needs. LEAs and schools were expected to give 'due regard' to this code of practice. A new rigour was introduced to the whole process of identifying and meeting special educational needs, with clear timescales for statutory processes of assessment and statementing. The roles and responsibilities of schools in carrying out the staged model of assessment were also introduced.

Detailed consideration of the requirements of the code of practice is given later in this chapter. Before moving on to this, however, it is important to explore the concepts and methods that underpin effective professional practice in meeting the needs of children with learning disabilities.

INDIVIDUAL NEED AND SPECIAL NEED

Changing the emphasis of teaching, from an approach based upon a child's handicap to an approach based upon special educational need, has important implications for professional practice. All those concerned with the child should share a common perspective of how best to help with the child's individual and special educational needs.

At first it may seem difficult to separate these two concepts: surely individual needs are the same as special needs, particularly if the child has a learning difficulty? Difficult as it may seem to draw a distinction between the two, however, it is important to develop a clear picture of both.

A definition of individual need

All children, regardless of ability, have individual educational needs. All children have a need to:

- acquire the skills and knowledge that will give them effective access to the world
- gain access to a curriculum that will provide the experiences necessary to enable learning of these skills and knowledge.

For most children, access to ordinary schools and the National Curriculum will provide for their individual educational needs. With effective teaching and classroom management schools can respond effectively to most children's educational needs, and provide an environment and curriculum which enables children to make the most of what is on offer.

However, for some children this is not the case, particularly where there is a degree of learning disability or difficulty.

Defining special educational need – a model for practice

Special educational needs can be defined as those that arise from a child's difficulty in accessing the curriculum ordinarily offered in mainstream schools. These special needs will, of course, be highly individualized and require a very sensitive approach to assessment and teaching. Later in this chapter we describe how the 1993 Education Act and the code of practice provide a framework for effective assessment, intervention and teaching of children with special educational needs. First, however, it is important to consider the general processes involved in defining the special educational needs of the individual child.

It is tempting and easy to ascribe a child's difficulty in accessing the ordinary curriculum solely to factors 'within' the child. In other words, it is possible to 'blame' the child for not learning effectively on the grounds of, for example, limited cognitive ability, lack of motivation, physical difficulties or emotional and behavioural difficulties. This may lead to an exclusive impression that there is something 'wrong' with the child that is preventing access to the curriculum. This may then lead to the belief that a 'cure' for 'within-child' problems might overcome the learning difficulties. This is not to say that within-child factors are unimportant: of course they are, but cures are extremely rare. As yet there is very little understanding of the neurological processes involved in learning that might lead to an understanding of how to cure learning disabilities.

Special education is a far more complex and interactive process than merely diagnosing a within-child problem and prescribing a cure. It must involve not only the within-child factors, but also factors in the child's learning environment.

It is possible to describe the educational process as an interaction between the child; the teacher/adult; and the curriculum. This interaction can be portrayed as a triangle (Figure 7.1.), where the relationships or dimensions between each of the points are seen to be vital to the effectiveness of the educational process. Effective education relies upon the integrity of the relationships or dimensions between each of the three points.

Dimension (a) in Figure 7.1 describes the relationship between the teacher and the child. The teacher's understanding of the child will involve some knowledge of within-child factors (e.g. medical conditions or physical disabilities which may affect learning). The teacher will also need to have a clear picture of the child's current levels of attainment and past progress in learning. In

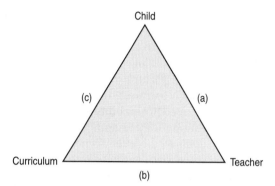

Figure 7.1   The interactive nature of the educational process.

some cases it may be important for the teacher to have some awareness of the child's past emotional and behavioural responses to certain learning situations. An understanding of all the above will enable prediction of the child's likely response to planned teaching. For the planned teaching to be effective, it is also vital that the child understands what the teacher requires in response.

Dimension (b) in Figure 7.1 describes the relationship between the teacher and the curriculum. It is obviously important that the teacher understands the framework and content of the curriculum to be delivered to the child. However, it is also vitally important that the teacher understands how best to tailor teaching approaches in order to enable the child to access the curriculum effectively. This is commonly known as the 'differentiation' of teaching approaches, and will rely upon the teacher's understanding of both the child and the curriculum.

Dimension (c) in Figure 7.1 describes the relationship between the child and the curriculum. The curriculum provided for the child must recognize both individual and special educational needs. The child must be able to access the curriculum effectively and demonstrate learning through appropriate response to the demands of the curriculum.

The child's assessed or measured response to the curriculum, in terms of learning progress and attainment, completes the relationships in the learning triangle. In other words, the quality and integrity of the relationships in the triangle are tested by the child's assessed progress in learning.

This interactive model, therefore, enables the analysis of all the factors involved in effective learning. A child's learning disability cannot be exclusively ascribed to inability or within-child limitations. The model demands that consideration is also given to the effectiveness and sensitivity of the assessment and teaching approaches provided for the child. Where a child's learning disability is causing concern, the model enables detailed analysis of not only what is 'wrong' or 'right' with the child, but also what might be 'wrong' or 'right' with the learning environment. Parents, teachers and support professionals can then contribute to the analysis of the factors in the learning environment which are vital for learning progress.

Assessment and intervention

An important aspect of good teaching is that the teacher is continuously assessing the child's response to the teaching. This enables the teacher to plan and adjust approaches to the child's learning on the basis of a developing picture of his or her special educational needs. In this way intervention and assessment become one and the same process.

This is an important issue when considering ways in which to help with the education of children with learning disabilities. The special educational needs of such children demand far more than a process of 'teaching first and assessing later' in order to see how the child has progressed. Any intervention designed to meet a child's learning need must be very sensitive to the child's response, otherwise the teaching may not achieve its aims.

The successful integration of assessment and intervention into one complete process relies upon the analyses made possible by the learning triangle described above. In other words, successful education of children with learning disabilities must take into consideration all the factors, both child-centred and in the learning environment, that might need attention and change.

For many children with learning disability this process of assessment and intervention needs to be a daily aspect of teaching. As the education progresses small changes may be required in the direction and emphasis of the teaching in order to respond adequately to the child's needs. If a child appears to be 'getting stuck' in the learning of a skill or knowledge, then consideration should be given to the ways in which the teaching might be changed to help the child to progress. It may also be that the assessment is not enabling the child to demonstrate the newly acquired skill effectively. This approach is a far cry from one which assumes that the child's failure to learn is solely a within-child problem.

If the teaching approach is based upon the concept of the learning triangle and an integrated process of assessment and intervention, then the input of outside professionals (support teachers, medical professionals, psychologists, learning disability nurses etc.) can be focused upon how to help with the teaching, rather than simply upon diagnosing what might be 'wrong' with the child.

Syndromes and conditions – educational implications

Many children with learning disabilities may also have been diagnosed as having some form of medical condition or syndrome (e.g. Down syndrome, autism, attention deficit disorder, cerebral palsy etc.). There is not the scope in this chapter for a detailed consideration of the implications of such diagnoses (see Chapter 2); however, it is important to look at the general implications of the existence of syndromes and conditions.

These diagnoses often cause teachers great concern in terms of their planning of effective teaching. There may be a fear that the condition or syndrome may require a specialist approach, and that there is a danger that the 'wrong' approach may be adopted. It is vitally important, therefore, that any such diagnosis should (where appropriate) be communicated to the educational professionals concerned in terms of the implications that conditions or syndromes may have for teaching and learning; this is especially so of the learning disabilities nurse.

A word of warning, however: there is the danger that diagnoses of conditions may imply limitations in the child's ability to learn, which might reduce expectations in the teaching approach. This is commonly referred to as the 'self-fulfilling prophecy', and can result in a reduction in people's expectations of the child's capacity to learn. There are many examples where children with conditions or syndromes which might have severely restricted their capacity to learn have responded positively to effective teaching (e.g. Feuerstein 1980). Such approaches have been based upon the sensitive assessment of need within the learning triangle, not solely upon the within-child factors which a diagnosis of a condition or syndrome might imply.

The concepts and methods outlined above are significant features of the educational approaches described by the code of practice, to which all schools and LEAs must have due regard. We turn now to a detailed consideration of the requirements of the code of practice.

APPLYING THE CODE OF PRACTICE

The code of practice provides schools and local education authorities with clear information regarding their responsibilities for all children considered to have learning disabilities. The basic principles are founded upon the Warnock recommendations and the 1981 Education Act. The code of practice should be considered as a valuable working document designed to guide the practice of all those involved with the education of children with special learning needs.

 Activity 7.1

The learning triangle
Select a skill or area of knowledge which you have attempted to learn but with which you have experienced difficulty. Now consider the three dimensions of the learning triangle. How might changes be made along the three dimensions in order to enhance the quality of your learning?

The 1993 Act and the code of practice require all schools to publish a policy document relating to the meeting of special educational needs. This should give clear information as to how resources are allocated to special needs, and how the schools' systems respond to the demands of the code of practice. The schools' governing bodies have responsibility for all pupils with special needs, and should appoint a governor whose role it is to oversee the operation of the special needs policy. Schools are also required to have a designated member of staff with responsibility for special needs, known as the 'special needs coordinator' (SENCO).

A school having regard to the code of practice will be using a staged approach to meet the needs of pupils with learning difficulties. This is based upon the principles of early identification and intervention, initially emphasizing the school's role in these processes. The involvement of parents in these processes is considered to be of vital importance.

The staged approach to assessment and intervention

Stage 1: Teacher, parent and child

The code of practice promotes early identification of need, and at stage 1 special need is usually noted by the class teacher. However, parents may express a concern regarding their child's progress, and this must be considered as being equally important. If a child is identified as having a need, their name should be entered on the school's special educational needs register at this stage. If the identification of a need has come from the class teacher, the parents should be informed immediately. Records of action and intervention should be kept, together with records of strategies adopted to meet the identified need. It is also considered appropriate to place a child at stage 1 if concerns have been expressed by health or social services professionals, if these concerns are considered to be affecting educational progress. Close liaison between parents and schools is vital here, as medical and other professionals should not disclose such information without parental consent.

Stage 2: Teacher, parent, child and SENCO

If the strategies of intervention used at stage 1 appear to be failing to meet the child's needs (i.e. satisfactory progress is not being made), then the class teacher may decide to proceed to stage 2 of the code of practice. At this stage, the class teacher seeks the involvement of the school's special needs coordinator (SENCO) in the planning and provision for the child's needs. The child is registered at stage 2, with the agreement of the SENCO. The teacher and SENCO review the evidence from stage 1 and any information from outside professionals already involved with the child, and from the parents. The SENCO and the teacher then draw up an individual education plan (IEP) for the child, and the parents are informed. (A detailed description of the structure and format of IEPs is given later in the chapter.)

The IEP will focus upon the skills and knowledge to be developed by the child, and upon the strategies to be employed by the school to help the child. The IEP will usually run for approximately one school term (although at stage 2 this could be longer) before being reviewed. Parents should be involved in these reviews.

It is important to note that at stage 2 the school will use its own resources to run the IEP. In reality this means that the class teacher continues to take responsibility for the education of the child, perhaps with additional teaching input from others, and with the continuing advice of the SENCO.

The child's response to the IEP should yield important information as to the appropriateness of the strategies being used by the school, and about the child's continuing quality of need. Queries may arise regarding, for example, the child's vision, hearing, language or physical development which might need to be checked by outside professionals (e.g. by referral to medical professionals, speech therapists or physiotherapists). The results of such checks will then inform future IEP planning.

The review of the IEP may result in:

- a return to stage 1
- continuation at stage 2 with a revised IEP
- consideration of stage 3 involvement.

Stage 3: Involving outside support agencies

A decision to move to stage 3 is taken when the teacher, SENCO and parents feel that the child's needs require the input of specialist professionals in order to contribute to the implementation of the IEP. The responsibility to compile, implement and review the IEP remains with the teacher and SENCO, but the contribution of outside professionals should be formally noted.

A range of outside professionals may be called upon, according to the nature of the child's needs. Specialist teachers with skills in the areas of learning disability, sensory impairment, emotional and behavioural difficulty and so on are often involved in advice or direct specialist teaching. Educational psychologists may also play a key role in the assessment and intervention of special need. Such people are usually employed by the local education authority and provide a service to schools as part of their routine delivery at stage 3. (Note, however, that grant-maintained schools, who receive their funding from central government and not the LEA, may have to provide such input from their own budgets. This does not apply to educational psychologists, who have a responsibility to provide a service across all schools in the state sector.) In addition to the services provided by LEAs, schools may also call upon the advice and guidance of medical and other professionals, according to the nature of the child's needs. School medical officers, learning disabilities nurses and therapists, along with social services personnel, may all have relevant inputs to make. The availability of such support will, of course, be affected by local policies of provision and funding, and it is vital that the SENCO is fully aware of the extent and quality of available help. Reviews of IEPs at stage 3 should be carried out on a termly basis, involving the views of parents, school and involved outside agencies. The review of the IEP at stage 3 may result in:

- a return to stage 2
- continuation at stage 3 with a revised IEP
- a decision to request a move to stage 4 (formal multidisciplinary assessment).

Stage 4: Multidisciplinary assessment

The decision to move to stage 4 must be taken in light of the evidence of the child's progress at stage 3. If there is concern and evidence that the child's needs place demands upon the school's resources which the school cannot fully meet, then a decision is taken to approach the local education authority to request a multidisciplinary assessment of those needs. The LEA will make this decision in the light of all the available evidence of assessments and interventions made thus far. If the LEA feels that there is a case for initiating a full statutory assessment, the case will be registered in school at stage 4 on the special needs register. IEPs should still continue to be devised and implemented while the statutory assessment is being made.

The code of practice and the 1993 Act impose time limits on the statutory assessment process, requiring that the whole procedure be completed within a 6-month period. Once the LEA agrees to proceed at stage 4 the parents are formally consulted, and written advice regarding the nature of the child's special educational needs is sought from those professionally involved.

There is a fundamental requirement for the LEA to formally seek the views of:

- the parents
- the school
- other educationalists involved with the child
- educational psychologists
- medical professionals: the child will be required to be medically examined, and reports should be submitted from those medical and therapeutic professionals involved in ongoing support
- social services personnel
- any appropriate independent agency requested by the parent.

Once these reports are received the LEA has a duty to consider all the advice and to determine whether a statement of special educational needs is required in order to meet the identified needs appropriately.

Statement of special educational need

A statement is a statutory document compiled by the LEA which

- outlines the nature of the child's special learning needs
- identifies the special educational provision which the LEA considers to be necessary to meet these needs. This provision is described in terms of the learning objectives for which the provision is intended, the quality of provision (e.g. details of school-based support, special school placement etc.) and arrangements for monitoring progress
- names the place where education is to be carried out
- lists non-educational needs agreed by social services, health professionals etc., and how provision for these is to be made.

Parents are consulted about the contents of the statement and the received professional advice before the statement is finally issued. If parents disagree with any aspect of the advice they can discuss their concerns with the professional in question. This is particularly important if the parents feel that an aspect of advice has led to decisions about resourcing in the statement with which they disagree. Likewise, if the parents disagree with the outlined provision then they have recourse to arbitration from the Special Needs Tribunal system provided by central government.

Notes in lieu of a statement

There may be occasions where the statutory assessment process has contributed evidence to the LEA that the child's needs can continue to be provided for within the existing resources of the school. If this is the case the LEA may issue a note in lieu, which indicates that strategies for provision need to developed in light of the advice received, without the provision of enhanced or additional resources. Again, should the parents disagree with this perspective they have the right of appeal to the Special Educational Needs Tribunal.

Stage 5: Annual reviews and transition plans

Annual review Once the statement is issued it is the responsibility of the school to review the appropriateness of the provision at least once a year. This is known as the annual review process, where the school, with the advice of appropriate outside agencies and parents, reassesses the child's progress and the effectiveness of provision. Should there be significant changes in the level of need or appropriateness of provision during the year, then the LEA should be informed in order to request a revision of the statement.

Transition plans The annual review of a statement in the period following a young person's 14th birthday is a significant event in the process of statutory provision for special educational needs. In order to ensure that effective plans are made for the young person's future beyond school age, the LEA must convene a meeting to review any special needs and provision. The aim of the meeting is to compile a transition plan, which will help to meet the needs of the young person in the final years of school and beyond. The meeting must be attended by LEA representatives, parents, appropriate school staff, social services personnel and representatives of the careers service. Consideration should be given to statutory assessments which may be necessary under legislation other than the 1993 Education Act (i.e. the Chronically Sick and Disabled Persons Act 1970, the Disabled Persons Act 1986 and the NHS and Community Care Act 1990). The transition plan should incorporate the views of the young person, the school, appropriate outside agencies and the family as to the young person's needs and appropriate resources for the future.

Preschool assessment

Much has been written in this chapter so far relating to school-based assessment and intervention in the area of special educational needs. However, many children have special needs that are identified long before their eligibility for full-time education at the age of 5. This may have been the result of health or social service interventions and involvements, or from parents' own observations and assessments. The code of practice outlines the roles and responsibilities of LEAs, social services departments, health authorities and trusts and voluntary organizations in meeting the special needs of preschool children. However, a preschool child has no statutory right of access to education or special education. Arrangements and provision for preschool education vary according to regional boundaries, and access to provision for any individual child is fundamentally affected by these variations. The 1993 Education Act does require LEAs to carry out assessments of children below the age of 2 who are believed to have special educational needs (particularly if requested by parents), and states that 'the LEA may make and maintain a statement of the child's special educational needs in such a manner as they consider appropriate' (section 175). In reality this may mean that access to home-based specialist teaching may be provided, but this will depend upon existing resources.

For children under the age of 5 the 1993 Education Act requires LEAs to 'use their best endeavours to secure that appropriate special educational provision is made for all their registered pupils with learning difficulties' (section 161).

The Act also requires district health authorities and NHS trusts to inform parents and LEAs where they feel that a child has special educational needs. They are also required to indicate where these needs may be met by voluntary organizations. Again, however, 'best endeavours' does not imply statutory obligation for provision, and the range of provision will vary on a regional basis.

Effective preschool education relies heavily upon liaison between LEA, health authority, social services and voluntary organizations. The quality of provision identified in a statement for

Activity 7.2

Informing parents

Imagine that you have to explain to parents how their child's special educational needs will be assessed and met. Which key points will you emphasize in your discussion in order to inform parents effectively about this complex process? Remember that these key points should be easily remembered after your discussion, and should help the parents to help the child.

a preschool child will be largely a reflection of the quality of this liaison.

INDIVIDUAL EDUCATION PLANS

Target setting for children

As the term 'individual education plan' suggests, each child considered to be at stage 2 or above on the school's special needs register requires a detailed individual plan of how their special educational needs are to be met. The code of practice clearly outlines the information required at the various stages of intervention. The plan at stage 2 should set out:

- nature of the child's learning difficulties
- action – the special educational provision – staff involved, including frequency of support – specific programmes/activities/materials/equipment
- help from parents at home
- targets to be achieved in a given time
- any pastoral care or medical requirements
- monitoring and assessment arrangements
- review arrangements and date (Code of Practice, paragraph 2:93).

The requirements for a plan at stage 3 are similar but include a statement referring to the involvement of 'external specialists'. The statements relating to action, targets and monitoring require careful planning by the professionals involved. In setting out the targets to be achieved it is vital that appropriate action is taken in an attempt to meet the needs of the individual child.

A good individual education plan will set specific targets for the child to achieve. These targets can only be reviewed effectively if they are expressed in terms of learning behaviour, i.e. skills which can be directly observed and assessed. Precision in thinking and planning are important aspects of the process of setting realistic targets, therefore a target to 'improve reading' could be considered to be far too broad; it may be better to focus upon particular component skills involved with reading, such as letter recognition, basic sight vocabulary or blend use etc. To enable precise targets to be set it is important to consider the abilities of the child and know what they can already do in the selected targeted skill area. The class teacher or SENCO may have to carry out 'baseline' assessments to establish a starting point. It should be possible to identify specific skills to be targeted in all major areas of learning activity, both academic and social.

In choosing a precise target the professionals are setting out an expectation for the child to achieve within a certain time limit, usually by the next review date. The targets should be observable and assessable in order to establish whether the child has made progress. It is important to specify the activities that will be carried out during the plan, and the setting in which these will occur (i.e. the child may be in a small group situation for some activities, or even receive some individual tuition). If outside agencies are involved they should be part of the planning process and their involvement should be recorded as part of the individual education plan.

In the mainstream school a child will be educated for the majority of time in a larger class-based setting. It is important, therefore, to identify those subject areas where differentiation is required in order for the child to access the curriculum. Precision is also vital in the planning of how this is to be achieved. In a secondary school setting the subject teachers will be mainly responsible for this differentiation, but the plan should reflect how it will occur. A record should be made in the plan of the materials and approaches to be used in recognition of the individual child's skill level. In a primary school setting the class teacher will probably be responsible for differentiation in many curriculum areas, and will need to be aware of the levels of skills in order to do this appropriately for each individual child.

A review date should then be set; at stage 2 this might be within a term, but at stage 3 it must be termly. At the review it should be noted what the child has achieved in the previously targeted areas. These achievements should be recorded in as precise terms as the original targets – if the targets were not reached, it is still important to note what the child is now able to do in that area. Discussions at the review will lead to decisions about where to go next. All the professionals involved in the delivery of the plan should be invited to attend, as well as the parents. If the original targets were achieved then decisions should be made about making a new individual education plan. If a child has been at stage 2 for at least two review periods and appears to be making satisfactory progress, the outcome may be to move him or her back to stage 1. If the targets were not reached, questions need to be asked about the nature of the targets, the consistency of the delivery and demands being placed upon the resources.

Pupils who have been issued with a statement will have that statement reviewed annually. However, they will still need an individual education plan, with short-term targets that can assess the progress being achieved.

Target setting for professionals

The role of the professionals in setting precise and accurate targets for an individual child is a crucial aspect of assessing progress. The professionals involved must be fully aware of each individual child's abilities, and have a knowledge of strategies that may help the child to reach the learning targets. It is important to consider not only the child's apparent progress but also the factors listed in the individual education plan that relate to its professional delivery. An analytical and critical approach is required to determine whether all aspects of the plan were delivered as originally anticipated. For example, certain materials or equipment may not have been as readily available as initially planned. The plan cannot

then be considered to have been fully delivered, thus contributing to the child not having achieved the set targets. This reflects the notion of the triangular model described earlier, where the interaction between the child, the teacher and the curriculum is vital to the process of learning. An effective individual education plan is therefore dependent upon the relationship between the targets set for the learner, and the targets set for the deliverer.

Even where all aspects of the plan have been delivered, however, if the child has not reached the set targets there needs to be careful consideration of the quality and appropriateness of the strategies employed by the professionals in the operation of the plan.

As mentioned earlier in the chapter, it is all too easy to blame the child for failing to achieve the targets without carefully considering:

- whether the targets were appropriate in the first place
- whether smaller 'steps to targets' are required
- whether the strategies were appropriate for helping the child to reach the targets.

The professionals involved in the delivery of the IEP should therefore regularly consider whether the targets set for their own delivery were appropriate in the first place.

Careful management of the individual education planning process, which concentrates upon the effectiveness of the interaction between learning targets and delivery targets, should ensure sensitive and effective special educational provision.

Figure 7.2 presents a proposed outline for an individual education plan which follows the requirements of the code of practice.

CONCLUSION

Current approaches to the education of young people with learning disabilities focus upon the interactive nature of the educational process rather than solely upon what might be 'wrong' with the learner. There has been a change of emphasis in the latter half of the 20th century, from an approach based upon the 'categorization

INDIVIDUAL EDUCATION PLAN

Name: _____   Period of plan: _____

School: _____   Review date: _____

Date of birth: _____   Year: 1 2 3 4 5 6 7 8 9 10 11

Compiled by: _____

Specific skills to be delivered by this plan _____
_____
_____
_____
_____
_____

What can the pupil do in skill area (s) at beginning of plan? _____
_____
_____
_____
_____
_____
_____
_____

Details of specific teaching/assessment activities to be delivered in individual or small group setting (including parental involvement) _____
_____
_____

Who will carry these out? _____
_____

When will they be carried out? _____

Hours per week devoted to these activities _____
_____
_____

Details of class-based differentiation
List areas of National Curriculum where differentiation is necessary and identify how this is to be achieved _____
_____
_____

Curriculum area/ Subject area	*Differentiated approach (materials/teacher method)*
_____	_____
_____	_____
_____	_____
_____	_____

IEP REVIEW

Date of review: _____   People attending: _____

What can pupil do now in targeted skill area? _____
_____
_____
_____

Observations regarding the success of the plan:
Did the plan reach its targets? _____
_____

Were all aspects of the plan delivered? _____
_____

Is a new IEP necessary?   *yes/no*

Relevant comments arising from review (Include comments regarding effective strategies to be continued, possible medical investigations necessary, etc.) _____
_____
_____
_____

Signed: _____   *Special Needs Coordinator*

Figure 7.2   Proposed format for an individual education plan.

Activity 7.3

Compiling individual education plans
Using the IEP format presented in Figure 7.2, compile an IEP for a child with a learning disability. Remember to select observable learning targets which can be reviewed after one term, and consider how you as a health professional might be incorporated into the delivery of the IEP.

of handicap' to an approach which attempts to define special educational need. This has enabled all those who work with children with learning disabilities to consider how best to respond to individual learning needs by analysing the ways in which the learner responds to new learning targets. This chapter has presented a working model (the learning triangle) that enables the analysis of all the major features of the learning environment; this should help with the process of identifying individual *and* special needs in ways that lead to an effective meeting of those needs.

Recent educational legislation has recognized the importance of the interactive nature of learning, and the code of practice on the identification and assessment of special educational needs endorses the interactive model by outlining the professional responsibilities required to ensure that such needs are properly met. The individual education plan, as required by the code of practice, should be a practical reflection of the interactive processes involved in identifying and meeting the needs of a child with a learning disability.

REFERENCES

Audit Commission 1992 Getting in on the Act. HMSO, London
Audit Commission 1993 Getting the Act together. HMSO, London
Department for Education 1994 Code of practice on the identification and assessment of special educational needs. HMSO, London
Dessent T 1987 Making the ordinary schools special. Falmer Press, London
Feuerstein R 1980 Instrumental enrichment. University Park Press, Baltimore

Portwood P F 1995 An experience of integration. Children Nationwide Medical Research Fund
Sayer J 1983a A comprehensive school for all. In: Booth A, Potts P (eds) Integrating special education. Blackwell, Oxford
Sayer J 1983b Assessments for all, statements for none. Special Education 10:4
Warnock M (Chair) 1978 Special educational needs. HMSO, London

FURTHER READING

Advisory Centre for Education 1994 Special education handbook; The law on children with special needs, 6th edn. ACE, London

Department for Education 1995 Innovatory practice in mainstream schools for special educational needs. HMSO, London

Accessing services

G. Connolly

INTRODUCTION

Over the last few decades people with learning disabilities and their carers have had to confront radical changes that have affected their lifestyles. In particular this can be seen from the unprecedented shift in residential provision, from large hospitals to community-based services. Most recently, the NHS and Community Care Act (DOH 1990) has changed the way most caring services are provided within our society. It was heralded as the best way of providing services to the most needy, while enabling them to remain as independent as possible, living at home where feasible. Services would be provided according to an individual's assessed need, leading to needs-led service provision. This is a philosophy that has been discussed for many years, as the National Development Group (DHSS 1978) suggested in their report:

A systematic approach to assessment should be guided by certain basic principles:
1. It is essential to assess the needs of each person as an individual.
2. Assessment must always lead to a programme of action, designed to help the individual to make progress – assessment for assessment's sake is of little value.
3. Assessment should take place as far as possible in a "real life" situation.
4. Assessment should not be limited to casual observations but should be systematic, duly recorded, and regularly reviewed.

If we consider these ideas and compare them with what the NHS and Community Care Act has to say about individual needs assessment, there are many similarities. However, from April 1993 the Act had a profound effect on anyone seeking a service, from either social services or a residential or nursing home. Social services became the leading agent to assess the need and purchase services to meet it. As with many other Acts, the way this has been applied around the country has been variable, because of the different needs of each area. It follows, therefore, that the systems by which people access services may also vary, depending on where they happen to live, their age, and which of the welfare organizations provides the service. In this chapter access to services is examined from a developmental perspective, starting with the identification of disability through to service provision for adults with learning disabilities.

IDENTIFICATION OF LEARNING DISABILITIES

When do services begin for people with a disability? It could be argued that care services commence when a woman's pregnancy is confirmed by her general practitioner. Over many years the welfare services of this country have developed comprehensive health and social systems to ensure that each baby has the best chance possible of being healthy when it arrives. Mothers to be are encouraged not to smoke, to eat a well balanced diet and to take exercise. Some mothers are tested to find out whether the baby has a particular disability: this may be the only time in the pregnancy when the parents think about having a baby which is not perfect. If the test is positive the pregnancy may be terminated, possibly raising more questions for the family and society than it answers.

A baby born with a severe medical problem or a recognizable disability usually has access to the medical services immediately, although there have been some well publicized cases highlighting the difficulty of finding special care beds in some areas. As with all children, their care cannot be separated from care for the parents, and this is especially true when the child may have an ongoing disability. In these early stages the way the parents are treated could affect the way the child is cared for by the family. The questions the family may ask should be answered as fully as possible, 'in an open and honest way' but with 'sensitivity and tactfulness' (Jupp 1992). This is a challenge for professionals, as in the early stages they too will be guessing at the child's possible future development, unless the disability is degenerative and carries a poor prognosis.

Emotions are in turmoil when parents are told their child has a problem. This is often described as a state of shock, feeling numb, disbelief, or being in a dreamlike state. There have been many descriptions of the stages parents go through; Miller (1994) has described four: surviving, searching, settling in and separating.

Surviving

'Surviving is what you do to keep going when you feel completely helpless because something totally out of your control has taken away your child's equal chance of life.'

It is evident from such a description why professionals should try and ensure that parents feel involved with the child's care, even when the intervention is medical. At the very least, parents must be actively involved in any decision-making process.

Searching

'Searching is a time of moving forward, the beginning of a sense of control over your emotions and life, and a time for seeking understanding about your child, your family, and yourself.'

This stage may be recognized when parents are looking for answers to questions, such as what is the cause? Has it got a diagnosis or a label? At this time parents may seek out a diagnosis or help; professionals should not see this as a negative time and should perhaps encourage the parents to seek second opinions. The professionals have more information about the child's condition and should guide the parents to where they can find help and alternative services.

Settling in

'Settling in is seeing the world for what it is, seeing yourself for who you are, moving beyond the intense emotions of surviving, feeling less the sense of urgency or searching, gaining a greater sense of control and balance.'

This stage could be when the child's schooling is arranged, with the parents feeling they should have the best services available for their child. This state may last until the child reaches school-leaving age.

Separating

'Separating is normal, a necessary process in development. Each step of separation is a step towards independence as your child grows up and away from you.'

Families reach and travel through these stages at different times and different speeds, and as the child grows, incidents may bring the family back to an earlier stage. Learning disability nurses are often more involved with this last stage, as one of

their main aims is to help a person with a disability reach the highest level of independence possible. Henderson (1969) has pointed out that 'The unique function of the nurse is to assist the individual, sick or well, in the performance of those activities contributing to health, or its recovery (or to a peaceful death), that he would perform unaided, if he had the necessary strength, will or knowledge. And to do this in such a way as to help him gain independence as rapidly as possible.'

The ways families come to terms with having a child with a disability have been described by many people, but, as with all things in life, the experience will be felt and handled differently by different individuals and family groups. This places an onerous responsibility on services to be constantly adapting to serve their needs.

CHILDHOOD
Early years

The diagnosis of a disability may not be apparent until some time after birth, and therefore services are not involved until the child starts to fall behind the 'normal' milestones of human development. This failure may be picked up by doctors or nurses when the child has its regular check-ups. However, parents often have a feeling all is not well long before any professional is concerned, which may cause difficulties for them. It is not unusual to find parents who have found it very difficult to persuade their doctor that their child has a problem, and sometimes parents feel that they are being seen as neurotic and overprotective. Families often experience a sense of frustration and subsequently they may find it hard to trust professionals.

Child development team

Investigations to discover the reasons for disability are often carried out by a multiagency child development team, although this often has a medical focus. Child development teams in different parts of the country have slightly different aims and objectives, but the overriding principles are:

- To identify the child's specific problem including a diagnosis
- To identify interventions and services that could be used to minimize the effect of disability on the child's development
- To give advice and support to parents.

All of these are important areas. Jones et al (1989) has quoted one parent as saying, 'Not until we were referred to the DHT for paediatric assessment did any one actually consider how we were coping as a family' (DHT stands for district handicapped team, which in some areas have been replaced by child development teams).

Before child development teams, the child and family could spend a lot of time visiting clinics or being visited at home by one professional or another. This was both inefficient and confusing: one parent told the author of this chapter that in the early years the family kept a calendar just for their son's appointments and visits. 'We had no time for ourselves and Andrew had to perform on all these appointments. I really resented the time and invasion, although I knew they were only trying to help'.

This can still happen with multiply disabled children, because of their complex needs. However, it is up to the team to ensure that both child and family have a coordinated service that is sensitively organized to meet all their needs. The child development team helps the family access other services that are provided by different organizations, such as social services, education and the voluntary sector. These could include respite care, benefit advice, portage and advice on access to special education.

Legislation to help children

In October 1991 the 1989 Children Act came into force. This was widely welcomed, as it brought together most of the laws relating to children in England and Wales. For children with disabilities (section 2, para 6) the local authorities were given a leading role, in an attempt to prevent the confusing variations between local authorities and health services around the country. Within the terms of the Children Act any child with a dis-

ability is included in the category of 'children in need'. The Children Act mirrors the 1948 National Assistance Act definition of disability, which is: 'a child is disabled if he is blind, deaf and dumb or suffers from mental disorder of any kind or is substantially and permanently handicapped by illness or congenital deformity or such other disabilities'.

The Children Act also describes the services that local authorities will be expected to provide for children in need (section 2, part 1). These include accommodation for children, both longer term and respite care, advice, guidance and counselling, occupational, social, cultural and recreational activities, home help (including laundry facilities), transport or assistance to pay for it to access services, and assistance with holiday and day care (including after-school and holiday activities). However, the Act does not specify the nature of the services, nor how much should be offered (Robinson 1991), and there has been concern, since the Act came into force, about the funding of such provisions. It is the case that a local authority need not provide such services but should be able to access them through statutory, voluntary or private agencies, and in order to ensure that children get the right service comprehensive assessment is essential.

The Children Act tried to address the problem that some children with disabilities face, of having assessments by different agencies that cover the same or similar areas, although ongoing assessment could be argued to be a positive step towards ensuring that the child has the opportunity to reach their full potential. Parents all too often complain that they have to produce the same information over and over again, and some begin to see assessment as a necessary evil to gain access to the services their child needs.

Activity 8.1

With another student or in a group, discuss and decide on your own definition of need, and what assessment you would use to identify need.

School age

As school age approaches assessment becomes increasingly important if children are to access an appropriate educational service. Before the 1970 Education Act children with disabilities could be classed as ineducable and therefore not entitled to schooling through the education system. The 1993 Education Act and code of practice built on the foundations of the 1981 Education Act, which maintained that schools should use their best endeavors to make provision for pupils with special educational needs. The code of practice came into force on 1 September 1994, and emphasized the importance of early identification and assessment for any child who might have a special educational need.

In practical terms many children who have severe learning disabilities will be identified as needing special education some time before they enter full-time education. Many now attend either specialist nursery schools, or ordinary nursery schools with extra staff. Minor problems are often identified in ordinary schools, and the children end by attending special schools and having statements of special educational need issued. The 1993 code of practice states: 'If it is decided that the child's needs are such that he or she will require a statement prior to entering primary school at 5, careful attention should be paid to the parents' views and to information available from the full range of assessment arrangements within all the relevant agencies making provision for young children with special needs'. All parents have difficult decisions to make: if your child has a learning disability they may seem endless. Which of the conflicting philosophies should they choose: integration or special education? Should the child enter mainstream school, which will give him the opportunity to mix with other children, but where he may lag behind and not get the attention he needs. If he goes to special school he could be labelled for the rest of his life. The reader may find it helpful to refer to Chapter 7 for a more comprehensive account of educational provision and accessing such services.

TRANSITION TO ADULT SERVICES

As with any child, children with statements of special educational need will remain in school up to the age of 16. After this time they may move on, for example to a college of further education or day centre, or could remain at school until their 19th birthday. The time leading up to school leaving is an important stage – much of adult life is shaped by what happens during this period. For people with learning disabilities this time has extra problems, because many have to rely on the multitude of different professionals to access the services they will need. The challenge to these professionals is to ensure that the transfer of information is accurate and timely.

The annual review of the statement becomes more significant after the young person's 14th birthday. Subsequent reviews should assist the services by developing a transitional plan that should pull together information from a wide range of individuals, including the young person and their family. Under section 5 of the 1986 Disabled Persons Act local education authorities must obtain an opinion from the social services department as to whether a child is or is not disabled, as part of the first annual review or assessment or reassessment after their 14th birthday. LEAs are required to notify social services departments 8 months before the date when a young person with a disability is likely to leave full-time education, and to keep this date under review. Social services departments are required to carry out a multidisciplinary assessment within 5 months of the LEA notification, unless the family do not want it.

The code of practice suggests the most important areas to be included in a transitional plan by the school:

- What will happen to enable the pupil to get the best out of the school before leaving?
- Which professionals will do what to ensure a smooth transition to adult services?
- What does the family feel about the future and what services should be provided?
- What does the young person want to do when they leave school?

Transitional plans should be a development of the previous annual reviews, and 'should focus on strengths as well as weaknesses and cover all aspects of the young person's development, allocating clear responsibility for different aspects of development to specific agencies and professionals'. These responsibilities will probably be focused on the school, and as the child becomes older the balance of responsibility will shift to outside agencies.

The careers service has an important role to play here, and a representative should be invited to the first and subsequent reviews after the child's 14th birthday. The code of practice suggests that the career service should provide 'continuing oversight of and information on the young person's choice of provision, and assist the local education authority and school in securing such provision and providing advice, counselling and support as appropriate'. However, the reality is that the more disabled people are, the more limited their choices will be. This tends to result in less input from the careers service, as a local authority day centre placement will probably be deemed more suitable.

The code of practice also makes clear that the young person's views should be obtained whenever possible. It suggests that the 'young person may wish to express his or her views through a trusted professional, family member, independent advocate or advisor'. The young person should also be involved on a regular basis in the annual review. Schools and other services should ensure the young person's full involvement in the decision making by 'information, careers guidance, counselling, work experience and the opportunity to consider a wide range of options'. The sentiment is fine, but putting it into practice is another thing; the real challenge to professionals is to ensure that all young people get the same opportunities no matter what their disability.

YOUNG ADULTS

Attempts to encourage employment of disabled people

After school all young people need time to adjust to their new environments, which for some will last for several years. If they do not go on to further education, then some form of employment is the expected goal of our society. However, obtaining employment often proves problematic for people with learning disabilities. Since 1919 social policy, through legislation, has been designed to help disabled people find employment (Topliss 1982). This was due, in part, to the large number of men who were disabled during the first world war. Training centres were set up, and a system to encourage firms to employ disabled ex-service men. The 1944 Disabled Persons [Employment] Act also aimed to help war victims, but entitled all adults of working age who were substantially handicapped by mental or physical disabilities to register for employment. It provided a quota system whereby employers of 20 or more workers were required to recruit 3% of their workforce from the registered disabled. In practice many employers ignored the quota, and in the early days often encouraged employees to register if they had some form of minor disability that did not affect them or their employer. These measures have never been particularly effective at getting disabled people to work.

Employment schemes

Employment is an important issue in anyone's life, and not just for financial reasons. Society still sees work as a central activity in adult life, and it is one of the major ways whereby individuals are valued, social status is measured and self-esteem influenced. Employers, however, quite naturally select people who will do a good day's work for a day's pay, and do not need support or careful supervision. Also, in the past some local trade unions did not look kindly on small payment schemes for supported placements for people with learning disabilities. Across the country there are many different employment projects to enable such people to access some form of working environment: sheltered workshops, specialized vocational college courses, and recreational and occupational projects. However, once again, access to these facilities depends on where you live, and in many areas little choice is offered.

One special scheme reported on by Beyers and Kilsby (1996), called 'supported employment', has helped some obtain jobs in the open market. The ethos of this scheme is based on the philosophy that anyone can hold down a job if enough attention is paid to finding the right job and provided the right level of training and support is given. Up until 1991 this scheme had helped some 1500 people find work.

Barriers to employment

Barriers to finding work are not only a result of the ways in which society views learning-disabled people, but also the way such people view themselves. Economics also play an important part, as taking a low-paid job, after taking into account expenses such as tax and travel, may well leave the person financially worse off. If a person loses their job the problem of reapplying for benefits also then exists to create anxiety. The Disability Working Allowance, introduced in 1992, was intended to overcome these difficulties. To qualify, the disabled person must work for at least 16 hours a week, and have recently received one of the disablement benefits, for example invalidity benefit or severe disablement allowance. The person's disability must also put them at a disadvantage in finding a job; they should also have less than £16,000 savings. However, good advice is necessary, as it may be better for the disabled person to stay on invalidity benefit and earn a 'therapeutic' wage.

ACCESS

Is it getting better?

The most literal form of access has not so far been considered. In recent years people with disabilities have become more outspoken in their quest for equal access to the most basic services, and in some cases have caused disruption by chaining themselves to buses, for example, in an attempt to bring to public notice their desire for equal opportunities. The many reports and Acts of Parliament have had little effect on improving access, especially for people with mobility difficulties.

The Chronically Sick and Disabled Persons Act of 1970 made provision for improving access in a number of ways. It required all property developers constructing new buildings or making major alterations to existing ones, to which the public have access, to give consideration to people with disabilities. The problem with such Acts is that they contain no mechanism for enforcement, and therefore, if after consideration it is decided that to make the building accessible for disabled people would be too costly or difficult, there is no way of compelling developers to do so. This Act also required local authorities to provide the 'orange badge' scheme to help parking for disabled people who drive or use a car regularly. Many authorities have also made special provision for car parking for disabled car users at amenities, although this varies from area to area. As discussed by Topliss (1982), there have been several reports and committees formed which have criticized the Act, but little action has been taken. The Silver Jubilee Committee made several recommendations on how to improve the performance of the Act, resulting in yet another committee called the Committee on Restrictions Against Disabled People, whose remit was to consider the whole issue of discrimination, whether intentional or not, that prevented the full participation of disabled people in community life.

Disability Discrimination Act (1995)

Although services have moved on since the 1970s when these committees were formed, it is not difficult to understand the frustration that has led to demonstrations and protests. It is perhaps through this pressure and political embarrassment that the 1995 Disability Discrimination Act received Royal Assent and became law. Some disability action groups have already dismissed it as another Act with little provision for enforcement, and it has been described by Valios (1996) as a 'toothless poodle'; however, history will show whether it will be effective at improving access to the facilities that the able-bodied currently enjoy.

LEGISLATION

Although there have been different types of legislation throughout this century that have affected disabled people, only the more significant Acts will be considered here. This is in addition to those that have already been mentioned.

The 1948 National Assistance Act

The 1948 National Assistance Act had a profound influence on the way services were delivered to people with disabilities. The Act defined who disabled people were and the types of housing and services the local authority should provide. Local authorities were also charged with a duty to maintain a register of disabled people. However, this was voluntary and therefore did not show the true number of people with disabilities, or the nature of their needs.

The 1970 Chronically Sick and Disabled Persons Act

The 1970 Chronically Sick and Disabled Persons Act made it a statutory duty for local authorities to inform themselves about the disabled people in their area and their needs. However, for want of a clear definition of disability, and because the procedures identified for this duty were so vague, few local authorities carried out a comprehensive survey. In 1980 the number of people on the local authority registers was estimated at only 119 800, many of whom were elderly. A report in 1971 estimated the figure to be nearer 3 million, although Townsend's (1984) survey of a sample of households produced a figure of around 9 million. With such a wide variation how is it possible to estimate the real level of services needed and therefore the true budget requirements?

This Act made it a duty of local authorities not only to provide services, but to publicize them, so that disabled people would be enabled to lead a fuller life in the community. Social services could provide aids and adaptations for disabled people living at home, varying from simple things such as a special telephone, to more com-plex, for example a building extension. It should be noted that the recipient may have had to meet part of any incurred costs. Other services included home helps, and holiday and day centre provision. The Act also provided for increased access to public places, even if this was ineffectual.

When the Act came into force there was a feeling of optimism that it would significantly improve the lot of disabled people. Unfortunately, its implementation has been fragmented and patchy and many of these services have been vulnerable to cuts. Indeed, as public spending in the 1970s was reduced because of the economic climate, this led to some local authorities being unable to meet even their statutory duties.

The 1986 Disabled Persons [Service, Representative and Consultation] Act

This Act gave local authorities a duty to assess people for services that might be available to them under the Chronically Sick and Disabled Act. It required that an authority must be asked by a disabled person or their representative to complete an assessment, and defined who could be the authorized representative of a disabled person. It also gave powers to local authorities to appoint a representative if a person appeared to them to 'be unable to represent themselves by reason of any physical or mental incapacity.' This part of the Act has not been implemented.

When an assessment is carried out it should look not only at the needs of the disabled person but also those of the carers. The assessment must be in writing and include a statement of what services are suggested to meet any needs identified. If a local authority cannot or will not meet these identified needs, an explanation must be given; there is also an inbuilt right to have a decision reviewed. The assessment process was extended to include any disabled person who was leaving full-time special education.

This Act also required local authorities to inform disabled people of services available to them, either provided by the local authority or by other agencies, which may be voluntary or statutory and outside the immediate area. It also required the Secretary of State to lay before Parliament a report on the development of services for people with disabilities or mental health problems. This also was not implemented. Many parts of this Act were superseded by the legislative changes of the 1990s.

The 1989 Children Act

The 1989 Children Act brought together much of the legislation relating to children and established a new way for social service departments to work with children. Any provision in the Act does not stand alone and must be considered within a wider context of provision for all children. Safeguards were included for children with disabilities, which included having to review cases of children living away from home, consideration given to a child's welfare, and consulting with parents and children before decisions are made. Another basic tenet of the Act was the introduction of a partnership principle between the parent, child and the services. It might be thought that the above should have already been in place, but in some areas it was customary to make plans for children with disabilities and only then inform the parents. The Guidance and Regulations Volume 6: Children with Disabilities (DOH 1991) identified five basic points concerning working with families:

- The family home is the natural and most appropriate place for the majority of children.
- Families are already caring for children, and supporting them to do so is, in most cases, in the best interests of the child and best allocation of resources.
- Children are individuals with their own needs, wishes and feelings.
- The family has a unique and special knowledge of a child, and can therefore contribute significantly to that child's health and development – albeit often in partnership with a range of service providers.
- Families provide continuity for children throughout their childhood, and, in the context of the Children Act, families are

recognized as being more widely defined than parents and brothers and sisters. Other relatives often play an important part in the life of a child.

The Act identified a number of responsibilities for social service departments. For example, Schedule 2 paragraph 2 required a local authority to open and maintain a register of children with disabilities; this has been implemented in a variety of ways around the country. However, agreeing to be placed on a register is voluntary, and services are not dependent on being registered. The main aim was for the register to be a planning tool. Also in Schedule 2, paragraph 3 was a requirement that a the local authority should provide services that were designed to minimize the effect of the disability, thus enabling the child to lead a life which was as 'normal as possible'. Unfortunately, the Act gave little guidance on what such provision should be, or how much should be available. The Act also gave power to local authorities to undertake an assessment of the child's needs in conjunction with other assessments required under other Acts, such as the 1981 Education Act, the 1986 Disabled Persons Act and the 1970 Chronically Sick and Disabled Persons Act.

After the child's needs had been assessed, a plan of the best service provision was to be made. When these services are to be either provided or paid for by a social services department, the plan must include 'an estimate of how long the service may be required, what the objectives of the service should be and what else others are expected to do' (Children Act 1989). The Act and guidance notes make it clear that there is an expectation for all service provision to be made in partnership with the child and family. Furthermore, whichever organization provides the services they should be coordinated by the social services department.

This Act, along with the guidance notes, also specified that where the family have other children their needs should also be considered. It might be necessary for brothers and sisters to have separate assessments carried out.

Much of the Act was welcomed by professionals, but although some additional funding was provided by central Government, some would argue that too little has been available to implement the Act fully. Social services, health, education and voluntary agencies are even now still trying to implement some of the changes brought about by the Act, and some social services departments are left in the unenviable position of having to prioritize and deal with child protection cases first. Clearly, this leaves few resources to meet the demand for services for children with disabilities.

The 1990 NHS and Community Care Act

This Act was introduced in response to reports by Griffiths (1988) and the White Papers *Caring for People* and *Working for Patients* (see the Appendix for an overview of legislation policies and reports), which made recommendations on how health and social care should be provided. The Government had decided that the reforms were necessary for many reasons, but one of the main considerations was the continuing rising cost of care, especially long-term care. The four main reasons stated by the Government for the changes were:

- To make the best use of public money
- To encourage authorities to set priorities
- To ensure that local authorities check on the quality of care which is being provided
- To encourage local authorities to use other organizations to provide services (Meridith 1995).

With these aims, the Government focused on ensuring that taxpayers' money should be spent on only those actually in need, while recognizing that there will never be enough resources to cover everything.

Objectives of the Act

The White Paper *Caring in the Community*, in paragraph 1.12, introduced six key objectives. These were to:

- promote the development of domiciliary, day and respite services to enable people to live in their own homes wherever feasible and sensible
- ensure that service providers make practical support for carers a high priority
- make proper assessment of need and good case management the cornerstone of high-quality care
- promote the development of a flourishing independent sector alongside good-quality public services
- clarify the responsibilities of agencies and so make it easier to hold them to account for their performances
- provide value for money.

It was also proposed to set up new systems for complaints against local authority social services departments.

Duties, powers and responsibilities

By changing the law, the Act allowed the recommendations within the White Paper to be achieved. It gave local authorities the required powers and duties. Duties are those things that must be done by the local authority; however, quantity is not included in the Act, and the proviso 'within available resources' is usually included. Powers are given to local authorities to provide a service if they are able to, but they do not necessarily have to.

The responsibilities of local social services departments include:

- Carrying out assessments of an individual's need for social care. This includes working with health professionals to consider all options, including residential and nursing home care, before deciding which services will be provided. A case manager should design a package of care to meet assessed needs. The social services department should become an 'enabling authority' to purchase and contract for services, and not simply act as a direct provider.
- Identifying procedures for receiving

comments and complaints from service users

- When appropriate, receiving advice from health professionals to monitor the quality of services
- Assessing the client's ability to contribute to the cost of the service they will receive.

The Government believed that, in order to undertake these new responsibilities, local social services departments would have to strengthen their management systems, especially in planning, financial, purchasing and quality control. Staff training was also an area that was identified as needing careful consideration, as staff roles would change fundamentally.

CARE IN THE COMMUNITY

What is care in the community?

Confusion often arises concerning the subject of *care in the community* and *community care*. Are they the same, and if not, what is the difference? The community has always provided care of one form or another, although large institutions are now recognized as providing inadequate care. Arguments against institutions include the tendency for the needs of the system to take precedence over the needs of the individual. There is also a tendency for the system to be authoritarian, leaving residents feeling inadequate and more dependent. This type of care often takes people away from their own community and could carry a stigma; however, it must be said that these negative effects can also be a feature of other types of care provision.

Care in the community defined

Care in the community may be in hostels, group homes, or institutions such as hospitals. *Care by the community* is an optimistic concept that rests on a possibly false assumption that the community is prepared to provide care and support for disabled and needy people. The Barclay Report (1982) recognized that the 'bulk of social care is carried out not by statutory or voluntary agen-cies, but by ordinary people. In many cases this, in reality, means women at home becoming responsible for caring without pay, training or support'.

Care by the community requires careful assessment of need and a planned and coordinated network of services to make it a realistic possibility. This will not necessarily make this type of care a cheaper option.

Care in the community has been defined by the Social Services Select Committee (HC13 1984/5) as meaning:

- Enabling an individual to remain in his or her own home wherever possible, rather than being cared for in hospital or residential homes
- Giving support and relief to informal carers (family, friends and neighbours) coping with the stress of caring for a dependent person
- Minimizing disruption to ordinary living
- Providing the most cost-effective package of services to meet the needs of those being helped
- Integrating all the resources of a geographical area in order to support the individuals within it. The resources might include informal carers, NHS and personal social services and organized voluntary effort, but also sheltered housing, the local social security office, the church, local clubs etc.

ASSESSMENT

Assessment as a tool to access service provision

Like the 1989 Children Act, the 1990 NHS and Community Care Act required an assessment of individual need to ensure access to service provision. The legislation and guidance from Government intended that social services departments should adopt the leading role, but working closely with health services according to the health needs of the client. Some felt that this legislation would help them to get more services in their local area, because if an individual's needs had been assessed and required a service, then the authorities would have to provide that service. However, right from the beginning the Government's agenda appeared somewhat transparent:

Assessments will therefore have to be made against a background of stated objectives and priorities determined by the local authority. Decisions on service provision will have to take account of what is available and affordable (Newsletter in November 1989).

Within the context of this statement the emphasis in any assessment shifts from establishing needs and deciding what services are required to the services that are available, and how much can be spent for that person. In some cases the presenting problems are not sufficient to warrant the time and expense of an assessment.

Assessment under the 1990 NHS and Community Care Act

The Act and guidance placed the responsibility for defining the assessment process they would use on local authorities. They were also required to monitor the outcomes of the assessment procedures, as they would have implications in the future planning of services. Local authorities were also given the task of defining a person's needs. The summary of practice guidance defined need as 'the shorthand for the requirements of individuals to enable them to achieve, maintain or restore an acceptable level of social independence or quality of life, as defined by the particular care agency or authority' (paragraph 11).

As with any definition there is a risk that any part, or even single words, of it may be interpreted differently, as the definitions are open to individuals' personal values, attitudes and perceptions. Clearly, this leaves the way people access services open to the possibility of wide variation around the country. Not all authorities have the same definitions or criteria to identify an individual's needs. Not surprisingly, this means that there is not even uniformity in determining whether an assessment of needs is necessary.

HOW THE 1990 NHS AND COMMUNITY CARE ACT HAS BEEN IMPLEMENTED

Case history: two geographical areas, before and after implementing the Act

Before the Act both these areas worked in a similar way: both had multiagency teams working with people with learning disabilities. The teams covered similar geographical areas, comprising a mixture of urban and rural locations. Both of the teams had open referral systems, and each used a referral meeting to allocate work to the most appropriate professional from the team. An initial visit would then be made to the identified person and an assessment completed to find out the presenting problems, and any other relevant background information. This would then be taken back to a team meeting for discussion. If the initial decision of the allocated professional was correct, this person would become the key worker to implement any ongoing schemes. This often included help in accessing services, sorting out benefits, behaviour management, training programmes and many other areas of intervention to help the person with learning disabilities.

Since implementation of the Act the two teams work in very different ways. Following agreement between the local health and social services departments, the first team agreed that all members should take part in care management training. This enabled all the team to carry out community care assessments, which would then be sent to the team manager (the care manager), who would make the decision about funding. In this way the team has managed to continue working in a similar pattern. In the second team only social workers were allowed to undertake such training, and they now occupy positions as assessment officers and care managers. The vast portion of their work is now purely assessment and any decision about funding services is carried out at the local area office. This has caused the team to review the way it works; it also considered disbanding the team by withdrawing the social workers back into their local area office. The possibility of breaking up a team which has helped to develop many local services is a difficulty local social services and health departments need to address, but it may be a result of the authorities trying to define what is health care and what social care. The Audit Commission (1992) has identified the importance of agreement at local level in defining health and social care, as failure to do so will lead to difficulties when individual care packages are being created.

This brief case history illustrates how two areas differ in how they have interpreted the Act, but how effective has the Act been at achieving the Government's aims? Has there been an improvement in getting services to the most needy? This is a difficult question to answer. As Meridith (1995) has explained when the Act was introduced 'there was no national standard for implementation', and as a result of this 'local authorities have used many different ways to bring about the reforms' (Meridith 1995). Meridith also points out the difficulties in measuring improvement, as before the reforms, 'there was little baseline information about the provision of services'.

Has the Act improved access?

Smith (1996), in the third Audit Commission bulletin on community care, has reported that the majority of local authorities have overspent on community services by 7% compared to the Government's 1995/96 limits. With the limitations on community care funding it has been suggested that local authorities should devise ways of prioritizing who qualifies for care and at what level. Eligibility criteria should be used to translate these priorities into a working tool. The criteria need to be 'simple and flexible on the one hand, and complex and precise on the other', and according to Department of Health recommendations they should be published in community care plans. The bulletin points out that many local authorities are finding this a problematic area to deal with. Some authorities, because of financial difficulties, have to adjust the criteria as the financial year progresses. This adds to the geographical variations in eligibility criteria, assessment systems and service provision. Chris Vellenoweth of NAHAT (National Association of

Activity 8.2

Use the library to find out what the 'Oregon Experiment' is. Could a similar system be used to prioritize need in this country and, if so, who should receive services?

Health Authorities and Trusts) (Caring Times 1996) emphasized this when speaking at a recent conference: he said, 'There is no unanimity of view among local authorities as to what constitutes a referral nor yet what constitutes an assessment'. With statements like this from the Government's own department it is perhaps hard to see where improvements can have occurred.

CONCLUSION

Access to children's services

Access to services is affected by a multiplicity of factors, as has been demonstrated throughout this chapter. Why this should be so is a question that causes considerable debate. When age is the criterion we can argue that a child should be seen as a child first, any disability being a problem that services should adapt to. Their difficulties should also be considered in the context of their family, and it should be remembered that parents will most usually be the child's most fervent advocates. When the child becomes an adult the parents may continue to have a great influence, as many continue to live with their parents for much longer than was the case in the past. Professionals may on occasions find themselves in conflict with parents as they try to ensure that the person with a disability achieves their full potential. The conflict may be about where they want to live, or relationships they may wish to have. When parents refuse to give their consent this in many cases denies access, because the adult with learning disabilities has often relied completely on their parents to access services for them. The challenge, therefore, is to help the adult with learning disabilities to access services in their own right, and if possible to help the family adjust to the new situation, over which they have less control. Counselling may be needed by the parents at different stages in their lives to help them adjust to the changing needs of their children.

As children grow and develop most families worry about their need to become more independent (Roper et al 1990), and their own inability to protect them from the ups and downs of life. It is unfortunate that society continues to perpetuate the myth that people with learning disabilities never grow up, and although adult in size they remain childlike and in need of protection.

Variations in access and provision

Access to services is also influenced by place of residence, and there is a great variety in service provision around the country. This is due to many factors: for example the services the area had before the policy of closing hospitals, and later the NHS and Community Care Act; how strong parents' groups in the area are; what voluntary support groups there are; and how the local authorities and health service work together and the priorities they set. Perhaps even more important than any of the above is how densely populated the area is. An urban area may have more services but there will be competition for places. In a rural area the services may be fewer and access more difficult because of transport difficulties; for example, some children in Lincolnshire have to travel for over an hour to get to their special school.

Who decides?

The difficulty is to decide whose need is greatest. This is problematic in services as diverse as special care beds for neonates, heart transplantation, support groups for families of children with a disability, or a place in a day centre for people with learning disabilities. Which of these should be funded? Whose need is greatest? How do we ensure that everyone has equal access to the services provided?

Access to services is controlled by health purchasers and social services departments. Therefore, it follows that these key players have to decide what they will pay for. Health authorities were required, by April 1996, to provide the Department of Health with criteria according to which patients will be entitled to long-term care provided by the health service. Any one who is not so eligible will have to apply to the local social services department for help, and this will be means tested. This will inevitably lead to different health authorities having different access criteria for funding, and to arguments between authorities about who will pay for services.

These problems have existed for some time, though at present, with budgets under threat, they are exacerbated and there is the possibility that some clients will fall through the care net. Coordination must therefore be a high priority for any professional working in the caring services. Discussions should be about the suitability of a service to meet a need, rather than who should fund it. Nurses will be involved in these discussions, advocating for their clients, and this role will on occasions bring them into conflict with their employers; this is not a comfortable position to be in (Gates 1994). The UKCC Code of Professional Conduct (UKCC 1992) helps in this situation, as the first few lines stress that the best interests of the individual should always be the nurse's primary consideration: 'Each registered nurse, midwife and health visitor shall act, at all times, in such a manner as to: safeguard and promote the interests of the individual and clients' (UKCC 1992).

The 1990 NHS and Community Care Act attempted to address some of these problems

Activity 8.3

With their permission, interview two sets of parents. The first set should have a child under the age of 10; the second set should have a son or daughter over the age of 30. Compare and contrast the services they have been offered and how easy or difficult it was for them to access those services. NOTE: This activity has to be handled with sensitivity, and advice should be taken from professionals to find out which families may agree to taking part. Confidentiality has also to be considered a priority.

and based services on a needs-led system; however, the resources available are finite. Access to services is, then, dependent on what is available in the area, and how many users there are; this is when prioritization becomes all-important to the person trying to access a service, as health purchasers and social services departments have to balance the many and varied needs of the whole community.

The last words of this chapter are reserved for a parent who has a child with learning difficulties. Johnson (1995) has written:

Valuable resources will continue to be wasted until agencies providing community care set up a network system that competently services those who need it. Agencies must work in unison. Professionals need to realise how valuable carers are and how much they have to offer.

REFERENCES

Audit Commission 1992 Making a reality of community care. HMSO, London

Barclay Report 1982 National Institute for Social Work Training. Social workers: their role and tasks. Bedford Square Press, London

Beyers S, Kilsby M 1996 A good job, independent living, community care. Reed Business Publishing, Sutton.

Caring Times Incorporating Care Concern, 1996 No place for rigid rules, Hawker Publications, London

Department of Education 1994 Code of practice on the identification and assessment of special educational need. HMSO, London

DHSS 1978 Helping mentally handicapped people in hospital. A report by the National Development Group for the Mentally Handicapped. DHSS, London

DOH 1989 Caring for people, community care in the next decade and beyond (White Paper). HMSO, London

DOH 1990 National Health Service and Community Care Act. HMSO, London

DOH 1991 The Children Act 1989 Guidance and Regulations, Volume 4. Children with disabilities. HMSO, London

DOH 1991 The 1989 Children Act: Guidance and regulations, Volume 6. Children with disabilities. HMSO, London

Gates B 1994 Advocacy: a nurses' guide. Scutari Press, Middlesex

Griffiths R 1988 Community care: an agenda for action. HMSO, London

Henderson V 1969 The basic principles of nursing care. International Council of Nurses, Geneva

Johnson M 1995 Lone voice, community care. Reed Business Publishing, Sutton

Jones I H 1989 Helping hands. Macmillan Education, Basingstoke

Jupp S 1992 Making the right start. Open Eye Publications, Godly

Meridith B 1995 The community care handbook: the reformed system explained. Age Concern, London

Miller N B 1994 Nobody's perfect: living and growing with children who have special needs. Brooks Publishing, Baltimore

Robinson L 1991 Home and away: respite care in the community. Venture Press, Birmingham

Roper N, Logan W, Tierney A 1990 The elements of nursing. Churchill Livingstone, Edinburgh

Smith N 1996 Care home briefing: balancing the care equation: progress with community care. Croner Publications, Kingston upon Thames

Social Services Select Committee 1984/85 Care in the community. Health Circular 13, HMSO, London

Topliss E 1982 Social responses to handicap. Longman, Harlow

Townsend P 1984 Poverty in the United Kingdom: Social Trends. Central Statistical Office, London

UKCC 1992 Code of professional conduct for the nurse, midwife and health visitor, 3rd edn. UKCC, London

Valios N 1996 Community care: challenges likely as new law fails disabled people. Reed Business Publications, Sutton

Behavioural difficulties

9

B. Gates

INTRODUCTION

In the field of learning difficulties, there can be no area which so profoundly challenges our assumptions, beliefs and value systems, as the planning and providing for those individuals who confront us with desperate, destructive and self injurious behaviours (Myers 1995).

These wise words of Mary Myers make an admirable introduction to this chapter, which is concerned with those people with learning disabilities who demonstrate some form of behavioural difficulty. This may manifest itself as being aggressive, abusive or destructive, and may be directed inwardly to the person themselves, or outwardly to others or the environment. The cause of such behaviour may be multifactorial and may be explained from a number of differing theoretical perspectives. Either way, the manifestations of behavioural difficulties present a challenge to commissioners and purchasers of services, as well as care practitioners, whether they be nurses or another professional group. Behavioural difficulties may be found in both children and adults who have learning disabilities, and not surprisingly this may have a tremendous impact upon the family (Qureshi 1993, Russell 1995, Gates & Wray 1995). Clearly, along with a theoretical account of the nature of behavioural difficulties, it is necessary for the reader to see how to manage such behaviours.

Defining behavioural difficulties

A necessary starting point for this chapter concerns the nurse being able to adequately define the meaning of the term behavioural difficulties (Gates 1996, Slavin 1995). Some might argue that the use of the term is unacceptable because of the potentially negative image it portrays; this is interesting, because whatever term is used, this area is extremely sensitive to the overtones of political correctness. Therefore, many professionals use an alternative term, challenging behaviour, which itself is not without its problems. Blunden and Allen (1987) have said:

The term challenging behaviour is used to emphasise the fact that the issue is a challenge to those who provide services, and to the rest of society, not just a problem carried around by the individual. The challenge is ours to find effective ways of helping people to behave and express themselves in ways which are acceptable to society (Blunden & Allen 1987).

In a relatively recent report from the Department of Health (DoH 1992) it was said:

People with learning disabilities who have challenging behaviour form an extremely diverse group, including individuals with all levels of learning disability, many sensory or physical impairments and presenting quite different kinds of challenges. The group includes, for example, people with mild or borderline learning disability who have been diagnosed as mentally ill and who enter the criminal justice system for crimes such as arson or sexual offences; as well as people with profound learning disability, often with sensory handicaps and other physical health problems, who injure themselves, for example by repeated head banging or eye poking (DoH 1992).

Emerson et al (1988) have said:

Severely challenging behaviour is behaviour of such intensity, frequency or duration that the physical safety of the person or others is placed in serious jeopardy, or behaviour which is likely to seriously limit or deny access to the use of ordinary community facilities (Emerson et al 1988).

It would appear that definitions of challenging behaviours may be grouped into two categories. The first of these uses the term to identify a collection of behaviours and a state of being that challenges both purchasers, commissioners and providers of services. The second appears to be reserved to refer to people who present with behavioural difficulties. The use of the term is therefore particularly problematic because it

means different things to different people. Clearly, the implications of this are particularly important to providers and purchasers of health care, where the management of challenging behaviour predominantly rests. This point has been made by Clifton and Brown (1993), who suggested that the term challenging behaviour had become so general that in practice a wide variety of definitions were being used, and that this would be particularly unhelpful when a purchaser sought to provide training to meet clients' specific needs. In addition to this there is an issue here concerning confusion between providers and purchasers about services for people with challenging behaviour. A provider might offer a service that included provision for people with profound learning disabilities with additional sensory and motor disability, whereas the purchaser might think they were buying services for people with behavioural difficulties. Evidently it is important that healthcare professionals speak the same language, and are clear about what they are referring to. This chapter is concerned with the broad range of behavioural difficulties that comprise one or more of the following:

- Violence and destructiveness
- Antisocial behaviour
- Rebelliousness
- Untrustworthiness
- Withdrawal
- Stereotyped behaviour and odd mannerisms
- Inappropriate interpersonal manners
- Unacceptable or eccentric habits
- Self-abusive behaviour
- Hyperactive tendencies
- Sexually aberrant behaviour and psychological disturbances.

These domains are those identified in the American Association for Mental Retardation's Adaptive Behaviour Scale (Nihira et al 1993). This is based upon an extensive survey of the social expectations placed upon people with learning disabilities in both residential and community settings. Extensive research on reliability has been undertaken on this scale, including internal consistency, stability, reliability and interscorer reliability; the authors also report on content, criterion and construct validity (Nihira et al 1993). Issues of reliability and validity of measurement are extremely important to nurse practitioners and/or researchers because they enable them, with some confidence, to be clear about the degree of 'trust' they can place in the data generated. However, a caveat to this statement is a need for caution because of a number of threats to and tensions associated with the measurement of behavioural difficulties.

Incidence and prevalence

It must be said at the outset that it has been estimated that people with learning disabilities are more likely to present with behavioural difficulties than others in the population (Qureshi 1994), although this assertion will be discussed in detail later. Also, there appears to be some agreement that behavioural difficulties in a child tend to improve as the child develops (Qureshi 1994). It would also appear that males are more likely than females to present with behavioural difficulties (Duker et al 1986). Whether this difference between the sexes may be explained by cultural expectations of male behaviour, or by biological factors, is not well understood. According to the Office of Population and Censuses Survey concerning the 97 000 children under the age of 16 with learning disabilities, (OPCS 1989) the proportion of children with behavioural difficulties is estimated to be higher than in the rest of the population (Saxby & Morgan 1993). Quine (1986) studied a sample of 200 children aged 5–18 years of age with learning disabilities and identified a range of behavioural difficulties. These included:

- Attention seeking   29%
- Overactivity   21%
- Tempter tantrums   25%
- Aggressiveness   21%
- Screaming   22%
- Wandering off   18%
- Destructiveness   14%
- Self-injurious behaviour   12%.

Evidently behavioural difficulties are common in children with learning disabilities, and this can be a major source of parental stress (Quine & Pahl 1985) with parents reporting a sense of powerlessness and lack of support in their problems. Concerning adults with learning disabilities, Mansell (DoH 1992) has suggested that between 25 and 50% have additional mental health needs, 12–15% have significant impairment of sight, 8–20% have impaired hearing and at least 50% have significant impairments of communication or social ability. His report calculated that 20 per 100 000 total population of adults with a learning disability present a significant challenge.

The prevalence of behavioural difficulties in learning disability is calculated on the basis of measurement, and there is considerable scepticism concerning the reliability and validity of claims concerning prevalence. For example, Kiernan and Moss (1990) found that 40% of people with learning disabilities at a large hospital exhibited moderate or severe behavioural difficulties. How appropriate the use of such a measurement is to other settings is debatable: there is an issue here of ecological validity, i.e. the generalizability of findings to other settings.

Theoretical explanations for behavioural difficulties

One of the most fascinating and challenging areas of enquiry concerning behavioural difficulty is its causation. This is especially so because, depending upon one's theoretical explanation of behaviour, there may be a prescribed solution to the correction of behavioural difficul-

 Activity 9.1

Spend some time reflecting on your experiences of working with people with learning disabilities. Did a significant number of these people have behavioural difficulties? Do you feel that the people you worked with formed a representative sample of people with learning disabilities? Do you think that the number of people you encountered with behavioural difficulties was greater than in the wider population of people you have encountered?

ties. For example, if it is believed that the cause of behavioural difficulties is biological, then curing the biological malady might correct the behaviour. Unfortunately, causation cannot be explained so simply. Behaviour is a manifestation of the unique interactions of a person with his or her environment. This person comprises a number of dimensions, and hence their behaviour is affected by emotional, spiritual, intellectual, biological, political and/or educational factors (Gates & Beacock 1996).

Biological explanations

The cause of severe learning disabilities can often be traced to some form of genetic or chromosomal aberration. Two classic causes of learning disability that have a very clear relationship with behavioural difficulties are Prader–Willi syndrome and Lesch–Nyhan syndrome. Both of these conditions are extremely rare. It is thought that all those affected with Lesch–Nyhan syndrome will present with self-injurious behaviour, including biting the lips and hands (Christie et al 1982). A particular problem in those with Prader–Willi syndrome is overeating, which often requires carers to keep food well away from affected individuals. There are other manifestations of learning disability where it would appear that there is an increased prevalence of behavioural difficulties, and these include epilepsy (particularly temporal lobe), mental health problems, phenylketonuria and autism. However, it is not clear whether the behavioural difficulties found in this second category are really the result of a biological abnormality, or of some other factor. It has become increasingly popular in recent years to reject biological explanations for behavioural difficulties, but there is growing evidence that a biological explanation can provide valuable insights into some of the causes. Readers are advised to refer to Oliver (1993).

Behavioural explanations

Behaviour, in part, originates from the things we learn during our development. From our earliest days we are reinforced either negatively or positively for particular behaviours that are thought by our carers to be either undesirable or desirable. For example, smiling, laughing and being kind are all thought to be desirable behaviours in our society, and therefore tend to be reinforced positively, for example by parents saying such things as 'You are a good boy for drying up the dishes', or 'You are a good girl for helping daddy in the garden'. The likelihood of the behaviour recurring is thereby increased. Conversely, one also hears remarks such as 'You naughty girl, you must not punch Thomas like that', or 'You really are a very unkind little boy, can't you see that you have hurt Jane's feelings?' It is suggested that because the child is denied the positive reinforcement of parental approval (i.e. negative reinforcement) and has to cope with disapproval, they will seek to avoid such behaviour in the future. There is evidence that behavioural difficulties in learning disability are learnt and reinforced through this process. Sometimes undesirable behaviours are unwittingly reinforced by parents or carers. For example, Lovaas et al (1965) found that responding to self-injurious behaviour in kind and gentle ways brought about an increase in the frequency of such behaviour.

Evidently, if behaviours can be learnt they can also be unlearnt, and this is where behavioural approaches may be particularly useful (see following sections).

Environmental explanations

Having looked at biological and behavioural explanations for behavioural difficulties, this final section will briefly explore how people's environment may also affect their behaviour. It would be difficult to sustain an argument that rejected the environment as having nothing to do with our behaviour. From the moment of our conception we begin to interact with our environment, and as we develop some of us learn to manipulate certain aspects of that environment. However, for some people the environment effectively controls them; this was the case in the old long-stay learning disability hospitals. At the end of the last century and the beginning of this our society saw an unprecedented increase in the building of asylums. Originally these were built to humanely segregate people with learning disabilities from society. However, as time progressed overcrowding, lack of resources, poor staff morale and a range of other factors led to a crisis in these hospitals (see Chapters 1 and 3). In effect, they ceased to be asylums and instead became environments of abuse – not deliberately, but as a result of years of neglect and desensitization to the effects of such environments on people with learning disabilities. A whole generation of such people grew up in environments that were the antithesis of 'ordinary living'. It is not therefore surprising that they failed to learn how to live ordinarily.

DIFFERENT APPROACHES TO THE MANAGEMENT OF BEHAVIOURAL DIFFICULTIES

In the literature on learning disability a range of non-chemical approaches are advocated in the management of behavioural difficulties. This section will briefly explore two very different approaches: behaviour modification and gentle teaching. It is suggested that these represent the extreme ends of a continuum of theoretical positions and their attendant practical application. At one end lies the theory that all behaviour is learned in response to the reinforcing properties of the environment; that behaviour must be observable and therefore measurable; that behaviour is the central focus and there is a downplaying concerning feelings and the nature of self. At the other end of the continuum lies the humanistic theory that the person is of central interest; that the quest for fulfilment and self-actualization is important; that subjectivity is more important than objectivity; and that great value is placed upon the integrity and uniqueness of the person. Each of these perspectives is very briefly explored before the practical application of behaviourism is considered.

Behaviour modification

This is a collection of therapeutic techniques based on learning theory. In the context of learning disability, most behavioural interventions operate according to the principles of operant conditioning, which involves the manipulation of behaviour through the systematic application of rewards or punishments. As a general therapeutic strategy behaviour modification is thoroughly investigated and well supported in the literature (Yule & Carr 1987). In the field of learning disability this approach forms the core of much teaching and instruction, particularly in teaching self-care skills to the more profoundly disabled person. Behaviour modification techniques have been used successfully in home settings to manage behavioural difficulties of children both with and without learning disabilities (Sehult 1985).

Gentle teaching

This is an approach of being with people with learning disabilities as well as helping those who also exhibit behavioural difficulties. Its use has increased in popularity over recent years, particularly among nurses, psychologists and occupational therapists (Jones & Connell 1993). The aim and specific focus of gentle teaching is not only on eradicating unwanted behaviours, but also on promoting meaningful 'complex dyadic interactions' between the person and their carers (McGee 1990, 1992). The general philosophical approach of gentle teaching claims to emphasize the intrinsic worth of the person more than that of behaviour modification. In this context, all the strategies used are non-aversive and seek to develop a bond between the individuals concerned. For a full account of gentle teaching see McGee et al (1987).

A psychological approach

There are a number of ways of identifying behavioural difficulties in order to work with the individual or their carer to bring about more desirable behaviour. One such approach is known as functional analysis. This has been defined as an attempt to understand the relationship between the various stimuli from the environment and the reinforcement or maintenance of behavioural difficulties. This is probably best understood as a process whereby an assessment measures and records behaviours and also takes into account the antecedents and consequences of those behaviours.

- **Antecedents** Here, carers, nurses or parents are required to retrospectively account for those factors that occurred immediately prior to an episode of behavioural difficulty. Factors of interest are the time of occurrence, people in the vicinity, location – in fact, any variable that might partly or fully account for the subsequent behaviour of an individual.
- **Behaviour** Here the carers, nurses or parents are required to retrospectively account for the manifestation of the behaviour. It is important that the behaviour is described in precise terms that are both accurate and complete. Therefore, the frequency, intensity and duration of the behaviour are important. So too is the topography of the behaviour: recalling exactly how a behaviour manifested itself is more difficult than might be imagined.
- **Consequences** Finally, the carers, nurses or parents are required to retrospectively record the consequences of the behaviour. This part of the functional analysis is vitally important, as it helps in determining either partly or fully the possible function of the behaviour. Figure 9.1 shows an example of an ABC chart for an individual who has presented with behavioural difficulties. The examples given represent the *antecedents*, i.e. events prior to the *behaviour*, followed by the *consequences* of that behaviour on the person and/or carers involved.

Evidently, functional analysis depends on observation and measurement: the nurse or carer is attempting to observe and undertake some form of measurement of a particular phenomenon and, not surprisingly, this is not without its problems. Some of the issues affecting measurement are outlined in the next section. However, it is important to acknowledge that functional analysis is more than simply completing a chart (see Activity 9.2): it is concerned with understanding the function or functions of a behaviour. This implies a need for careful assessment of a whole range of factors that may directly or indirectly affect a person's behaviour, and may include such diverse variables as constitution, medication, diet, genetic predisposition, childhood trauma, or indeed anything in an individual's past or present. For a comprehensive overview of this approach refer to Emerson (1993).

Measurement

Three methods of measurement are advocated in the literature (see, for example, Yule & Carr 1987, Iwata et al 1990). These are indirect, descriptive and experimental.

Observation time	Antecedents	Behaviours	Consequences
19.05	Mary's mother prevented Mary from pinching her sister Emily	Mary began screaming and banging her head with her fists	Mary's mother became very distressed by Mary's behaviour and gave her a cuddle
19.10	Mary's mother prevents her from taking a biscuit out of the biscuit barrel in the kitchen	Mary commences biting her hands and rocking back and forth whilst banging her head on the wall	Mary strikes out and hits her mother and continues with her behaviour
19.15	Mary's mother puts on her favourite music tape	Mary sits quietly, having eventually relaxed	Mary's mother tells Emily to stay well away from Mary because she is quiet and she doesn't want her annoyed

Figure 9.1   An ABC chart of the behaviour of Mary and family members.

Activity 9.2

Spend some time looking at the ABC chart for Mary. What sort of conclusions might you draw from these observations? Is there enough information for the nurse to devise an intervention? Do you think the ABC chart provides enough breadth of detail to devise therapeutic interventions?

- **Indirect** This style is probably the simplest approach used to obtain data. Carers are interviewed by a nurse or researcher concerning the frequency or absence of a predetermined list of behaviours. Such an approach is clearly dependent upon the carer being able to answer the questions posed, and also having sufficient knowledge of the subject to answer fully and reliably.

- **Descriptive** This is a more objective approach undertaken through systematic analysis of behaviour following naturalistic observation. This is achieved by developing interval-based observation procedures, gathering objective data and calculating for interobserver reliability. Although time-consuming, Iwata et al (1990) have stated that the descriptive approach is superior because it is more objective than verbal reports, and that as it is quantitative it allows for correlation calculation between variables. Lastly, it is thought to be superior because observation is conducted in a natural environment, where a wide range of events can be observed and studied.

- **Experimental** In a sense this is a very pure form of functional analysis, where the person with a behavioural difficulty is observed in a 'laboratory'-type situation where a clinician, usually a clinical psychologist, attempts to control for a number of variables while observing. The approach is experimental because at least one variable, of interest to the clinician, is manipulated in a highly controlled environment in order to bring about a reduction in an undesired behaviour. The purpose of measurement is therefore to demonstrate a cause and effect relationship between a variable in a person's environment and the behaviour they demonstrate.

Where direct observational analysis is used then one or more of the following types of measurement are commonly found:

- **Frequency** This form of measurement requires the clinician or researcher to identify the number of times a target behaviour is observed within a predetermined period. The total of observed targeted behaviours can be divided by the period of observation to arrive at a mean calculation of frequency of that behaviour.

- **Duration** If a target behaviour occurs infrequently, but for long periods of time, then observation may be required for extended periods. An example here may be bouts of screaming that occur relatively infrequently but with such intensity, and over such a long period of time, that the behaviour is extremely distressing for both individual and carers. It then becomes more appropriate to measure the total amount of time spent on such behaviour. This approach is necessary to obtain a reliable measure of targeted behaviour.

- **Interval recording** In this form of measurement the nurse and/or researcher divides the observation period into predetermined intervals. This is useful when behaviours are of variable duration, for example head banging, which may last only a few seconds or for several minutes. Each occurrence of the targeted behaviour that falls within the time interval is recorded. Such measurement provides relatively accurate information on the frequency of a behaviour, but only limited insight as to its duration or intensity.

- **Time sampling** The last type of measurement explored here is that of time sampling, which involves specific periods when the target behaviour is to be measured. If the behaviour occurs during the sampling period it is recorded. A major strength of this approach is that it is less time-consuming than other approaches. Clearly, however, the measure may not be reliable in that target behaviour may occur outside the sample frame and would therefore not be recorded.

With respect to these differing methods of measurement, Iwata et al (1990) have stated that 'Although designed to serve the same purpose, these methods vary considerably in terms of both precision and complexity, and each method contains inherent strengths and weaknesses'.

The methods described here are not exhaustive but they do serve to illustrate that, whichever measurement is taken, there are a number of issues that the nurse or carer should consider. First, the reliability of the measurement process is entirely dependent upon the observer rating the behaviour. This issue was discussed by Yule and Carr (1987), who said: 'Observers are human, and human beings process their observations before recording them [therefore] simple observational measures of behaviour can become unreliable'. In addition to this a number of studies have pointed to anomalies in rater reliability. For example, Taplin and Reid (1973) found that raters behave differently when they are observed in reliability studies, than when they are on their own. There is a simple formula for establishing the extent of reliability of raters' observations:

$$\frac{\text{Number of agreements (66)}}{\text{Number of agreements (66) and disagreements (13)}} \times 100 = \text{Inter-rater reliability (83.54\%)}$$

In this formula it can be seen that two raters agreed on 66 separate occasions concerning the behaviour they observed; on 13 occasions they disagreed. The number of agreements is divided by the number of agreements and disagreements and multiplied by 100 to arrive at a percentage. Generally speaking, a result of above 90% is desirable, although above 80% is acceptable.

In addition, the choice of the measures that are taken can also affect the reliability of any findings. For example, time sampling, although both convenient and less demanding of resources, may well provide unreliable data as to the frequency or severity of behavioural difficulties. Given that behavioural difficulties and their management in the field of learning disability present care problems for both parents and professionals, therapeutic interactions or research studies that attempt to measure the efficacy of different interventions, and their effect upon outcomes, are vitally important. With carefully conducted measurement the nurse practitioner or researcher can:

- Evaluate treatment against therapeutic goals
- Compare results achieved with others using the same treatment methods
- Explore self-reporting of improvements in measurement.

Within the context of limited resources for health care, and the consequent need for effective targeting of those resources, evidence-based nursing is necessary to ensure that the most appropriate therapeutic strategies are adopted in the management of people with a learning disability who exhibit behavioural difficulties. The importance of outcome studies in this area is very clearly articulated in two recent publications by Emerson et al (1994) and Wright et al (1994).

Obtaining desired and eliminating undesired behaviours

If we pursue the behavioural approach outlined above, then based on the fundamentals of behaviourism it is possible to increase a particular behaviour because it is desired, or to decrease or extinguish it on the basis that it is undesirable. The basis of this belief can be traced back to the turn of this century, when a Russian neurophysiologist described a chance observation of a relationship between unconditioned responses and unconditioned stimuli. The response was called unconditioned because it was reflexive in nature, meaning that it was an integral component of the organism's repertoire of behaviour. The most famous example of this was salivation by a dog in the presence of food. Pavlov found that if an unconditioned response was paired with a conditioned stimulus, then it would be possible, eventually, to elicit a conditioned response. This is demonstrated in Table 9.1 as occurring in three stages. First, in stage 1, the unconditioned stimulus of food causes the dog to respond by salivating. If this unconditioned response (stage 2) is paired for a sufficient period of time with a conditioned stimulus (in this case a bell), then it will be possible for the response of salivation to be

Table 9.1 The process of classical conditioning		
Stage 1	UCS (food)	UCR (salivation)
Stage 2	UCS (food)	
	CS (bell)	UCR (salivation)
Stage 3	CS (bell)	CS (salivation)
UCS, unconditioned stimulus; UCR, unconditioned response; CS, conditioned stimulus; CR, conditioned response		

obtained with the conditioned stimulus on its own.

This early work helped shape the thinking of a group of American psychologists now referred to as the behavourists; of these, Watson and Skinner are probably the best-known. John Watson, credited as the father of behaviourism, believed that for psychology to become a science its data had to be objective, observable and measurable. He rejected the introspective, hypothetical causes of behaviour, arguing that behaviour was a direct result of conditioning, originating in the individual's environment, and that this environment would shape behaviour by reinforcing specific behaviours. The extent and depth of his beliefs is evidenced by the following:

Give me a dozen healthy infants, well-formed, and my own specified world to bring them up in and I'll guarantee to take any one at random and train him to become any kind of specialist I might select – lawyer, artist, merchant, chef and yes even a beggar man and thief, regardless of his talents, penchants, abilities, vocations, and race of ancestors (Watson 1924).

From the early work of Watson, and based upon the notion of conditioning, emerged the work of B.F. Skinner. Skinner postulated a behavioural explanation for the acquisition of all behaviour through the making of a connection between a stimulus, the elicited response and subsequent rewards or punishments. The assumption, at a simplistic level, is that if a behaviour is reinforced positively then the frequency of that behaviour will increase. Conversely, if a behaviour is negatively reinforced the incidence of that behaviour will decrease. The appeal of this theory, which became known as operant conditioning, and later behaviour modification, was enormous, because it was thought that all sorts of desirable

as well as undesirable behaviours could be modified by the practical application of behaviourism. Clearly, in the context of working with people with learning disabilities who present with behavioural difficulties, the thought of modifying undesirable behaviour is appealing. On the other hand, the teaching of new behaviour was seen as just as possible. The thought was that people with learning disabilities, through operant conditioning, could be taught new skills to enable them to live more independently. The teaching of new behaviour is clearly dependent upon the use of factors that reinforce particular behaviours. Two main categories of positive reinforcer can be identified:

- Primary: These meet a physical need, therefore food, sweets, fruit, water are all examples of primary reinforcers.
- Secondary: These are reinforcers that are used to meet primary needs. They include such items as tokens and money, which in themselves are not reinforcing but which can be exchanged for something that is. Also within the category of secondary reinforcers are the social reinforcers, such as smiling, stroking or other kinds of sensory reinforcers.

The systematic application of such reinforcers has the potential to bring about an increase in a desired behaviour. If they are appropriately withheld, they can bring about a reduction in undesired behaviour.

In order to reinforce a particular type of behaviour it is necessary to establish a schedule whereby a target behaviour is reinforced using either a primary or a secondary reinforcer. There are some important general principles concerning the administration of reinforcers:

- Always administer the reward as soon as is practically possible after the target behaviour has been demonstrated: the closer the reinforcer is to the target behaviour the stronger the association between the two.
- In the initial stages it is often desirable to reinforce on each occasion the target behaviour is demonstrated.
- Reduce the frequency of reinforcement for

the target behaviour as it becomes more established (intermittent reinforcement); strangely, the
properties of intermittent reinforcement are surprisingly powerful.

For a comprehensive account of how operant
conditioning may be used in learning disability
see Bellack et al (1982) and Ager (1989).

A final note in this section concerns the concept of punishment as a negative reinforcer.
Unfortunately, during the early development of
behaviourism a range of aversive punishments
were used by care staff in the belief that their use
would eradicate undesired behaviours. Such
strategies included noxious smells and tastes, the
use of electric shocks and the like. Such procedures are inhumane, and it is suggested that the
majority of practitioners from a range of professional backgrounds find them unacceptable.

Aversive and non-aversive techniques

It is not sufficient that nurse practitioners, in
either clinical practice or research, confine themselves to purely methodological issues of validity
concerning different therapeutic interventions in
the management of behavioural difficulties. Any
question of validity should be placed within the
wider context of societal values. The issue of
social validity developed from the disaffection
and ideological distaste that arose from the use of
aversive methods in the management of behavioural difficulties (Murphy 1993, Wolery and Gast
1990) have contributed significantly to the debate
on studies of behavioural difficulties, and cite
Wolf's (1978) classic paper that called for studies
to address the following issues:

- Are specific behavioural goals really what
  society wants?
- Do the ends justify the means?
- Are consumers satisfied with all the results,
  including any unpredicted ones?

Wolery and Gast (1990) have suggested that
these issues do not simply represent points on
the spectrum of the argument about aversive and
non-aversive interventions; rather, they are

mooted as being necessary considerations,
regardless of which approach is to be used. Goza
et al (1993), in a recent study, pointed out that the
social validity of the argument developed by
supporters of non-aversive approaches was
based upon selective review of the literature, and
that the argument is vague, philosophical in
nature and lacks operational definitions of the
terms used, thus making empirical scrutiny
difficult.

ROLE OF THE LEARNING DISABILITIES NURSE IN THE MANAGEMENT OF BEHAVIOURAL DIFFICULTIES

In Chapter 1 the role of the nurse in the specialism of learning disabilities was defined. In the
case of people with learning disabilities who present with behavioural difficulties, the role of the
nurse is very clear. Evidently, the skills of nursing
in being able to conduct reliable and valid assessments are of paramount importance. In the case
of people who engage in self-injurious behaviour
health surveillance is important, to monitor for
infection, loss of function and/or additional disabilities (Emerson 1990, Blair 1992). Developing
personal competence is also important because if
we are to eradicate undesired behaviour then we
must replace it with alternative behaviours that
help the individual lead a more valued life. The
successful eradication of undesired behaviour is,
in the author's experience, entirely dependent
upon the collective expertise of the multidisciplinary team. Although it is not always the case that
it should be a nurse coordinating services, it is
sometimes necessary because of their sustained
and intimate relationship with the clients and/or
their families. People with learning disabilities
who present with behavioural difficulties, or
their carers, often need help in accessing the
types of services they require. Nurses have an
incumbent responsibility to assist in enabling and
empowering parents and/or people with learning
disabilities to receive the services they are entitled
to. As was said at the beginning of the chapter,
people with learning disabilities who also have
behavioural difficulties challenge our beliefs and

value systems. Nurses must respond to this by ensuring that these people receive good-quality services based on humane principles that reflect our common commitment to the integrity and uniqueness of each individual. Pre-registration education on its own will not prepare nurses to meet the needs of this group of people. There is a need for specialist nurse practitioners, who can develop their knowledge base and skills to help this client group in the best possible way. It may be that this extension of knowledge and skills will require nurses to adopt, adapt and use the knowledge and skills of other disciplines and professional groupings; nurses must not be precious about this but recognize the valuable contributions colleagues from other disciplines can make in this area (McGill & Bliss 1993).

The final part of this section is devoted to the case history of a young man the author has recently worked with in clinical practice. The reader should spend some time reading Case study 9.1 and then attempt to undertake Activity 9.3. Also spend some time reflecting on the key roles of the learning disabilities nurse (Figure 9.2) and imagine how you might have worked with this young man.

Case study 9.1

Robert is a 37-year-old man who lives in a group home run by social services. He has a sister who is 30 years of age and has a mild learning disability; she is currently being cared for in a unit for people with learning disabilities who have a mental health problem. According to the records of both health and social work professionals, their parents did not cope very well with bringing up the children. During his childhood both Robert and his sister were sexually abused by their father and physically and verbally abused by their mother. Eventually, through interventions from an interdisciplinary team from the statutory bodies and child agencies, the father was sent to prison for his abuse. At this point Robert was admitted to a long-stay learning disabilities hospital because his behaviour was uncontrollable. His sister remained at home with her mother, who was supported by social services. Robert spent some 15 years at this hospital before finally being discharged when it closed in 1992. At this point his care formed part of the re-provision of services in his area, and he moved into a social services-run group home; he shares this with three other people who also have learning disabilities. In the home Robert is verbally abusive: he swears, shouts and gestures at both staff and residents. He also frequently punches and slaps another resident: staff feel that he perceives this person to be weak. He refuses to take part in most group activities, and at times even refuses to eat his meals with the others, who always eat together. He attends a social education centre 3 days a week, spends 1 day on an outreach project and 1 day back at the home working with his key worker. He is currently prescribed 200 mg of Clopixol (zuclopenthixol deconate), administered by intramuscular injection every 4 weeks; he also takes Kemadrin (procylidine hydrochloride) 5 mg three times a day by mouth to counteract the extrapyramidal effects of the Clopixol.

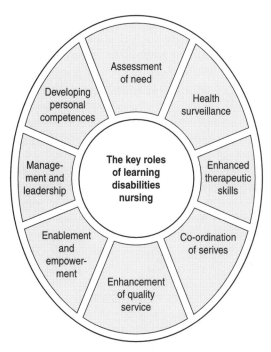

Figure 9.2   The key roles of learning disabilities nursing.

Activity 9.3

Spend some time reflecting on the case history of Robert. What do you think might have contributed to the development of his behavioural difficulties? Staff at the home have asked for input from the 'special support service', a team of learning disability nurses, clinical psychologists and occupational therapists from a health unit that provides support and advice for such people. What kinds of therapeutic interventions might the learning disabilities nurse engage in to bring about a healthier, valued and more fulfilling life for Robert?

CONCLUSION

This chapter has outlined a number of issues concerning behavioural difficulties in learning disability. It has been identified that the measurement of behavioural difficulties is particularly problematic because of the difficulty of ensuring reliability and validity. Also, the use of the term challenging behaviour, as an all-embracing term to include behavioural difficulties, is inadequate and has led to the anomaly of not being able to accurately determine, or separate the prevalence of, behavioural difficulties from a range of other phenomena. It is for this reason that the term behavioural difficulties has been used throughout this chapter. It is suggested that this term has the advantage of permitting a clear operational definition to enable behavioural difficulties to be more readily examined empirically. It has also been suggested that there are problems with the method of measurement used: it would appear that the most accurate method may not always be the most convenient or the most practicable. All measurement in this field evidently places heavy emphasis upon observer reliability, and it has been established that in this area there are potential threats to such reliability. In addition, a criticism of a number of existing measures is that they have often only been studied for inter-rater reliability, and that other measures of reliability and validity have largely been ignored. Given the reservations discussed in this chapter, nurse practitioners should use a battery of scales and types of measurement of behavioural difficulties, that will enable them to be more confident about the reliability and validity of assessment, for the purpose of evaluating their therapeutic interventions.

There are also some very practical issues that nurses must address. The first of these is a need for nurses to critically examine their own value base and attitudes towards the people they care for, who demonstrate behavioural difficulties. Nurses in this specialty need to learn new ways of 'being' with people with learning disabilities. We need to learn new postures that are not perceived as threatening. Some need to refrain from abusing the professional power that makes their relationship with others inequitable. Learning disability nurses need to learn how to provide unconditional regard and warmth, and we have much to learn about people with learning disabilities who present with behavioural difficulties. It is to be hoped that the professional and academic disciplines of nursing, psychology, medicine, speech and occupational therapies, together with social workers, will continue to learn, work and research this area collaboratively, in order to bring about real health gains and wellbeing for this group of people.

REFERENCES

Ager A 1989 Behavioural teaching strategies for people with severe and profound mental handicaps: a re-examination. Mental Handicap 17: 56–59

Bellack A, Hersen M, Kazdin A 1982 International handbook of behaviour modification and therapy. Plenum Press, New York

Blair A 1992 Working with people who self injure: a review of the literature. Behavioural Psychotherapy 20: 1–23

Blunden R, Allen D 1987 Facing the challenge: an ordinary life for people with learning difficulties and challenging behaviour. Kings Fund Paper No 74. Kings Fund Centre, London

Christie R, Bay C, Kaufman I A et al 1982 Lesch–Nyhan disease: clinical experience with nineteen patients. Developmental Medicine and Child Neurology 24: 293–306

Clifton M, Brown J 1993 Learning disabilities, challenging behaviour and mental illness. Research Highlights. English National Board for Nursing, Midwifery and Health Visiting, London

DoH 1992 Mansel report on services for people with learning disabilities and challenging behaviour or mental health needs. HMSO, London

Duker P, Van-Druenen C, Jol K, Oud H 1986 Determinants of maladaptive behaviour of institutionalised mentally retarded individuals. American Journal of Mental Deficiency 91: 51–56

Emerson E 1990 Severe self injurious behaviour: some of the challenges it presents. Mental Handicap 18: 92–98

Emerson E 1993 Challenging behaviours and severe learning disabilities: recent developments in behavioural analysis and intervention. Behavioural and Cognitive Psychotherapy 21: 171–198

Emerson E, Cummins R, Barrett S et al 1988 Challenging behaviour and community services: 2. Who are the people who challenge services? Mental Handicap 16: 16–19

Emerson E, McGill P, Mansell J (eds) 1994 Severe learning disabilities and challenging behaviours: designing high quality services. Chapman & Hall, London

Gates B 1996 Issues of reliability and validity in the measurement of challenging behaviour (behaviour difficulties) in learning disability: a discussion of implications for nursing research and practice. Journal of Clinical Nursing 5: 7–12

Gates B, Beacock C 1996 Dimensions of learning disability. Baillière Tindall, London

Gates B, Wray J 1995 Support for carers of people with learning disabilities. Nursing Times 91(46): 36–37

Goza A B, Ricketts R W, Perkins T S 1993 The social validity of an argument supporting a ban on aversive procedures. Journal of Intellectual Disability Research 37: 449–458

Iwata B A, Vollmer R, Zarcone J R 1990 The experimental (functional) analysis of behaviour disorders: methodology, applications, and limitations. In: Repp A, Singh N (eds) Perspectives on the use of non aversive and aversive interventions for persons with developmental disabilities. Sycamore Publishing Company, Illinois, USA

Jones R S P, Connell E 1993 Ten years of gentle teaching: much ado about nothing? The Psychologist 6: 544–548

Kiernan C, Moss S 1990 Behaviour disorders and other characteristics of the population of a mental handicap hospital. Mental Handicap Research 3: 3–20

Lovaas O, Freitag G, Gold V J, Kassorla I C 1965 Experimental studies in childhood schizophrenia: analysis of self-destructive behaviour. Journal of Experimental Child Psychology 2: 67–84

McGee J 1990 Gentle teaching: the basic tenet. Nursing Times 86: 68–72

McGee J 1992 Gentle teaching: assumptions and paradigm. Journal of Applied Behaviour Analysis 25: 869–872

McGee J, Menolascino M D, Hobbs D, Menousek P 1987 Gentle teaching: a non-aversive approach to helping persons with mental retardation. Human Sciences Press, New York

McGill P, Bliss E V 1993 Training clinical practitioners. In: Kiernan C (ed) Research to practice? Implications of research on the challenging behaviour of people with learning disability. BILD, Avon

Murphy G 1993 The use of aversive stimuli in treatment: the issue of consent. Journal of Intellectual Disability Research 37: 211–219

Myers, M 1995 A challenge to change: better services for people with challenging behaviour. In: Philpot T, Ward L (eds) Values and visions: changing ideas in services for people with learning difficulties. Butterworth-Heinemann, Oxford

Nihira K, Leland H, Lambert N 1993 AAMR Adaptive behaviour scale – residential and community. Examiner's manual, 2nd edn. Pro ed, Texas, USA

Oliver C 1993 Self injurious behavior: from response to strategy. In: Kiernan C (ed) Research to practice?

Implications of research on the challenging behaviour of people with learning disability. BILD Publications, Avon

O P C S 1989 Survey of disability in Great Britain. HMSO, London

Quine L 1986 Behaviour problems in severely mentally handicapped children. Psychological Medicine 16: 895–907

Quine L, Pahl J 1985 Examining the causes of stress in families with mentally handicapped children. British Journal of Social Work 15: 501–517

Qureshi H 1993 Impact on families: young adults with learning disability who show challenging behaviour. In: Kiernan C (ed) Research to practice? Implications of research on the challenging behaviour of people with learning disability. BILD, Kidderminster

Qureshi H 1994 The size of the problem. In: Emerson E, McGill P, Mansell J (eds) Severe learning disabilities and challenging behaviours – designing high quality services. Chapman and Hall, London

Russell P 1995 Supporting families. In: Philpot T, Ward L Values and visions – changing ideas in services for people with learning difficulties. Butterworth Heinemann, London

Saxby H, Morgan H 1993 Behaviour problems in children with learning disabilities: to what extent do they exist and are they a problem? Child Care Health and Development 19: 149–257

Sehult C 1985 Using parents as their children's therapists. Behaviour Modification 15: 309–318

Slevin E 1995 A concept analysis of, and proposed new term for, challenging behaviour. Journal of Advanced Nursing 21: 928–934

Taplin P S, Reid J B 1973 Effects of instructional set and experimenter influence on observer reliability. Child Development 44: 547–554

Watson J B 1924 Behaviourism. In: Stevanson L 1974 Seven theories of human nature. Oxford University Press, Oxford

Wolery M N, Gast D 1990 Reframing the debate: finding the middle ground and defining the role of social validity. In Repp A C, Singh N N Perspectives on the use of non aversive and aversive interventions for persons with developmental disabilities. Sycamore Publishing Co, Illinois, USA

Wolf M M 1978 Social validity: the case for subjective measurement or how applied behaviour analysis is finding its heart. Journal of Applied Behaviour Analysis 11: 203–214

Wright K, Haycox A, Leedham I 1994 Evaluating community care. Services for people with learning difficulties. Open University Press, Buckingham

Yule W, Carr J 1987 Behaviour modification for people with mental handicaps, 2nd edn. Chapman & Hall, London

FURTHER READING

Brigden P, Todd M 1995 Behavioural approaches. In: Learning disabilities: practice issues in health settings. Routledge, London

Chamberlain L, Chung M C, Jenner L 1993 Preliminary findings on community and challenging behaviour in

learning difficulty. British Journal of Developmental Disability XXXIX, 2. 77. 118–125

Dagan D, Kroese B S 1993 The uses of a special needs register for people with learning difficulties. Mental Handicap 21: 10–13

DHSS 1980 Mental handicap: progress, problems and priorities. HMSO, London

Gates B, Wray J, Newell R 1996 Challenging behaviour in children with learning disabilities. British Journal of Nursing 5: 1189–1194

Harris P 1993 The nature and extent of aggressive behaviour amongst people with learning difficulties (mental handicap) in a single health district. Journal of Intellectual Disability Research 37: 221–242

Hastings R P, Remington S 1993 Connotations of labels for mental handicap and challenging behaviour: a review and research evaluation. Mental Handicap Research 6: 237–249

Kiernan C (ed) 1993 Research to practice? Implications of research on the challenging behaviour of people with learning disability. BILD Publications, Avon

Leedham I 1989 From mental handicap hospital to community provisions. Unpublished PhD thesis. University of Kent, Canterbury

Qureshi H, Alborz A 1992 Epidemiology of challenging behaviour. Mental Handicap Research 2: 130–145

Scorer S, Cate T, Wilkinson L, Pollock P, Hargan J 1993 Challenging behaviour project team: a six month project evaluation. Mental Handicap 2: 49–53

Complementary therapies

J. Wray

INTRODUCTION

In recent years there has been a considerable increase in the use of, and interest in, complementary therapies, both by the general public and by healthcare professionals. An estimated £60 million is currently being spent by the general public on over-the-counter 'alternative' medicines (Which 1996), and increasingly patients with chronic and intractable diseases are seeking alternative healthcare options as conventional medicine fails to provide a cure, or even relief, for some conditions. Reasons for this dissatisfaction include:

- The unpleasant side effects of some conventional drug treatments
- A wish to have more choice about treatment
- The failure of orthodox medicine to provide satisfactory healthcare (Guardian Educational Supplement 1996).

Treatments such as acupuncture, homoeopathy, aromatherapy and herbal medicine, which were once considered 'fringe' therapies, are now gaining widespread acceptance, and many doctors are prepared to refer patients to alternative practitioners. Recent reforms in the health service have provided an opportunity for purchasers and providers to reconsider alternative options for the provision of healthcare. The National Association of Health Authorities and Trusts (NAHAT 1993) reported that complementary therapies were being regularly paid for and offered to patients by the Family Health Service Authorities (FHSA), the District Health

Authorities (DHA) and the newly formed hospital Trusts, and recent figures have suggested that as many as 93% of general practitioners are prepared to refer patients to a complementary practitioner (Perkin 1994).

Demand for alternative healthcare is both patient and practitioner generated, and in the case of the nursing profession the opportunities to improve individualized patient care through the appropriate use of such therapies appears to be the driving force.

Within the nursing profession a similar escalation of interest appears to be developing. An estimated 75–80% of aromatherapy courses aimed at healthcare professionals are being taken up by nurses (Tattam 1992). This growing interest is demonstrated by the number of articles on complementary therapies currently available in the nursing press. Professional bodies such as the United Kingdom Central Council for Nursing, Midwifery and Health Visiting (UKCC) and the Royal College of Nursing (RCN) have been compelled by the extent of this interest to provide guidelines to document the role that complementary therapies will play in nursing, health visiting and midwifery in the future.

With the growing acceptability of these therapies the need to ensure safety and guidance has become paramount, and this control and regulation has been achieved individually for each of the therapies in terms of legislation. The professional bodies for each therapy have been applying for professional recognition and regulation through Parliament. The health service view on individual therapies appears to be varied: homoeopathy, acupuncture, osteopathy, chiropractic and, to a certain extent, herbalism have a perceived current legitimacy and acceptability to healthcare purchasers and providers. Homoeopathy has been available on the NHS since 1948, and there are five homoeopathic hospitals in the United Kingdom (in London, Tunbridge Wells, Bristol, Liverpool and Glasgow). A limited number of other therapies, such as aromatherapy, reflex zone therapy, hypnotherapy, shiatsu and meditation, are being used and have developed a degree of perceived legitimacy, but are seen by some healthcare professionals as being representative of 'new age' or 'fringe' therapy. This seems to reflect the differing perceptions healthcare professionals have regarding the potential role of each therapy within their practice. It would appear that nurses are prepared to embrace these other therapies, but medical colleagues generally are not, citing concern over lack of proven effectiveness, lack of proven cost-effectiveness, resource constraints and priorities and fears about uncontrolled demands for such therapies (NAHAT 1993) as reasons for their reluctance.

It is becoming evident that nurses, midwives and health visitors will have an important role to play in the future use of complementary therapies within both the public and the private sectors of healthcare provision. If this role entails undertaking training in a therapy in order to offer it to patients as an integral part of healthcare provision, then this has obvious implications for the extension of the nurse's role and the scope of their professional practice.

WHAT DO WE MEAN BY 'COMPLEMENTARY'?

Unorthodox, unconventional, natural, fringe, alternative; these are all terms commonly used with reference to a complementary therapy. Many of these terms are used interchangeably, assuming them to be synonymous, but confusion is generated through inappropriate usage. The concepts may be similar, but problems arise when we attempt to find an appropriate definition that encompasses a range of therapies as diverse as massage and iridology (a diagnostic method which uses the iris of the eye with which to diagnose). As many therapies become more acceptable, both to the general public and to healthcare professionals, the descriptive term used has become less 'alternative' or 'fringe', and more 'complementary', the therapies themselves being considered by many patients and practitioners as complementary to mainstream or orthodox medicine.

For clarity, the term 'complementary therapy' as used here will be taken as meaning 'The adoption and use of unorthodox treatments that are used to complement (not replace) orthodox treatments in health care' (Gates 1994).

An orthodox treatment is one which conforms to the established and widely accepted treatment standards used by healthcare professionals. 'Complementary' defined in this way describes a therapy which aims to work in conjunction with orthodox methods of treatment, rather than offer an alternative or substitute treatment option. This distinction becomes important when we consider the types of complementary therapies it would seem that nurses are wanting to introduce into their practice. They do not seek to replace the selection of treatments available to patients and healthcare practitioners, but to develop and enhance their own role and their range of professional skills by incorporating a range of additional therapeutic skills and techniques. Using complementary therapies nurses can offer a range of treatments which offer patients choice and reflect the fundamental principle of individualized patient healthcare which is at the heart of nursing theory and practice. It seems likely that, as such therapies continue to gain respectability within nursing and medical circles, they will become less 'alternative', more 'complementary' and increasingly part of the new orthodoxy of purchaser and provider healthcare.

COMMON THERAPIES USED IN LEARNING DISABILITIES

Much of the nursing literature refers to the use of complementary therapies in general hospital settings and clinical practice, and so the extent of its use by community nurses, and especially learning disability nurses, is difficult to estimate. However, as complementary therapies allegedly have some potential benefit to offer to clients, it is reasonable to consider the possible merit in using such therapies in the care of both adults and children with learning disabilities. Interest in complementary therapies in the field of learning disability nursing, notably the work of Sanderson and colleagues (1994), suggests that:

We find that the beneficial effects of aromatherapy and massage are the same for everyone . . . it therefore follows that we have no special "remedies" specific to

people who have learning difficulties, and the basic principles described here are applicable to everyone (Sanderson et al 1994).

Therapies considered to be of beneficial use in the care of people with a learning disability are those using a 'hands-on' approach, such as aromatherapy, massage and reflexology. It has been suggested that this current interest in complementary therapies reflects a movement away from the 'high-technology' no-touch care philosophy which has permeated nursing in recent decades (Sayre-Adams 1994). For nurses in the field of learning disabilities care this hands-on approach is fundamental to their core practice and an essential part of their relationship with their particular client group. The professional role of the learning disabilities nurse involves much functional touching, which is central to working with people with severe and profound learning disabilities, when communication through more conventional channels is not always possible or appropriate.

The 'big five' therapies commonly referred to in the literature are:

- acupuncture
- osteopathy
- homoeopathy
- herbalism
- chiropractic (NAHAT 1993).

These five therapies represent those generally considered acceptable by the medical profession and have a reasonably well established theory, practice and research base. The therapies generally being used by the nursing profession are those such as aromatherapy, shiatsu, reflexology, massage and therapeutic touch, that is, those therapies more recently described as 'fringe', which are currently developing their research and theory base. These particular therapies are on the whole, although not exclusively, being used by nurses as techniques, rather than whole systems of treatment. They are using them in the sense of an 'add-on' procedure, for example using one essential oil (lavender) to produce one treatment effect (sedation). Increasingly others within the profession are seeing such therapies not as techniques, but as 'windows through which the healing potential, the unconscious and the intention of the nurse can be expressed', (Sayre-Adams & Wright 1995). In this sense both the carer and the recipient of care become relevant to the therapeutic relationship. For the nurse it becomes not so much what one does but how one does it, and with what intent, and this attitude accurately reflects a holistic nursing philosophy.

Aromatherapy

Aromatherapy is the therapeutic use of essential oils extracted from petals, plants and trees, and is used to treat illness through the systematic application of the oils. The essential oils are volatile, highly concentrated and complex substances containing chemical properties, and each oil has its own individual properties, specific uses and actions. Many are used in conjunction with massage, but they can also be used in baths, inhalations, compresses and, in restricted cases, taken orally (diluted) and applied neat to the skin. Essential oils have their most rapid effect through the olfactory and limbic systems, so that inhalation is often the method of choice (for

Activity 10.1

Select a therapy that you are interested in using in your practice and identify the interest in, and attitudes to, that particular therapy in your clinical environment. Ask all members of the multidisciplinary team the following questions and record their responses:

- Have you had personal experience of this therapy (e.g. aromatherapy)?
- Are you caring for/have you cared for a client who uses this therapy?
- Are you interested in using this therapy within your clinical practice?
- Have you completed any training in this particular therapy? If yes, describe the training.

Put all the information together in the form of a presentation and display your findings to the rest of the team. If an interest in the therapy is established move on to Activity 10.3.

The same exercise can also be conducted to elicit client and carer experiences of, and attitudes to, a particular therapy. Present the information generated to the team managers.

example using an aromatherapy burner). Essential oils appear to interact with the body in different ways: they can act chemically, causing changes to occur when the oils react in the bloodstream with hormones and enzymes. They can also act physiologically, effecting stimulation or sedation depending on the oil used. On a psychological level they can have an emotional or affective consequence, the individual reacting to the smell of the oil and its associations, producing an uplifting or relaxing response. The oils are potent and in most cases must be diluted in carrier oil. Some are considered dangerous: for example, in pregnancy oils such as juniper, basil and clary sage are not recommended for home use because of their possible neuro-toxic, emmenagoguic, or diuretic effects.

Research evaluating the effectiveness of aromatherapy suggests that beneficial effects for the patient can be derived in certain contexts. However, many of the studies conducted by nurses are individual observations based on the authors' own clinical practices. Behavioural and emotional stress levels were reduced in post-cardiotomy patients when lavender oil was used in a randomized double-blind trial (Buckle 1993), and similar results were seen when neroli oil was used and combined with a foot massage in Stevenson's (1992) randomized controlled trial. The effect was considered to be more than just touch or placebo, but in the first study it did matter which type of lavender oil was used. There are three species of natural lavender and one hybrid, each with a differing chemistry, and therefore, its own particular therapeutic effect. (*Lavendula angustifolia, L. lanfolia, L. stoechas* and *L. burnatii* (hybrid)). In Buckle's study (1993) *L. burnatii* was more effective than the naturally occurring *L. angustifolia* which has a long history of therapeutic use. Aromatherapy has been shown to be more effective than massage or a 20-minute rest period in reducing patients' heart rate, blood pressure, respiratory rate, pain level and wakefulness when given as a foot massage with lavender essential oil (Hewitt 1992), although these results have not as yet been replicated. It appears that the psychological influence on the patient may herald the greatest effect, and this is confirmed by Dunn et al's (1995) study in which intensive care patients showed an improvement in mood and perceived anxiety when compared to a control in a study evaluating aromatherapy, massage and periods of rest, although the effect was not sustained or cumulative. The small amount of published research currently available is beginning to partially substantiate claims to treatment effect, but the question remains whether these findings can be generalized to all patient groups.

The International Federation of Aromatherapists (IFA) suggests that aromatherapy should only be used by practitioners who have an accepted qualification. Many practitioners are becoming concerned at the ill-informed ways in which some nurses are introducing aromatherapy into their practice. It is considered to be both a danger to patients and disruptive to the aromatherapy profession for non-qualified practitioners to 'dabble' in such practices if appropriate advice and consultation has not taken place.

Case study 10.1

Aromatherapy
Mary is 14 years old with a moderate learning disability, and suffers from eczema, predominantly on her elbows, arms, legs and trunk. Her mother was concerned about Mary's current treatment for eczema, as she had been using a variety of different steroid-based creams for several years with little or no success. Mother decided to consult an aromatherapist. Following a full assessment a treatment plan was decided, and Mary was given a full body massage with essential oils. Following the first session, Mary's mother did not notice a pronounced treatment effect, only a slight reduction in the redness of some of the patches. However, her daughter had enjoyed the experience, especially the smell of the oils. By the third consultation many of the angry red patches were less obvious, and 4 months later Mary is reducing her contact time with the therapist as her eczema has much improved. The essential oils, mixed with massage oil, are prepared by the therapist and her mother now massages Mary as directed before bedtime.

Massage

This involves the touching, kneading and stroking of muscles, tendons and ligaments of the body with varying degrees of pressure. The basis of massage is touch, and this has a number of physiological and psychological effects, including the release of stress and tension. The movements involved in massage can improve blood and lymph flow, loosen knotted tendons and relax muscles. There are, however, contraindications to the use of massage and situations in which it should not be undertaken, for example where there is acute inflammation, bruising or infection, circulatory problems such as varicose veins, when the client has had a heavy meal, and over skin conditions such as an open wound or recent scar tissue. It is believed that massage encourages the production of endorphins, and these can reduce pain and create a feeling of wellbeing (Oldfield 1992). The most commonly used massage is 'effleurage', an ordered and systematic sequence of stroking; however, there are more sophisticated forms of massage treatment, such as shiatsu, which is a form of healing using moderate physical pressure to attend to the quality of energy perceived in the body and adjust the tension found. The advantage offered by massage is that its principles and applications are known and understood by a variety of different medical cultures. It can be explained to western orthodox medicine in terms of anatomy, biology and psychology, and therein lies its perceived legitimacy to the medical profession.

Massage is used predominantly as a form of relaxation, and this can have a positive effect on the behavioural difficulties (verbal, aggressive and movement) of adults with learning disabilities (McPhail and Chamore 1989). Children with anxiety, depression or behavioural disorders have also been found to benefit from the combined use of yoga exercises, massage and progressive muscle relaxation (Plantania-Solazzo et al 1992). However, the published explanatory research remains equivocal in its findings. Dunbar and Redick (1986) found that a 1 minute back rub produced little physiological effect, although they did acknowledge a positive effect in terms of the massage as a 'comfort measure'. Bauer and Dracup (1987) replicated this study using a 6-minute massage and found no significant differences in physiological parameters. Other studies evaluating

Case study 10.2

Massage
Richard is 6 years old and lives with his mother and two sisters. He is diagnosed as being autistic and has been having some problems settling down to sleep at night. His mother was looking for a way of dealing with this without resorting to medication, and a friend suggested contacting a massage therapist. At the first session it was difficult for the therapist to begin as Richard did not wish to sit down and be massaged. A progressive introduction to massage was begun: at first Richard was praised if he sat down, and gradually over a period of 3 months the therapist and his mother were able to introduce small back rubs, building up to a neck, shoulder and back massage. His mother then began introducing the massage as part of Richard's bedtime routine, and found that, although initially resistant to this, he settled quite quickly into the routine. Now his mother no longer takes Richard to the therapist: she gives Richard a back and neck rub before bed, which she feels settles him down for the night. He does not sleep for longer periods, but will settle down and go to sleep more quickly.

the effect of massage have found that a 10-minute back rub, by a nurse, alleviated anxiety and helped the healing process by stimulating the production of antibodies (Groer et al

1994). Such studies seem to support the psychological effect of massage as a positive therapeutic intervention, although ambiguities in the research profiles suggest the need for further evaluation.

Before a massage is offered to clients the International Therapy Examination Council (ITEC) suggests that a recognized qualification, such as the one awarded by its professional body, should be obtained.

Reflexology

Also known as reflex zone therapy, this a method of treatment where reflex points in one part of the body are massaged in a particular way to produce beneficial effects in other parts of the body. Usually the feet are used, but it is also possible to use the hands and face. The method is based on the idea that the body is divided into 10 longitudinal zones, from the toes to the head and down the arms to the fingers, through which energy pathways pass (Figure 10.1). This is similar but not identical to the concepts underlying Chinese medicine. Exactly how reflexology works is unknown, but

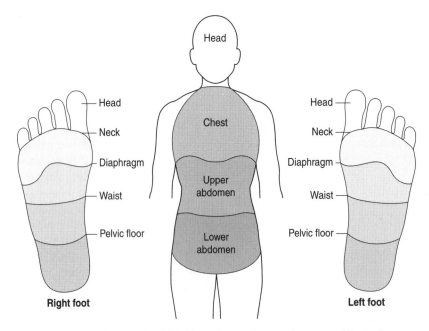

Figure 10.1   The feet can be divided laterally to correspond to areas of the body.

it has been suggested that malfunctioning of any organ, gland, or part of the body causes crystalline deposits of uric acid and calcium to form on nerve endings in the feet (Thompson 1994). Massaging the reflex zone corresponding to the malfunctioning part of the body breaks down these crystals, creating an optimum environment for the body's inherent healing capacity.

Reflex zone therapy can be used to treat a number of conditions, including back pain, digestive disorders and stress-related problems. People with progressive disorders such as multiple sclerosis may find that control of muscle function is improved by reflexology (Booth 1994). Also, this therapy is said to provide relief for women suffering from postnatal problems such as urine retention and wind following caesarean section (Evans 1990). However, Thomas's study (1989) suggested that there was no different treatment effect between a foot massage and a cosy chat with a member of the nursing staff. The current published research conducted by nurses exhibits some ambiguities, the worst of which suggest a poor treatment effect, with some studies being poorly conducted and badly controlled. Some positive treatment effects have been established, but their general scarcity makes it difficult to make a sound clinical judgement regarding the appropriateness of reflexology for use in the care of people who have a learning disability.

Therapeutic touch

The practice of therapeutic touch (TT) within nursing was originally explored by Dolores Krieger (1975), and is the modern-day derivative of the ancient practice of laying on of hands. However, it differs from this practice in that it is not done within a religious context and it requires no professed faith or belief. Also, it requires no direct physical contact between the practitioner and the patient. As a nursing intervention the practitioner's hands are used to direct energy to the patient with the intent of helping. The process initially involves 'centring', or assuming a meditative state or intention to help the patient. The hands are then used as sensors or scanners to move over the patient's body,

assessing their energy flow and energy needs. Using the hands, areas of accumulated tension and energy are identified and redirected to restore the patient's energy balance. TT has been described as a special kind of caring because of the intense focus of concentration required, which is considered by some to be often absent during routine daily nursing care. The essential components of TT are empathy and a desire to help on the part of the therapist, thus making use of one of the most fundamental communication skills of the nurse. TT represents a 'practical demonstration of the nurse's desire to care for and heal the individual, while recognising the interrelatedness of mind, body and spirit' (Rankin-Box 1988).

Krieger's (1975) original exploratory studies revealed some degree of effect; however, these studies, although experimental, were poor in design. Later studies have shown that TT is a fulfilling therapeutic experience for patients (Samarel 1992) which can reduce pain (Randolph 1984) and the time needed to calm children after stressful experiences (Kramer 1990). Keller and Bzdek's (1986) study showed a positive therapeutic effect in the treatment of tension headaches, although the researcher conducted the experiment herself, indicating the possibility of experimenter bias. These results were not substantiated by Meehan's (1993) study, in which little statistical significance was obtained when comparing the effects of TT with acknowledged and accepted pain relief treatments. He did conclude the existence of a mild treatment effect, but suggested that this was placebo in nature.

Healing using TT is non-invasive and has few side effects, and this natural potential can be used by anyone. It is therefore an ideal tool for use by learning disability nurses, as professionally we have permission both to touch and to use touch pervasively in our practice. Advocates of TT see it as an appropriate modality for a nursing intervention that does not require a doctor's order or supervision, although sceptics have suggested that it is merely a placebo.

Concluding comments

An examination of the empirical evidence available suggests that many of the therapies currently being used and promoted by nurses lack an established research base. Systematic evaluation of these therapies has been insufficient, the studies conducted being poor in design and representing case studies and anecdotal evidence. The ambiguity of such research findings provides an important starting point for discussion, but within learning disability nursing they do not provide an adequate impetus to justify their implementation into practice. Nevertheless, some of the better-designed and controlled studies do highlight a psychological treatment effect, which is subjective in nature but is a treatment effect all the same. Supporters of these practices are failing to evaluate them comprehensively, and poorly validated results make it difficult to generalize the findings to the different healthcare settings, as research provides the most compelling means by which a treatment effect can be validated.

USING COMPLEMENTARY THERAPIES IN LEARNING DISABILITY NURSING

The increase in the use of and interest in complementary therapies in nursing has been ascribed to the rise of holism and the movement towards individualized patient care. Within the field of learning disabilities nursing this interest can also be explored in terms of the role that touch and the client–therapist interaction play in the provision of care. Nursing theory and practice has in the past been dominated by the 'biomedical model', a model which attempts to explain care provision in terms of disease and illness. The rise of holism within nursing has been a theoretical and philosophical development, incorporating a belief in the importance of individualized nursing care emphasizing the treatment of the patient as a whole being. 'Increasingly in the West, account is being taken of the fact that in both health and illness, people have to be assessed in their individual physical, psychological, socio-cultural, environmental and politicoeconomic context' (Roper et al 1990).

Holistic health and nursing

This change has been seen directly in the movement from a task-oriented nursing care model to a team-based care model, through to the current emphasis on primary nursing care and individualized care provision. The 'whole person' approach to care planning and provision is multidisciplinary in nature, and although the learning disabilities nurse provides the fundamental part of that care, input from other healthcare professionals is essential. The biomedical model has contributed an increasingly technological dimension to patient care, and the hands-on caring and nurturing role of the nurse has been devalued. The holism central to complementary therapies restores the concept of caring for the whole person at an individual level, thus embracing a patient-centred approach. Holistic nursing advocates the care of people on a physical, psychosocial and spiritual level. The interplay of the mind, body and spirit is recognized and explained, with reference to how holism 'directs individuals towards a greater understanding of the way in which social, emotional, physical and spiritual aspects of our lives interrelate to influence personal well-being' (Rankin-Box 1988).

The nursing profession's notion of a holistic model of care provision rejects the biomedical model and represents a paradigm shift within healthcare. A paradigm shift is said to have taken place when an old set of assumptions is rejected in favour of a new explanation of the world; this new explanation reflects the available information more appropriately or realistically at a particular point in time. Within healthcare philosophy we are seeing a movement away from a mechanistic western orthodox medical model to a more holistic concept of health.

Holism is represented within nursing science by Rogers' Theory of Unitary Human Beings (Rogers 1970), which developed from ideas first produced in the 1960s. Rogers' theory provides an explanatory framework in which all persons are highly complex fields of various forms of life energy. This energy is coextensive with the universe and in constant interaction with surrounding energy fields. Rogers' theory provides a functional basis for understanding therapies such as therapeutic touch, in which the direction of life energy moves through the hands of the therapist to the recipient. Holism evolved (or re-evolved, as it was never dead) because it represented a desirable option over the biomedical model in caring for the nursing needs of the whole individual. Within the field of learning disability care the biomedical model has been inadequate in providing an appropriate care philosophy. The movement from hospital- to community-based care reflected the philosophical movement from a medical model to a social and educational model. Quite simply, people with a learning disability are not 'ill' in a biomedical sense: they are affected by the same healthcare problems as the rest of the population, although the variety and extent is greater. An estimated 4000–6000 people with a learning disability require specialist services for healthcare problems, which may be physical, behavioural, emotional or psychological in nature (Sines 1992). The provision of community care for people with learning disabilities can be seen in terms of a movement towards holistic healthcare provision. The legislative changes brought about by the 1989 White Paper and the NHS and Community Care Act of 1990 focused on care for people with learning disabilities in a much wider sense, including the carer and the family unit.

Complementary therapies also offer the client a range of therapeutic benefits, which orthodox medicine has been slow to recognize. These important aspects of caring, such as support, personal involvement from the practitioner, empathy and empowerment in treatment, are predominantly psychological and emotional in nature, although their influence on health and wellbeing is accepted, and they are essential ingredients of a positive therapeutic relationship.

The role of touch

The most appropriate therapies for community nurses with the necessary training to incorporate into their nursing practice are those involving touch (Thompson 1994).

It is difficult to separate the social, physical and psychological aspects of touch. However, touch can be described in terms of tactile sensations differentiated by different properties, such as duration, intensity, location and other characteristics specific to the source of stimulation. Jackson (1995) suggests that there are four types of touch performed by nurses:

- Instrumental touch (bathing, giving of injections)
- Expressive touch (empathetic promotion of compassion and understanding hand-holding)
- Systematic touch (deliberate manipulation of soft tissues, e.g. massage)
- therapeutic touch.

The importance of using appropriate touch in the provision of care of people with learning disabilities is well documented in the nursing literature (Harrison & Ruddle 1995). The absence of touch and the withdrawal of physical affection in early life can have profound effects on both the physical and the psychological wellbeing of the individual (Ward 1990). For the person with severe or profound learning disabilities, who may have a limited range of communicative abilities, touch can become vitally important. Touch, considered a second sense to many, may act as a first or primary sense for those who are unable to communicate through the more conventional channels. Up to 30% of people with a severe learning disability have additional sensory or physical impairments (Sines 1992), and the prevalence of additional impairments is far greater than in the general population. The information this client group receives from non-verbal channels thus acquires a greater significance.

A client with learning disabilities often has little or no choice about how often and in what ways they are touched by those who care for them. Much of the touching behaviour carried out by the nurse can be instrumental and functional in character, and massage can offer a different kind of experience (Sanderson et al 1992). The client can be involved in choosing the oils as well as determining the nature and extent of the massage. The basis of many of the complementary therapies is touch, and this has a number of physiological and psychological effects, includ-

Activity 10.2

For one working day, monitor and record how often you touch the clients in your care. Using Jackson's (1995) classification of:

- Instrumental touch
- Expressive touch
- Systematic touch
- Therapeutic touch,

observe and categorize each of your touching experiences for that day and reflect on your particular use of touch within your practice. Are you satisfied with the way you use touch? Is your client satisfied? Would you like to change the way you use touch? How would you change your current practice?

ing release of stress and tension. The various movements can improve the blood and lymph flow, loosen knotted tendons and relax muscles. Such therapies, therefore, can be used in the care of a client with physical and motor problems to relieve muscle tension and spasm. Proponents of both massage and therapeutic touch claim that it can help with problems such as high blood pressure, arthritic and rheumatic pain, asthma, colds, constipation, depression, muscular strain and sciatica (Trevelyan 1993). Touch can bring significant benefits to patients at minimal cost. Using touch has always been an integral part of how nurses relate to the people in their care, using it to soothe, reassure and communicate. It is essentially a part of the nurse's professional skills, and the resulting experience for the person with a learning disability can be beneficial, stimulating, relaxing and communicative.

Touch as communication

Touch can be used to convey feelings of encouragement, concern and emotional support. It can also communicate emotional warmth and, used in a therapeutic way, can help reduce clients' distress, anxiety or difficulty in articulating feelings. Touch provides us with a form of communication which can help to facilitate and encourage the therapeutic process, helping the person with a learning disability to have contact with the social

world, to receive information and to convey it. Some of the complementary therapies also make use of other senses, such as taste and smell, which can also be used to communicate information.

Therapies such as massage, reflexology and aromatherapy, which incorporate touch, can be used as a means of communicating care and comfort to patients experiencing isolation and vulnerability. A person with learning disabilities may be isolated thorough sensory or physical impairments and/or challenging behaviour, and touch can provide a point of contact for them. Holistic health practitioners use touch to enable the client to become more aware of themselves by fostering a 'helping–healing' relationship (Sanderson & Carter 1994).

There is evidence to suggest that poor communication skills are correlated with challenging behaviour (Stansfield & Cheseldine 1994), as is the absence of social contact (Durand & Crimmins 1987). Behavioural difficulties are an effective way of obtaining social contact, and some self-injurious and self-stimulatory behaviours can be explained in terms of attempts to seek more accessible tactile stimuli (Hogg et al 1990). People with profound learning disabilities seldom have high levels of social contact (McGill & Toogood 1994) and touch can therefore provide an opportunity for such contact within the client–therapist relationship. Normal experiences of touching and being touched can be denied the person with learning disabilities because of the profession's concern with the sexual implications of using touch.

Client–therapist interaction

Fundamental to the practice of complementary therapies is the concept of client-centred work, allowing the provision of one-to-one attention and close interpersonal contact between client and therapist. One of the important psychological effects of, for example massage, is the establishment of a relationship between the therapist and the client, where touch is used both as a social and a therapeutic medium through which non-verbal communication can also be derived.

Traditionally within the nurse–patient relationship an element of distance has been maintained. This has been considered professional, and prevents the nurse becoming too involved with the patient or client. Withholding social contact and touch is one way of communicating this distance (or power) within the relationship.

The traditional view has, perhaps unconsciously, taken heed of this potency [of touch] by insisting on keeping an emotional distance between carer and patient (Ellis 1994).

The intimacy of the client–carer relationship within the field of complementary therapies is altogether different and reflects the holistic philosophy at its centre. The interaction that takes place during a massage permits the establishment of a relationship which can contribute to an appropriate and beneficial healing environment. Time, opportunity and confidence to share are provided, allowing the client to share problems with the assurance that they will be considered sympathetically, without the rush and hurry that too often characterizes medical interviews. One of the reasons people choose to visit a complementary practitioner is the increased amount of time and attention given to the client during a consultation (Sharma 1992).

Concluding comments

For people with learning disabilities the combination of these factors – oils, touch and the therapist–client interaction – can provide a beneficial therapeutic experience. Using such therapies within the context of care provision for this client group can help create a supportive and stimulatory atmosphere. These experiences, which make use of both touch and smell, can enhance the individualistic care provided for the person with a learning disability. Although different in nature, the Snoezelen rooms provided in many care facilities attempt to stimulate the client in much the same way, that is, to provide a multi-sensory experience, and in the case of complementary therapies this is coupled with high-level one-to-one contact. Relaxation is often difficult for some of our clients to achieve, and it has been

shown that teaching clients with learning disabilities an individual relaxing posture can reduce noise and disruption levels in a ward (Deakin 1995). The management of behavioural difficulties is just one area of possible use for complementary therapies: already relaxation training is commonly used and is a potentially effective component of any treatment plan aimed at resolving behavioural difficulties.

Increasingly within nursing literature the need to recognize the importance of touch and to incorporate such therapeutic interventions into our care planning is being acknowledged and valued. A person with physical limitations and/or additional sensory impairments can be helped to explore a range of different sensory encounters, thus providing them with a rewarding therapeutic experience. The scientific backlash against complementary therapies can be seen by the accusation that their effectiveness can be explained in terms of the placebo effect, i.e. a response that cannot be explained on the basis of actual drugs or treatment. The effects produced are generally considered to be psychological in nature, with the patient's expectation to get better coupled with the beneficial effects of extra attention and a desire to 'please' the doctor producing the effect rather than the drug or treatment itself. Whether the therapeutic change can be attributable to the oils, the massage or the placebo effect, what is important is whether or not the person with a learning disability experiences it as beneficial or life enhancing.

I've worked with people who are deaf and blind with severe mental and physical handicaps who would not understand the concept "placebo" and who are very different after a combination of oils and touch (Hanse 1990).

Within the constraints imposed upon us when practising complementary therapies, if we can safely say they enhance the quality of care we provide for our clients, then there is no reason not to consider using them. In terms of costs, there is little to consider except the cost of the oils and the nurse's time, and if it can have a beneficial effect on the health and wellbeing of the person with a learning disability then these costs are low indeed.

ESTABLISHING THE EFFECTIVENESS OF COMPLEMENTARY THERAPIES

Less than 10% of lay people who use a complementary therapy have based their decision to use that particular therapy on scientific evidence (Jackson 1995). However, as healthcare professionals we have a responsibility to conduct and use research to validate and endorse our nursing decisions. Despite our enthusiasm to implement these practices, it remains imperative that we ensure that client care is based upon sound research evidence.

Within the literature there are primarily anecdotal accounts of the effectiveness of complementary therapies, and the overall paucity of sound research evidence is a stumbling block for nurses wishing to implement such therapies in their practice. The current research picture suggests that a range of different therapies are being explored by nurses, and that some evaluation is being conducted. Aromatherapy in particular has received attention from nurse researchers, and the profile is slowly developing; however, some of the studies have not involved controls, and uncontrolled observations do not allow for systematic evaluation. We must not be content with the introduction of these therapies until their value and potential contribution to the care of our client group can be reliably established.

Activity 10.3

Select a therapy that interests yourself and/or the other members of the multidisciplinary team and gather as much information and research on the subject as possible. Divide the information you gather into the following categories:

● Well conducted and controlled studies
● Case studies and anecdotal evidence
● Background information, including contact numbers and addresses.

Use the information gathered to produce a 'resource' file on the subject for the team members. The information can be presented at a team meeting or displayed in the form of a poster exhibition.

The need for research and evidence-based practice

There is evidence that nurses in all settings, including learning disabilities care (hospital and community), are either interested in or currently using complementary therapies. However, the lack of appropriate research in this area can only impede the progress of this developing area of nursing expertise.

For therapies to become part of professional nursing practice we must also be prepared to undertake research in order to justify that our actions are based upon knowledge rather than belief (Rankin-Box 1992).

The need to evaluate the effects of complementary therapies through well-designed studies using appropriate research methods is considerable. It has been argued that when evaluating complementary medicine, it is difficult to devise a research protocol which is able to sensitively measure treatment effects using the current (orthodox) rules for research practice (Patel 1987). This is not necessarily the case: the nursing profession and related health disciplines have a wealth of different research methods at their disposal, and as more studies emerge we find that practitioners are using a combination of quantitative and qualitative methods to measure treatment effect. What is becoming increasingly important is that the method chosen is appropriate to the study, and that the measurement tools are reliable and sensitive enough to detect treatment effects. It is necessary for nurses to explore the range of research methods available, and there are solid arguments for the devising of more creative methods (Osborne 1994) in which the individual response of the client will be reflected in the research protocol. Box 10.1 highlights the practicalities of introducing complementary therapies into nursing practice.

As a result of escalating interest in complementary therapies it is encouraging to see that research moneys are gradually being earmarked to undertake study into their efficacy. As a profession we must take advantage of all opportunities to develop the research base of our practice. However, funding research into complementary therapies is not likely to be considered a high pri-

Box 10.1   Practicalities

If you are considering introducing a complementary therapy into your practice there are several issues worthy of consideration prior to implementation.

Information and research. Gather as much information and knowledge as you can about the therapy you wish to introduce, including critiques of the available research literature.

Advice. If you are not appropriately qualified as a complementary practitioner yourself, seek specialist advice and help from a reputable and qualified therapist in that field.

Collaboration. Discuss the use of complementary therapies with the doctor and other healthcare professionals involved in the care of a particular patient. Seek their support and discuss with all members of the multidisciplinary team your intention to introduce that therapy into your practice. Therapies must always be appropriate to the patient's assessed needs, and should not conflict with other aspects of care management.

Establish guidelines. Devise a team strategy and produce guidelines on how you intend to implement and monitor the complementary therapy within your practice. Include accountability and safety measures reflecting the multidisciplinary nature of the service provided. The UKCC encourages employers to establish local policies to provide a framework for the use of complementary therapies by practitioners in their employment.

Evaluation. An evaluative framework is necessary in order to monitor the patient's response to and experience of the therapy. The evaluation should be systematic and ongoing, with regular information sharing and dissemination among the team and to others wishing to implement a therapy.

Consent. The UKCC suggests that it is worth considering obtaining the client's formal consent to such a treatment. Where appropriate, both clients and their relatives should be consulted and appropriate information given to ensure informed decision making by the client. Following consultation and authorization, all information should be recorded in the appropriate documentation.

ority in a system of finite resources, as there are already difficulties in funding therapies of proven effectiveness.

REGULATION OF COMPLEMENTARY THERAPIES

As complementary therapies find an increasingly more substantial role within healthcare, it is important to ensure that their introduction is supported by sound regulatory bodies. If they are to be fully integrated into contemporary nursing practice then some regulatory framework becomes necessary to protect both the client and the practitioner. The 'big five' therapies have, over time, gradually achieved an acceptable level of regulation in the eyes of the general public and the medical and healthcare professions. Nevertheless, others, such as aromatherapy and reflex zone therapy, have yet to achieve such standards of control and management.

UKCC regulations

In January 1994 the UKCC produced a position statement on complementary therapies, recognizing their growing popularity within the nursing profession. This position statement refers to various other documents produced by the council that govern the use of complementary therapies by nurses, midwives and health visitors. The UKCC refers to the standards set in the Code of Professional Conduct, and in particular to the application of principles set out in paragraphs 8–11 of the UKCC's document *The Scope of Professional Practice*, which is concerned with developing practice. Specific mention of complementary therapies is made in *Standards for the Administration of Medicines* (Articles 38 and 39). The UKCC's position is illustrated by the recurrent theme which states that the nurse is responsible for her or his actions:

It is the responsibility of the individual practitioner to judge whether a qualification obtained in a complementary therapy has brought the practitioner to an appropriate level of competence to use that skill in patient or client care (UKCC 1994).

In this way the UKCC seeks to regulate nursing practice in relation to complementary therapies by re-emphasizing the boundaries set by other regulatory documents. This places the degree of responsibility firmly with the individual practitioner.

RCN guidelines

The RCN has also considered the implications for nurses, midwives and health visitors with the imminent introduction of complementary therapies into the practice arena. The College has formed a special interest group from which has evolved the RCN Complementary Therapies Forum, whose priorities are: 'UKCC recognition of courses, standardisation of education in general, development of and distribution of principles and guidelines for practice, networking, research, increased funds (for courses/research)' (RCN 1993).

The RCN has also constructed guidelines on choosing an appropriate course in a complementary therapy, and a 'consumer checklist' (RCN 1993) to allow nurses to give patients advice on how to choose a therapy or therapist. 'One of the great dangers of complementary therapies is that people become interested in one field and rather than take an accepted training course, simply become knowledgeable "dabblers"' (Frost 1992).

Within the profession nurses are practising these therapies with a range of expertise, training and qualifications. Some are gaining formal qualifications, whereas others are practising after a much shorter course of training, in some cases as little as 10 weeks. Trevelyan (1995) describes these different types of practitioners as 'experts', 'dabblers' and 'facilitators'. The 'experts' are those who hold a recognized qualification; 'dabblers' are those who may have a personal and professional interest in a therapy and have usually attended workshops or a short course, and then introduce some aspect of that therapy into practice, for example using an essential oil. The 'facilitators' are those who are suitably informed about complementary therapies and are able to give information to the client regarding the most appropriate therapy or practitioner for them to consult; they do not practice themselves, but ensure informed decision making by the requesting client.

It remains the responsibility of the individual practitioner to judge whether a qualification obtained in a complementary therapy has brought them to an appropriate level of competence to use that skill in patient care. Where a practitioner is working independently, self-evaluation of competence and accountability becomes particularly important.

Precautions

All therapeutic interventions, whether they are designated as being western, orthodox, complementary or alternative, carry their own set of contraindications, side effects, warnings and special applications. As with the provision of orthodox treatment and care, precautions should be taken when practising a complementary therapy.

THE IMPLICATIONS FOR NURSING

If it is accepted that nurses will continue to use complementary therapies in their practice, there are several considerations to be reflected upon. These can be summarized as follows.

Education and qualifications

There is a need for standardized training courses in complementary therapies, and courses should aim to receive accreditation by the ENB and the UKCC. A proposal for a Council directive states that individuals supplying a service, including medicine, nursing and complementary therapies, will have to justify their actions should a malpractice suit be brought against them. This being the case, adequate professional training must be undertaken prior to the inclusion of a complementary therapy into nursing practice, to safeguard both the practitioner and the client. The need for information regarding minimum training guidelines is becoming progressively more urgent, and the appropriate training levels need to be decided by the professional bodies governing nursing practice. Competence to practise can only be established if standards are set that determine both training and educational levels.

Regulation

Alongside a system of standardized education is the need for regulation. When choosing a course in a complementary therapy it should be a professionally validated one, but also the therapy itself should be regulated by one of the two central organizations, the British Complementary

Medicine Association or the Institute for Complementary Medicine.

Regulation ensures standard setting, organizational codes of conduct and disciplinary procedures. It seems likely that the UKCC will be compelled to make a decision regarding those therapies that are acceptable in nursing practice and those that are not. Nursing autonomy, accountability, health, safety and legal liability all need to be addressed more stringently if complementary therapies are to be integrated into orthodox nursing practice.

Research and development

There is an acute need for the development of a substantive research base in order to critically evaluate and rationalize the use of complementary therapies for specific disorders. Effective evaluation is necessary to ensure that evidence-based practice is achieved and that sound clinical judgements are made regarding appropriate usage of such therapies. A critical review of all currently available evidence on the effectiveness of complementary therapies needs to be undertaken by credible and independent researchers. Following the critical review a research and development strategy needs to be decided in which additional research is conducted, including looking at the cost–benefit analysis of such therapies. All research information should be published and widely disseminated so that informed decisions can be made by practitioners. The opinions of local populations and health professionals need to be determined to assess the potential demand for such therapies, so that joint policies in funding and commissioning complementary therapy services can be determined.

CONCLUSION

Nursing is currently engaged in discussions regarding its future role in healthcare provision and the possible extension of its professional role boundaries. It could be that nurses seek to expand this role by using these simple techniques, and so add to their range of professional skills and enhance the quality of care given to clients. The general public will continue to demand alternative and complementary healthcare, and these demands provide the opportunity for both the client and the practitioner to have additional choice. However, before any decisions are made regarding complementary therapies, their effectiveness and appropriate usage need to be determined if we wish to accept that they have a place in the care of people with learning disabilities. Appropriately designed research studies are needed which are well controlled and designed, using a relevant method and measuring tools. The popularity of complementary therapies stems from their easy incorporation into practice, but the question remains whether the profession should be embracing a therapeutic intervention without using sound evidence-based clinical judgement. 'There is little doubt that the incorporation of complementary therapies within community nursing practice will continue to gain ground' (Thompson 1994).

REFERENCES

Bauer W, Dracup K 1987 Physiological effect of back pain in patients with acute myocardial infarction. Focus on Critical Care 14(6): 42–46

Booth B 1994 Reflexology. Nursing Times 90(1): 38–40

Buckle J 1993 Aromatherapy: does it matter which essential oil is used? Nursing Times 89(20): 32–35

Deakin M 1995 Using relaxation techniques to manage disruptive behaviour. Nursing Times 91(17): 40–41

Dunbar S, Redick E 1986 Should patients with acute myocardial infarctions receive back massage? Focus on Critical Care 13(3): 42–46

Dunn C, Sleep J, Collett D 1995 Sensing an improvement: an experimental study to evaluate the use of aromatherapy, massage and periods of rest in an intensive care unit. Journal of Advanced Nursing 21: 34–40

Durrand V M, Crimmins D B 1987 Identifying the variables maintaining challenging behaviour. Journal of Autistic and Developmental Disorders 18: 99–115

Ellis R B 1994 Defining communication. In: Ellis R B, Gates R J, Kenworthy N (eds) Interpersonal communication in nursing: theory and practice. Churchill Livingstone, Edinburgh

Evans E 1990 Reflex zone therapy for mothers. Nursing Times 86(4): 29–31

Frost J 1992 Herbalism: an overview of ancient art. Professional Nurse January: 47

Gates B 1994 The use of complementary and alternative therapies in health care: a selective review of the literature and discussion of the implications for nurse practitioners and health care managers. Journal of Clinical Nursing 3: 43–47

Groer M, Mozingo J, Droppleman P et al 1994 Measures of salivary secretory immunoglobulin A and state anxiety after a nursing back rub. Applied Nursing Research 7(1): 2–6

Guardian Educational Supplement 1996 Back to our roots. January 10

Hanse M 1990 Points of view. Nursing Standard 4(48): 43

Harrison J, Ruddle J 1995 An introduction to aromatherapy for people with learning disabilities. British Journal of Learning Disabilities 23: 37–40

Hewitt D 1992 Massage with lavender essential oil lowered tension. Nursing Times 80(25): 8

Hogg J, Sebba J, Lambe L 1990 In: Sanderson H, Harrison J, Price S (1992) (eds) Aromatherapy and massage for people with learning disabilities. Hands On Publishing, London

Jackson A 1995 Alternative update. Nursing Times 91(8): 61

Keller E, Bzdek V M 1986 Effects of therapeutic touch on tension headache pain. Nursing Research 35(2): 101–106

Kramer N A 1990 Comparison of therapeutic touch and casual touch in stress reduction of hospitalised children. Paediatric Nursing 16(5): 483–485

Krieger D 1975 Therapeutic touch: the imprimatur of nursing. American Journal of Nursing 75: 784–787

McGill P, Toogood S 1994 Organising community placements. In: Emerson E, McGill P, Mansell J (eds) Severe learning disabilities and challenging behaviours: designing high quality services. Chapman & Hall, London

McPhail C, Chamore A 1989 Relaxation reduces disruption in mentally handicapped adults. Journal of Mental Deficiency Research 33: 399–406

Meehan T C 1993 Therapeutic touch and post-operative pain: a Rogerian research study. Nursing Science Quarterly 6(2): 69–78

National Association of Health Authorities and Trusts 1993 Complementary Therapies in the NHS. Research Paper 10. NAHAT, London

Oldfield V 1992 A healing touch. Nursing Standard 6(44): 21

Osborne S E 1994 The future of homeopathy and other complementary therapies as part of the British National Health Service [Guest Editorial]. Journal of Advanced Nursing 20: 583–584

Patel M S 1987 Problems in the evaluation of alternative medicine. Social Science Medicine 25: 669–678

Perkin M R 1994 A comparison of attitudes shown by GPs, hospital doctors and medical students towards alternative medicine. Journal of the Royal Society of Medicine 87(9): 523–525

Plantania-Solazzo A, Field T M, Blank J K et al 1992 Relaxation therapy reduces anxiety in child and adolescent psychiatric patients. Acta Paedopsychiatrica. 55(2): 115–120

Randolph G L 1984 Therapeutic and physical touch: physiological response to stressful stimuli. Nursing Research 33: 33–36

Rankin-Box D F 1988 Complementary health therapies: a guide for nurses and the caring professions. Croom Helm, London

Rankin-Box D 1992 European developments in complementary medicine. British Journal of Nursing 1(2): 103–105

Rogers M 1970 Introduction to the theoretical basis of nursing. F A Davis, Philadelphia

Roper N, Logan W W, Tierney A J 1990 The elements of nursing: a model for nursing based on a model for living, 3rd edn. Churchill Livingstone, Edinburgh

Royal College of Nursing 1993 Complementary therapies: a consumer checklist. RCN, London

Samarel N 1992 The experience of receiving therapeutic touch. Journal of Advanced Nursing 17: 651–657

Sanderson H, Carter A 1994 Healing hands. Nursing Times 90(11): 46–48

Sanderson H, Harrison J, Price S 1992 Aromatherapy and massage for people with learning disabilities. Hands On Publishing, London

Sayre-Adams J 1994 Therapeutic touch: a nursing function. Nursing Standard 8(17): 25–28

Sayre-Adams J, Wright S 1995 Change in consciousness. Nursing Times 91(41): 44–45

Sines D 1992 Caring for people with learning disabilities. RCN Nursing Update. Nursing Standard 25(7): 3–8

Sharma U 1992 Complementary medicine today: patients and practitioners. Tavistock/Routledge, London

Stansfield S, Cheseldine S 1994 Challenging to communicate. Learning Disability Bulletin. BILD. 98/1.

Stevenson C 1992 Measuring the effect of aromatherapy. Nursing Times 88(41): 62–63

Tattam A 1992 The gentle touch. Nursing Times 88(32): 16–17

Thomas M 1989 Fancy footwork. Nursing Times 85(41): 42–44

Thompson J 1994 Complementary therapy: increasing patients' options. Community Outlook September: 19–23

Trevelyan J 1993 Massage. Nursing Times 89(19): 45–47

Trevelyan J 1995 Incorporating complementary therapy into contemporary nursing practice. Conference Paper. Complementary Partnerships Conference, 1.11.95, York

Trevelyan J, Booth B 1994 Aromatherapy. Nursing Times 90(38): 3–15

United Kingdom Central Council for Nursing, Midwifery and Health Visiting 1992 Code of professional conduct, 3rd edn. UKCC, London

United Kingdom Central Council for Nursing, Midwifery and Health Visiting 1994 Complementary therapies position statement. UKCC, London

Ward A 1990 The role of physical contact in child care. Children and Society 4(4): 337–351

Which 1996 Healthy choice. November: 8–13

FURTHER READING

Journals
Churchill Livingstone produce two journals, *Complementary Therapies in Nursing and Midwifery* and *Complementary*

Therapies in Medicine. For further information contact Robert Stevenson House, 1–3 Baxter's Place, Leith Walk, Edinburgh EH1 3AF. Tel: 0131 556–2424

There is also the *Journal of Alternative and Complementary Medicine,* published by the Green Library, Homewood NHS Trust (DHQ), Guildford Road, Chertsey, Surrey KT16 OQA. Tel: 01932 874333

Nursing journals such as the *Nursing Standard* and the *Nursing Times* regularly run articles on complementary therapies.

Books

Booth B 1993 Complementary therapies. Nursing Times Macmillan, London

Rankin-Box D F 1988 Complementary health therapies: a guide for nurses and the caring professions. Croom Helm, London

Sanderson H, Harrison J, Price S 1992 Aromatherapy and massage for people with learning disabilities. Hands On Publishing, London

Sharma U 1992 Complementary medicine today: patients and practitioners. Tavistock/Routledge, London

---

USEFUL ADDRESSES

For general information contact:

The Alternative Health Information Bureau (a research database) 12 Upper Station Road, Radlett, Hertfordshire WD7 8BY.
Tel: 01923 469495

The British Complementary Medicine Association
39 Prestbury Road
Pittville
Cheltenham
Gloucester GL25 2PT

The Institute for Complementary Medicine
PO Box 194
London SE16 1QZ

The Research Council for Complementary Medicine
60 Great Ormond Street
London WC1N 3 JF

For therapy-specific information contact:

Aromatherapy Organisations Council
3 Latymer Close
Braybrook
Market Harborough
Leicester LE16 8LN

International Federation of Aromatherapists (IFA)
Stamford House
2–4 Chiswick High Road
London W4 1TH

For more information contact:

British Acupuncture Council
Park House
206–208 Latimer Road
London W10 6RE

Confederation of Healing Organisations
113 High Street
Berkhamstead
Hertfordshire HP4 2DJ

Faculty of Homoeopathy
Hahnemann House
2 Plowis Place
Great Ormond Street
London WC1N 3HT

Independent Register of Manipulative Therapists Ltd
106 Crowstone Road
Westcliffe-on-Sea
Essex SS0 8LQ

Society of Homoeopaths
2 Artizan Road
Northampton
NN1 4HU

Profound and multiple disability

E. Wake

This chapter aims to consider the holistic needs of the individual with profound and multiple disabilities, within the context of family-based care. It seeks to incorporate the recent publication from the Department of Health entitled *Continuing the Commitment* (Kay et al 1995a) and act as a catalyst for further study by the reader.

WHAT DOES 'PROFOUND AND MULTIPLE DISABILITY' MEAN?

This is a term that is often used yet difficult to define. Kay et al (1995a) state that it is important to move away from definitions that are 'static' and move 'towards a more person centred approach'. Using this approach, profound and multiple disability could be construed as referring to an individual who requires maximum assistance in all aspects of everyday life, in terms of 24-hour care and supervision. The person may have difficulty in communication, eating and drinking, continence and mobilization, for example. Multiple disability means that the individual has additional needs, for example in terms of physical disabilities and/or sensory impairment, and this often also includes a range of additional, complex health needs.

It is important that professionals working with people who have profound and multiple disabilities stop and reflect upon the meanings that are attached to such terms. As nurse practitioners, it is vital that we question such labels from a psychosocial perspective. Words that we invariably use in our schemas, and which create our view of everyday life, include a wide range of attributions about others in terms of our own attitudes, beliefs and values. It is important, therefore, that nurse practitioners involved in the care of people with profound and multiple disabilities examine and re-examine their attitudes, beliefs and values regarding this group of people. Nurses invariably state that they hold only positive beliefs with regard to such people, but it is possible to challenge this (see the questions in Activity 11.1).

To value the person with profound disabilities as a person first and foremost, involves our own implicit value systems, which means both consciously and subconsciously held values and beliefs regarding others.

It is essential that nurses working with people with profound and multiple disabilities act as advocates for their clients, and focus on their abilities and strengths, rather than concentrating on what they are unable to do. The medical model has a distinct tendency to focus upon what a person cannot do, and nurses should

Activity 11.1

- If you were offered an opportunity to change places with someone with profound disabilities, would you do it? If not, why not?
- Are there any specific aspects of that person's disabilities that you would rather not have? Why is this?
- When you think about a person with profound and multiple disabilities, what images does this conjure up for you?
- What is the basis on which you feel you have formed these images?

challenge this, celebrating the uniqueness of every individual and focusing care on their strengths. This does not mean that needs are not acknowledged, simply that the person's strengths should be used in helping to meet his or her own needs. This can involve a high degree of healthcare input, much of which is aimed at maintaining health and preventing ill health.

Every individual has a different health status in terms of what his or her usual health is. For example, if someone receives enteral feeding, it will be usual for that person to have a daily nutritional assessment to maintain good hydration and nutrition. However, for another person, who is able to eat and drink normally, either with or without help, such an intervention would be unnecessary. Yet the person who is having enteral feeding is not ill, they are just not able to have all their nutritional needs met by oral feeding. The enteral feeding therefore maintains their health. (This issue will be further explored when nutrition is discussed, especially as regards whether enteral feeding is a therapy or a treatment: this is a current ethical issue within learning disabilities nursing and the legal system in the UK – see Chapter 5 for further explanations.)

HOLISTIC CARE: A MULTIDISCIPLINARY APPROACH?

It is important that professionals recognize the boundaries of their knowledge and skills. The person with profound and/or multiple disabilities will have a wide range of needs, as will their carers. It would be wrong to assume that the client will need to be under the care of a consultant psychiatrist and not require the full range of services that the rest of the community uses. This is especially so as many people with profound disabilities live in the community; therefore, their care should be in and by the community (Brown & Smith 1992). The person with profound disabilities may require help from the primary, secondary and tertiary health sectors, as well as from social services and other statutory and nonstatutory agencies, which may cause difficulties. They may also find they have to deal with a multitude of professionals, and there can be a significant lack in consistency of approach by those professionals. Thus the 'key' or 'link' worker or 'named nurse' approach has been used to minimize the difficulties of multiagency working. This named individual acts as the main link with the client and his or her carers, and seeks to coordinate services with them, thus avoiding duplication. One problem that has been identified with this approach is that each agency will appoint a named person, who will work with the family; this is not a true key worker approach. The agencies involved should acknowledge that one person from the service that is most involved should coordinate services. Central to this arrangement is the need for this person to be someone with whom the client and the carer can identify, and who they feel will best act as a facilitator, advocate and enabler. Regular reviews of service input should be arranged, and these meetings must include the service users, i.e. the client and his or her carer(s).

Need for holistic and lifelong planning of care

This section aims to focus on how people with profound and/or multiple disabilities can be supported to maximize their quality of life. One of the ways in which this can be achieved is the maintenance of the individual's health. Health gains are also considered where appropriate, but it needs to be appreciated that health gains cannot be met if the individual is not being supported in the maintenance of health and in strategies

to avoid ill health. Thus the chapter considers the range of healthcare needs that the individual may have, although not everyone with multiple disabilities may have the same needs.

FEEDING ISSUES

People with profound and multiple disabilities often have a number of specific problems concerned with eating and drinking (see Chapter 12 for additional information). The reason for linking with the chapter on communication is that eating and drinking, and hence good feeding skills in carers, are important in terms of communication skills. This section considers specific feeding difficulties, as well as why they occur and basic management techniques.

Difficulties with eating and drinking

The disabled person may have problems related to muscle tone around the mouth and face, or in the body generally. A person with severe cerebral palsy, for example, may have a problem with all of these that will express itself in terms of general posture, i.e. seating position difficulties, as well as problems with their ability to suck, chew and swallow without aspirating (Rogers et al 1993). Important reflexes such as coughing and gagging may be limited, and the person may still have some of the reflexes that are present in infancy, such as the startle reflex. The implications of the startle reflex are commented on in the next section.

Such problems may be in addition to other problems common in the general population, such as food intolerance and allergies, malabsorption syndromes and specific oral/dental and skeletal problems. The implications on eating and drinking of conditions such as cleft lip and palate, Pierre Robin syndrome and Goldenhar syndrome, for example, cannot be underestimated. It is also important to consider the impact of underlying health problems, such as congenital heart disease and respiratory difficulties, both of which can greatly affect a person's ability to eat and drink. Gastrointestinal problems such as oesophageal reflux are relatively common in people with severe cerebral palsy, and cause a great deal of discomfort (Halpern et al 1991). Management of gastro-oesophageal reflux is usually via conservative medical treatment, initially using drugs such as cimetidine and cisapride, as well as advice to carers on techniques that may alleviate the symptoms, such as ensuring that the person is in a comfortable, upright sitting position during the meal, and is not laid down for at least 30 minutes afterwards. Close observation of the individual is needed after meals, especially if they are prone to reflux problems, as any discomfort or vomiting could have serious consequences (for example if the individual was lying down). The avoidance of drugs and food or drink that are linked with gastro-oesophageal irritation should be encouraged, and all who are involved in the person's care should be aware of what foods can cause such problems for him or her. Offering smaller meals more often, rather than the traditional 'three square meals a day' will also help, especially if there is an underlying medical condition such as cardiac or respiratory disease.

It may be necessary for a specialist in gastro-oesophageal problems to become involved if the condition continues despite conservative management, as the discomfort and distress of reflux and its potential complications, such as oesophageal erosion, should not be underestimated. It may therefore be necessary for surgery to be performed (the Nissen fundoplication) (Heine et al 1995) to lessen the likelihood of reflux. For some people this may be done as a precursor to insertion of a gastrostomy, in which case insertion will be part of the overall surgical procedure, rather than via endoscopy as described below (Jolley et al 1985, Langer et al 1988). However, the good feeding regimens should continue after surgery and the person will continue to require careful monitoring.

Another aspect of feeding problems to consider relates to the level of learning disabilities the person may have, as it may be that they have very immature feeding skills, such as sucking food rather than attempting to chew it, or even being unable to take food off a spoon correctly, except by tongue thrusting and licking movements. Some people with profound and multiple disabilities are unable to manage food even in a semisolid form.

Management of eating and drinking skills

It essential that the person with profound and multiple disabilities and his or her carers have regular access to a speech and language therapist with specific training in feeding difficulties and management. It is important to obtain advice and guidance from the therapist on, for example, feeding techniques, food consistency, and the management of problems specific to the individual. The therapist may advise that non-oral feeding is in the person's best interests (see below). The involvement of the physiotherapist and occupational therapist is also very important in the overall approach to feeding difficulties.

In residential and professionally run units/homes it is important to have specific policies with regard to the management of feeding difficulties of each individual who utilizes the service. The reader is advised to use the contacts, addresses and texts that are mentioned at end of the chapter for further information.

NUTRITIONAL NEEDS

This is an area in which there appears to be increased interest, perhaps because there are now more speech and language therapists available with specialist skills in feeding management. This is also perhaps currently the most controversial area of healthcare in the UK, with the issue of enteral feeding methods (i.e. nasogastric and gastrostomy feeding) being debated in terms of whether they are or are not treatments. To some they could be seen as an active medical intervention where families have requested that none be given.

Nutrition and feeding

There are many people with profound and multiple disabilities who have difficulty with feeding skills, particularly the ability to suck, chew and swallow, as well as drinking adequate volumes of fluids. The main issue here is the potential risk of aspiration (Gisel et al 1995). This is in addition to the difficulty of feeding onself, and thus being reliant on carers for food and drink. This raises the issue of the varying abilities of carers as regards appropriate and safe feeding techniques.

Before one can consider the actual feeding techniques used, it is essential that the physical handling and positioning of the person is correct, otherwise this will exacerbate the above problems as well as being uncomfortable for the individual. For this it is essential to liaise closely with the occupational therapist and physiotherapist. The correct seating position and equipment are essential. The person with severe muscle spasms due to cerebral palsy will, for example, require a seating system that enables the correct posture to be maintained and thereby minimize the impact of extensor spasms. If this is not achieved and the person experiences extensor spasms while eating or drinking, there is a high risk of choking and aspiration. However, carers also need advice about the whole environment in which the person will be having meals.

It is important to consider the opportunities available to enhance the quality of the individual's mealtime experience. A quiet period beforehand to reduce the impact of the mealtime activity itself can be useful, for example approaching the person gently, talking quietly

and massaging their face can help, and mealtimes should be unhurried. The carer should sit face to face with the individual, allowing better eye contact and ensuring that being fed is a sociable occasion, rather than something you have 'done to' you. Certainly with new staff it can be useful to spend time on role play, giving the carer the opportunity to find out how it feels to be fed, and how not to feed someone, before they engage in such an activity. It is vital that a new member of staff does not attempt to feed someone with feeding difficulties, owing to the increased risk of causing the person to choke and aspirate. In units or homes that care for people with extensive feeding difficulties it is recommended that there be supervision by a medical practitioner and a speech and language therapist trained in this aspect of care. It is also advisable that someone trained in the use of emergency suction techniques be always available at mealtimes.

When people with such difficulties are cared for at home, the main carers should be taught how to use suction equipment, and have appropriate portable equipment available. Supportive nursing services should also be available 24 hours a day where necessary, so that eating and drinking are not restricted to mealtimes only.

Severe swallowing difficulties – a management strategy

It is important to seek the advice and support of the speech and language therapist trained in feeding skills (Caudery & Russell 1995). If an individual has significant feeding difficulties it may be that they are not receiving their full nutritional and hydration requirements. Added to this is the problem that a person with severe cerebral palsy, for example, may have an increased energy requirement owing to increased metabolism and frequent involuntary movements. Thus it is important also to refer to the dietitian for advice and strategies that can be used to ensure that nutritional needs are being met. These strategies can include a wide range of nutritional supplements based on the person's age, weight, calorie needs and abilities, as well as their tastes. These

Activity 11.2

Consider the following scenario:
Paul is having his meal in the residential home for ten adults in which he lives. Paul has severe cerebral palsy, and as a result tends to have a lot of problems with extensor spasms and an exaggerated startle reflex. He is therefore easy startled, which results in involuntary movements. The dining room in which he has his meals has a heavy swing door into the kitchen, which is constantly in use. The door bangs shut each time it is used and each time this happens Paul is startled and starts to cough and choke. As Paul's main carer, what would you do to ensure that he is able to eat his meals with the minimum of difficulty?

can include fortified drinks such as juices and milk shakes, fortified puddings, whole meal supplements in drink form, and high-calorie powders that can be added to the meal and which do not alter its taste.

The use of the thickened drinks, meal supplements and puddings has an added benefit in that they are easier to swallow than fluids on their own. Fluid thickeners (with no calorie content) that promote easier swallowing are also available.

If it is felt that an individual is not taking adequate nutrition orally, it may be in their interests for oral feeding to be supplemented with enteral feeding, via a nasogastric tube or gastrostomy, the latter being much more suitable as a long-term approach. The benefits of this are that:

- it ensures that the person has adequate fluid and nutritional intake in a given 24-hour period
- it enables the person to take in orally whatever they wish and are able to, without the carer worrying about the amount taken that day.

The disadvantages focus mainly on the fact that enteral feeding may be viewed as an intrusion or 'unnatural', and the cost involved. However, it is a strategy that is increasingly being used. It could be argued that the benefits of such feeding techniques outweigh the difficulties in terms of reducing the risk of aspiration. Also, if oesophageal reflux is minimized the associated discomfort and potential distress of oesophagitis may be alleviated (Heine et al 1995).

Key professionals should work together with the person and their main carer(s) to assess particular feeding problems, and to ensure that any strategies implemented are regularly evaluated. As mentioned earlier, an individual with serious swallowing difficulties is at risk of aspiration, hence the importance of life-saving suction skills. There is a wealth of effective portable suction equipment available, and the community nurse will be able to offer advice, as well as access to an equipment loan scheme. In such cases it is important to question whether oral feeding techniques are really in the person's best interests. Videofluoroscopy is currently regarded as the

Activity 11.3

Christopher is 39 years old and has profound and multiple disabilities. He is unable to sit up properly even with the support of a seating system. He has all his meals and drinks orally. However, his father has noticed that Christopher is coughing more and more often when being fed, and is repeatedly suffering severe chest infections. After much discussion and consultation Christopher had a videofluoroscopy performed, which showed that he was aspirating a considerable amount. It was then decided by his father and the professionals involved that it would be best if Christopher had a gastrostomy, and no longer took food or fluids orally because of the significant risk of aspiration. A month after the operation Christopher's father said he was finding the new regimen difficult, because he felt that Christopher did not understand why he could not have any more drinks or food. He was now wondering whether the gastrostomy was best approach.

There are a number of issues within the above scenario that are important to consider.

- If the gastrostomy had not been performed there was a significant risk of aspiration-induced respiratory problems. Given that this is known, does it justify the approach taken?
- Although it can clearly be argued that the action taken was in Christopher's best interests, perhaps there is an alternative argument when making such a decision, given that Christopher has had oral feeds for 39 years. Does this make the decision more difficult, and why?
- In view of the current debate regarding enteral feeding and whether it is an 'extraordinary' treatment, what if Christopher's father later wished for feeding to be stopped?

best technique available for identifying a person's overall swallowing abilities (Morton et al 1993, Mirret et al 1994, Gisel 1995).

It may be considered that the risk of aspiration is too high: indeed, the person may have experienced episodes of aspiration resulting in respiratory difficulties or even aspiration pneumonia. In this instance non-oral feeding may be the best option, and for no oral feeding to take place.

The benefits of enteral feeding, especially gastrostomy feeding, cannot be ignored, especially as it is argued that up to 80% of children with profound learning disabilities are considered to be at risk of aspiration (Griggs et al 1989, Morton et al 1993, Mirret et al 1994). Techniques for gastrostomy insertion have become simpler and the equipment has become more user friendly. Gastrostomies can now be inserted via endoscopy, hence the term percutaneous endoscopic gastrostomy (PEG); this means that usually only a short general anaesthetic is needed for the procedure. Overall this has tremendous benefits for individuals with underlying respiratory problems.

After the gastrostomy tube has been used for approximately 6 months (the time element is very much based on individual needs) it may be changed for what is termed a 'button gastrostomy', which is almost flush with the skin. The button gastrostomy is easy to use and the design ensures that there are no free-moving parts that could be accidentally pulled or damaged (see Fig. 11.1). Each button will have its own attachments for feeding use. Several manufacturers provide a wide range of gastrostomy devices, and are usually very helpful with information, such as basic troubleshooting as well as aids and adaptations to make the system easier to use. Many manufacturers also supply portable electrical pump systems, which are small and lightweight and would enable a person to have a continuous feed over time if necessary, and yet not have to be dependent on a mains supply to operate the pump.

Access to the full range of equipment for gastrostomy feeding is usually via the dietitian and community nurse. The feeds to be used and the dietary regimen must be under the strict supervision of a dietitian, and the feeds are available on prescription. The equipment may also be available on prescription, but it is most often ordered via the dietitian, who liaises with the medical practitioner and community nurse. Many manufacturers provide a 'door-to-door' service to the individual's place of residence.

CARE OF A GASTROSTOMY
Oral hygiene

Individuals having all or some of their nutritional intake via a gastrostomy will still need regular

Activity 11.4

Consider how you would feel if you had no oral intake and were reliant on carers to provide your oral hygiene needs. How often would you like to have this? How would you like to have it performed for you?

oral hygiene. It is a common misunderstanding that if someone does not have fluids or food orally they will not suffer from dental decay; however, plaque continues to form on the teeth whether you eat or not. Also, if a person is unable to ask for a drink, they are likely to be given a drink whenever their carers feel they need one, rather than when they want one, so it is likely that their mouth will be more dry and the need for mouth care increased. This will be discussed more fully later in the chapter.

The gastrostomy itself

Gastrostomy care is reasonably straightforward and involves certain basic principles regardless of the type of tube used. There are additional guidelines which refer specifically to each gastrostomy design, which should be explained by the community nurse. Again, manufacturers provide specific information about their products that includes management advice.

Basic care principles include good hand hygiene and skin care around the gastrostomy site. The following should also be observed:

- Keep the site clean and dry.
- Gently wash around the site with cool boiled water or Normasol at least once daily. Pat gently dry, ensuring that the area is thoroughly dried.
- Watch for any leakage, excoriation or redness around the site. The advice of the community nurse or medical practitioner should be sought if any of these occur.
- The gastrostomy itself should not be covered by a dressing or taped down, unless specifically advised to do so by the medical practitioner.

Feeding techniques

- Always use the equipment specific to the type of gastrostomy being used.
- Only use the feeds and amounts of feeds that are prescribed for that person.
- The tube should be gently flushed with cool boiled water before and after feeds – the amount is dependent on the needs of the person and dependent on the dietitian's advice.
- When bolus feeding with a large syringe the feed should *never* be forced in using the syringe plunger – it must always be allowed to go in via gravity. The community nurse will advise on management if it appears that feeds are blocking the tube.
- A large syringe should be used for bolus feeding – ideally 50 or 60 ml syringes and no smaller than 30 ml.
- When continuous feeding is used the correct electrical pump for that type of commercial feed should be used, with its own giving set designed for single use.

Carers are advised to consult the relevant health professionals and appropriate texts for further information. There are also videos and leaflets that can be helpful.

It is important that, even if individuals have some or all of their meals via the gastrostomy, they do not miss the social experience of mealtimes, and are able to have the same care offered to others. Mouth care during the gastrostomy feed is essential, and for many people a range of small amounts of food in the mouth, if appropriate, can be very important in terms of oral stimulation. Mealtimes are part of the collective culture of the United Kingdom, and often a time of relaxed socializing. It is important that the person who is having gastrostomy feeds should not miss out on such occasions.

MOBILIZATION NEEDS

The importance of a correct seating position is something that carers tend to take for granted. For the person with profound learning and multiple disabilities being able to move around inde-

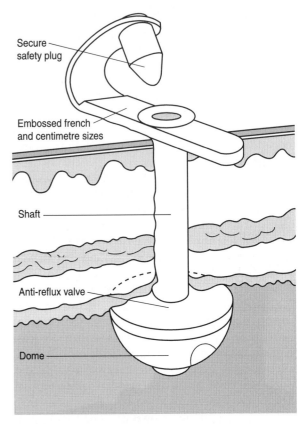

Figure 11.1 Button gastrostomy. (With permission from Merck Biomaterial, after illustration of button in Information Sheet on Corpak® Button.)

pendently is something that cannot be taken for granted, and many such individuals are completely dependent on their carers for their every move. Because of this carers need to stop and reflect on the full impact of what it means to be fully dependent on others. This requires a degree of empathy to consider ways in which the individual can be empowered to make their needs and wishes known, using the abilities they have. This may be facial expression, eye pointing or by verbal methods, for example. Communication is essential and must be valued, whatever method is used.

For the person with mobility difficulties the input of physiotherapist and occupational therapist is essential. These team members should be included in the planning of everyday care provision for all individuals with such problems.

The key areas considered in this section are:

- The promotion of an individual's potential in terms of everyday functional skills and the role of the therapists in this
- The minimization of additional physical disabilities
- The prevention of pressure sores
- Strategies to enhance mobilization/ensure optimum comfort and positioning for the individual.

Promoting the individual's potential

Perhaps the most important issue here is the inherent right of the individual to have access to therapists and resources that enable them to gain the most from their own motor and sensory skills. This not only means that the person has the opportunities to develop his or her own potential, and enhance their quality of life, it also ensures that therapists can identify potential mobility problems. Active measures can then be taken to minimize the impact of potential complications.

Role of therapist

As mentioned earlier, a good seating system is important. The physiotherapist and occupational therapist should therefore work with the person and their main carers to identify a seating system that is comfortable as well as providing the correct body posture in terms of hip alignment and limb and trunk positioning to minimize any potential further disabilities. Neck support is also important. Some people with profound physical disabilities may need a seating system that includes a body mould (i.e. an insert moulded to the shape of their body). The introduction of such an insert, to encourage a more upright position, must be very gradual, especially if the person has always previously been in a supine or prone position.

Safety in the use of seating and mobility systems is essential. The positioning straps and supports are there not only to encourage the best position, but also to provide safety for individu-als who cannot support themselves. Therapists spend a great deal of time with individuals and their carers considering the possible options, such as the ability of the system to help minimize the effects of involuntary movements, and to provide reliable and comfortable safety devices, which must also be easy to keep clean. For individuals who may be at risk of aspiration, or who have severe seizures on a regular basis, quick-release safety and positioning devices are essential.

The design of the seat must also be age appropriate, so as not to reinforce the negative view of individuals with profound learning and multiple disabilities as being 'eternal children'. Families may express concern that the seating system should not be cumbersome or significantly different from furniture in their homes. There is a wide range of systems available that seek to overcome these concerns, and most manufacturers endeavour to provide equipment that is not only therapeutic but also aesthetic, catering for the wishes of both the individual and their family. Also, most equipment nowadays is portable, thereby overcoming transport difficulties. However, it is important that services such as short-term breaks have access to the equipment used by an individual. Usually there is only one system for the individual to use in their usual care setting and one in their educational or day care setting. However, there is a need for one to be available in each care setting, because of the problem of limited transport facilities and the inconvenience for carers of having to transport equipment around.

Therapists' roles are diverse, and can be seen to have a demonstrable and positive effect on a person's quality of life in terms of posture, balance, coordination, and strengthening of function in the limbs. The use of tilting tables, for example, which encourage a more upright posture in a secure, supported standing position, has many benefits. These include:

- improvement of circulation
- promoting bone strength and limiting the impact of spontaneous fractures
- improving breathing, and also neck control

- the opportunity to see everyday life from a different perspective.

This may also enhance communication skills, as the individual has an opportunity to communicate at a different physical level, which can help limit the negative impact of being 'talked down to' which can occur when someone is in a wheelchair.

It is important that equipment is used with guidance from the physiotherapist, who will advise on how to ensure that the individual is comfortable, and in a safe as well as a beneficial position. They should not be left unattended while using the equipment, especially if they have a tendency for powerful involuntary movements that could affect their safety.

Physiotherapy can be provided in both formal and informal settings. Formal methods also include strategies such as conductive education, patterning and concentrating on specific movements. These methods can be very helpful, and are run in conjunction with an occupational therapist, focusing on movement as well as the prevention of problems such as contractures. It is important that children in particular are referred to therapists at an early stage. Informal methods can include activities such as horse riding, which is valuable in encouraging good posture and balance, as well as being an important social occasion. Swimming, as well as formal hydrotherapy sessions, also helps promote good breathing techniques and relax stiff and contracted muscles, as well as providing the obvious benefits of buoyancy and freedom of movement.

Minimizing additional physical disabilities

As stated earlier in this chapter, a great deal of the time spent caring for the person with profound learning and multiple disabilities is aimed at maintaining health, which is very important in terms of quality of life. This is particularly so given the survival rates of individuals in this client group (Evans et al 1990) and the debate surrounding the assessment of anticipated ortho function, i.e. limb flexibility. This is often described as being particularly poor in this client group, yet many of these same individuals are later argued to have better ortho function than that which was initially predicted (O'Grady et al 1995).

Physical disabilities can be exacerbated in many ways, and a range of strategies must be used to ensure that this is prevented, or at least minimized. Potential problems include:

- muscle atrophy
- contractures
- loss of limb flexibility (ortho function)
- increased difficulty in using seating, hoists and wheelchairs, necessitating more and more adaptations
- podiatry-related problems.

The above problems can also mean that an individual is more at risk of respiratory problems, pressure sores and perhaps even fractures. People with profound learning disabilities who are immobile are estimated to be most at risk of developing deformities (Bottos et al 1995).

Immobility-related problems are an issue for people with profound and multiple disabilities, because of muscle atrophy and reductions in muscle size, caused by lack of oxygen. As muscle contraction increases this further limits joint movement, and this can be difficult to prevent, even with high levels of physiotherapy intervention. For people with cerebral palsy, as well as those with Down syndrome, the risk of hip dislocation cannot be ignored.

Physiotherapy and occupational therapy devices such as splints and body braces can be invaluable in enabling the person to maintain optimal posture and limb positioning. However, surgery may become the main option to alleviate the discomfort of hip subluxation or dislocation as the person enters adulthood (McKinlay & Holland 1986). This problem is exacerbated in individuals with muscle contraction, in that at present the only reliable intervention for excessive muscle tone, particularly in the lower limbs, is surgery in the form of a tenotomy. Intensive physiotherapy as part of the individual's everyday activities is essential. Passive physiotherapy techniques can be particularly beneficial when used in conjunction with hydrotherapy, either formal or informal.

Medication can also be beneficial in helping to reduce potential muscle spasms, which can exacerbate contractures and the associated discomfort. Medications such as baclofen (Lioresal), the current drug of choice, and dantrolene (Dantrium), aim to reduce muscle tone and can be very beneficial. Diazepam (Valium), a benzodiazepine, is also used, but is associated with increased sedation and even occasionally extensor hypotonus. All drugs used for muscle relaxation, particularly those such as baclofen and dantrolene, must be introduced very gradually and the dose slowly titred to ensure the optimum effect with the minimal dose. These drugs must always be reduced gradually if they are being withdrawn. Dantrolene should *not* be used with children (British National Formulary 1996). However, medication should be an adjunct to other supportive methods rather than a single treatment option. As stated earlier, physiotherapy is essential, and one should consider the range of massage techniques that can be used to help reduce muscular spasms, as well as the use of complementary therapies such as aromatherapy and homoeopathy (see Chapter 10). The use of TENS – transcutaneous electrical nerve stimulation – should also be considered as a non-invasive yet very effective way in which the discomfort and pain of muscle spasm can be reduced.

Good seating and positioning are also essential to minimize muscle spasms, and can even inhibit the full extent of extensor spasms, for example, by enabling the person to be more in the midline, or perhaps even in a position of mild flexion. This would have to be maintained in any moving and handling techniques used.

There is a wide range of mobilization aids that the physiotherapist and occupational therapist may use to promote ortho function and thus enhance daily living. Arm gaiters, for example, can be very useful for support when sitting balance is being attempted. They can also help minimize involuntary muscle actions and thus enable the person to perhaps use an adapted motorized wheelchair. The recently developed lycra-based dynamic splinting suit (Blair et al 1995) has been publicized as promoting ortho function. The 'Upsuit', as it is termed, is made to meet the needs of the individual and is considered to be very effective. It is argued that an adaptation of this in the form of dynamic splinting on the limbs only may be easier to use, and is certainly better for the individual for whom lung function is a concern, or where carer compliance is an issue (Blair et al 1995).

Flotron therapy is also used to assist mobilization as it can alleviate muscle spasm and help prevent contractures. It is often used following the removal of plaster or delta casts, which may have been used after a tenotomy has been performed. Flotron therapy can be used, for example, for a specified period of time before the person is helped to get up after a night's sleep.

Prevention of podiatry problems

This is an area of care that is often forgotten, possibly because it is overshadowed by the other mobilization difficulties that are predominant. However, this does not mean that regular podiatry assessment and preventive care is not important. The simplest issue is the need to ensure that any footwear whether specialist or not, fits well and does not rub or irritate the skin (Prasher et al 1995). If an individual wears ankle/foot orthoses as well as specialist footwear, there is the chance that the orthosis may be put on incorrectly by carers, and cause sore areas on the feet. Carers should not attempt to apply orthoses without demonstration and supervision by the physiotherapist.

Regular podiatry assessment is an essential component of everyday care for the individual, and is readily available without financial cost for people with learning disabilities via local health authority trusts.

Prevention of pressure sores

People who are immobile are at high risk of potential skin breakdown as a direct result of their immobility. If they are left in the same position for long periods, with no attempt to change that position either by themselves or by others, then skin integrity will be compromised and may potentially break down. This can be so severe as to cause extensive tissue and muscle damage, as well as being a potential site for localized or systemic infection.

Prevention involves a range of strategies:

- Ensuring that the individual has the correct nutritional and fluid intake to meet their daily needs
- Ensuring that these nutritional needs are re-evaluated when the individual is unwell or having elective surgery, so as not to compromise their overall health status and hence promote their wellbeing
- Regular evaluation of the range of equipment used daily for the individual's comfort: checking for any areas where skin may come into contact with straps, fastenings and the general framework of the equipment is essential
- Ensuring that the person's position is changed regularly to maintain skin integrity, including while they are asleep. However, the practice of changing someone's position hourly or 2-hourly while they are asleep should be questioned, and the time period altered according to the individual's sleep pattern
- Specialist equipment such as alternating pressure mattresses can be of use, especially if the person has significant physical disabilities and limited movement. (Some individuals with severe muscle contractures are only able to lie or sit in a limited number of positions, and are therefore more at risk of pressure sores.)
- Daily calculation and recording of the potential risk of skin deterioration: if the individual is being cared for in a residential facility or by multiple formal carers, difficulties could arise in identifying potential skin integrity problems and taking action as soon as possible. Using an appropriate risk calculator, such as that of Waterlow (1992), can assist in identifying the level of risk as well as acting as a means by which to monitor the effectiveness of any related intervention

- Prompt action is important if there are any concerns regarding skin integrity in order to minimize skin breakdown.

Strategies to enhance mobilization

Caring for someone who is immobile, involves difficult and time-consuming activities, such as dressing, undressing, moving and bathing the person, which leaves less time for carers to spend considering the individual's leisure and recreational needs. Families should be encouraged to seek the best equipment available that will enable them to care for their relative, and occupational therapists can suggest a range of ways in which such routine activities can be made easier. Dressing and undressing someone with severe contractures and muscle spasms can be extremely difficult, and can be responsible for back and neck injuries in carers. The occupational therapist may therefore suggest loose-fitting clothing, so as to ease the difficulties of dressing and undressing. Changing the way in which a garment is fastened can also help, for example front-fastening bras can be useful for women with profound and multiple disabilities. There is a range of aids for assisted bathing, such as bath hoists, cradles, alternating-height baths, shower trolleys and other individualized adaptations. The cost of such equipment can be considerable, but the cost of providing extra carers to support the family is much greater, and thus helping families in any way possible is of benefit to all concerned.

Nurses must consider the following:

- Be aware of the impact of nutrition and fluids on maintaining health.
- Ensure that therapists such as physiotherapists and occupational therapists are involved in caring for the individual: their input is essential.
- Consider moving and handling strategies that maximize comfort and safety for the individual and carers at all times.
- Carers should never lift a person on their own if at all possible. Formal carers working in residential facilities, for example, will be

breaking the organizational rules for health and safety if they attempt to lift someone on their own.

- Do use the range of pressure-relieving equipment available to meet the individual's needs.

THE INDIVIDUAL WITH VISUAL IMPAIRMENT

There are many factors to which visual impairment may be attributed. Retinopathy of prematurity is stated to be a common cause of visual impairment, where retinal blood vessels spasm and complete retinal detachment can occur (Dodds 1993). The condition was first described in 1942, and was attributed to the high levels of supplemental oxygen given to neonates (Silverman 1980), although it is now argued that there are so many factors that can affect the preterm infant, that this condition has a multifactoral basis. It has a significant impact on the individual, and can affect general development in that the young child has to maximize the use of their other senses to explore their environment, and it also affects their spatial awareness (Dodds et al 1991).

Other causes of visual impairment include conditions that are generally associated with the elderly, although it should be remembered that this is not always necessarily the case. Macular degeneration, in which central vision deteriorates, is a common cause of significant visual impairment. Peripheral vision is often still present, and carers need to be aware of the need to maximize any residual peripheral vision that the person may have.

Glaucoma can also affect the individual's vision. This involves the build-up of aqueous fluid in the ducts of the eye, resulting in pressure on the optic nerve as well as on the retina. It can occur gradually, and thus not be identified until the individual expresses concern regarding their sight, or it can occur over a short period of time and is associated with pain and discomfort. Given that either form may develop, it is important that visual screening is regularly performed, especially if there is a known familial tendency to

the condition. The chronic form might otherwise not be noticed by carers, especially if the individual has limited communication skills. A key worker is important if the person is being cared for in a formal setting, so that any difference in the individual's behaviour can be identified and the cause linked to a deterioration in vision. A potential tendency to develop glaucoma can be identified in children: indeed, there is a form of glaucoma that occurs in young children known as buphthalmos (Klemz 1977).

Damage to the optic nerve and the areas of the brain associated with vision during pregnancy or postnatally owing to, for example, meningitis or trauma, is also an associated reason for visual impairment in people with profound and multiple disabilities.

Visual impairment in a person who is immobile is of particular concern, as their only means of independent 'mobility' within their environment is through sight. If an individual is dependent on visual cues as a means of non-verbal communication, when verbal communication is not possible, this could be seen as a fundamental need. Thus the promotion of optimal visual health is not an option but a necessity. This includes regular visits to the optician, and attendance at an ophthalmology clinic if appropriate. It is important that common conditions such as myopia (short-sightedness), hypermetropia (long-sightedness) and presbyopia (far-sightedness, which is more prevalent in older people) are screened for in people with profound and multiple disabilities, as correction of these conditions via the use of spectacles can be invaluable in ensuring that they have the best possible quality of life. However, there is a range of visual health issues that are more prominent in people with profound and multiple disabilities. These include, for example, tear production problems and resultant blepharitis, cataracts and hemianopia.

Tear production problems are common in people with Down syndrome, in that the tears contain excessively high amounts of protein. This causes a chronic eye infection known as blepharitis, owing to the eyelash follicles becoming irritated and inflamed. If the individual is susceptible it is important that carers perform eye care as part of their daily routine.

Cataracts can seriously impair an individual's vision. It is argued that up to 50% of people with Down syndrome have cataracts (Lane & Stratford 1985). Cataracts can be congenital, but are often not detected till young adulthood or can develop later in life. Given the significance of visual skills for people with profound and multiple disabilities, it would appear to be prudent to check their visual status at least annually.

Hemianopia usually presents as part of the person's overall physical disabilities, in that it is often associated with hemiparesis. This can be particularly difficult for an immobile person as it means that their visual field is often significantly impaired on the affected side of their body. As with all visual impairments, it is important that the extent of such a condition is known by carers, so that they can seek support and advice from therapists as to how the person's residual vision can be optimized. Advice from the local service for the visually impaired is invaluable, as is the range of equipment and advice available from support groups such as the Royal National Institute for the Blind (RNIB).

Caring strategies

It is argued that nearly 75% of people with cerebral palsy have some form of visual impairment (Black 1980). It is important that those involved in the day to day care of an individual with profound and multiple disabilities are aware of the significance of visual impairment. It is acknowledged that inappropriate self-stimulatory behaviour can be a result of significant visual impairment (Moller 1993); hence the need to ensure that any residual sight is maximized, and the emphasis on using the person's other skills must be paramount, in order to discourage the development of any such behaviour.

A range of strategies can be used to meet the needs such individuals. Multisensory techniques can be invaluable, but they must be used with care and understanding to prevent a distressing sensory overload. Techniques such as Snoezelen (Doble et al 1992, Laurent 1992) can be beneficial

to both individual and carers when used properly. The use, for example, of relaxation techniques and the gradual introduction of auditory and olfactory stimulation while maximizing the person's residual vision, can also be extremely satisfying.

Other strategies can also be used, such as tactile and auditory equipment that is age appropriate in design and use. Altering the lighting in an individual's home can help promote the use of residual sight, by using bright light and primary colours, for example in eating utensils and crockery. The development of a 'multisensory garden' or window box can be very worthwhile: this involves maximizing the use of the fragrances given off from flowers and herbs.

THE INDIVIDUAL WITH A HEARING IMPAIRMENT

Hearing impairment and visual impairment are among a range of health needs that have been acknowledged by the Department of Health (Kay et al 1995a). Carers, both informal and formal, need support in developing their understanding of the impact of hearing impairment given that it is suggested that as many as one in 10 people with learning disabilities have some form of hearing impairment (Ball 1991). Definitive statistics are difficult to obtain, possibly because the screening of such individuals is still inadequate. However, as more infants and young children are screened for hearing impairment, realistic statistical information should emerge. The interpretation of the statistics could be argued to be more important, in that it may enable more people with profound and multiple disabilities to access the range of hearing impairment services they require, which could help improve their quality of life. It is argued that currently approximately 0.16% of the general population of the United Kingdom have severe learning disabilities, and approximately 33% of these have sensory impairments (Harries 1991). However there is still ' . . . no current universally accepted definition of what constitutes a significant sensory impairment in a person with learning disabilities . . . ' (Hatton & Emerson 1995).

A study by Hatton and Emerson (1995) highlighted the problems in the provision of services for people with profound and multiple disabilities who have a hearing impairment, owing to the difficulty of identifying such people. The authors argued that, even though local authority service providers expressed a willingness to offer services, provision will remain patchy, as there are currently also no 'reliable assessment procedures and clearly defined service options to address service user needs' (Hatton & Emerson 1995).

Given the importance of actually defining what is meant by hearing impairment, there are a number of options that one could use to support the individual and the family which should assist service purchasers in reflecting on the need to develop service provision further. The advent of the multiagency Children with Disabilities registers as a result of the Children Act (1989) may be regarded as a means by which to highlight service provision needs within localities. Although registers are seen by some as further labelling individuals with learning disabilities, the need to overcome the problems highlighted by Hatton and Emerson (1995) perhaps tips the balance in their favour, if it means that service provision will ultimately improve. As with vision, it is important that residual hearing is maximized. A programme of positive approaches that professionals can use with the individual and the family include:

- screening of individuals who are seen as being at risk of hearing impairment
- early identification of any hearing difficulties
- prompt and systematic management strategies to minimize the impact of hearing impairment
- information for families regarding the diagnosis and management of hearing impairment, and the support networks and services available.

Risk factors would include prematurity, prenatal infection, maternal illness during pregnancy (e.g. rubella and herpes zoster), neurological impairment such as severe cerebral palsy (particularly athetoid linked), meningitis and other central nervous system infection, and trauma. Iatrogenic causes of sensorineural (perceptive) hearing impairment should also be considered, for example intravenous antibiotic therapy used to treat meningitis.

Serum otitis media, generally known as 'glue ear', is a form of conductive hearing impairment that should be suspected, particularly in people with Down syndrome (Lane & Stratford 1985).

Familial incidence of hearing impairment should also be regarded as a significant indicator to consider screening the child with profound and multiple disabilities. Hotchkiss (1989) argued that a genetic link could be found in a large proportion of people with profound hearing impairment.

Care issues

Treatment of any underlying medical cause of the hearing impairment is essential. With any other type of hearing impairment it is important that, as stated above, residual hearing is maximized. This may involve the use of appropriate hearing aids and adaptations to the person's environment, for example an audio loop to enhance hearing aid performance within the home. It is important that the effectiveness of any aids is regularly evaluated, particularly as compliance with their use may be a problem (Yeates 1995).

For the individual with profound hearing loss, as well as profound and multiple disabilities, verbal communication could be severely affected, and so the development of non-verbal communication skills is essential. If the individual has motor and mobilization difficulties the use of non-verbal signing systems, such as Makaton, may be more difficult to achieve. However, a personalized version of Makaton and/or the use of electronic touch-sensitive talkers can be of considerable benefit. It may be argued that personalized signing systems limit communication with others in the fullest sense, but the ability to use them with carers should not be disregarded, as it represents an opportunity for the individual to express their needs. In formal care settings care plans should reflect a person's own communication needs and abilities. Communication is explored in more depth in Chapter 12.

CARDIOVASCULAR PROBLEMS

Cardiovascular problems are cited as an important healthcare issue in the Governments' (1995) publication, *The Health of the Nation: a Strategy for People with Learning Disabilities*. It is not possible here to explore the range of cardiovascular disorders that may affect the person with profound and multiple disabilities: none the less, it is important to acknowledge the need for a better understanding of any underlying cardiovascular condition an individual has. There are a number of support groups for carers, which can be found through a general practitioner. The community learning disabilities nurse should also be able to provide further details.

The initial *Health of the Nation* document (1991) also highlighted cardiovascular problems as an area that should be targeted for action to reduce the incidence of cardiac disease. A range of strategies can be used by carers, for example offering a varied, nutritional choice of foods. Even if the person has to be fed by a carer and have their food chosen for them, it is important to encourage a varied and nutritional diet. Professionals working with carers are advised to use the guidance provided, for example by the Department of Health Committee on Medical Aspects of Food (DoH 1994) and NACNE (National Advisory Committee on Nutritional Education). Carers can also seek the advice of a dietitian regarding the nutritional and fluid needs of an individual. It is a common misperception that someone who is immobile needs fewer calories, as often an individual who has frequent involuntary movements and muscle spasms will require more calories to replace the energy expended.

Lack of physical mobility can predispose the individual to the risk of circulatory problems, such as peripheral vascular disease. There is therefore a need for a daily range of passive and/or active physiotherapy routines that will help maintain the cardiovascular system's effective functioning. Excess weight gain may be a difficulty for some individuals with profound and multiple disabilities, and if this is the case it is important to seek advice. The individual's general practitioner should be contacted prior to considering any weight loss programme, to ensure that any underlying cause such as thyroid problems are eliminated. The dietitian and physiotherapist can help in identifying strategies to promote weight control.

ORAL HYGIENE

This area of care has already been discussed in reference to individuals who are unable to manage food and/or fluids orally. However, there are some additional general guidelines that should be explored, as well as some specific issues of importance for carers of individuals with profound and multiple disabilities.

Oral hygiene is something we tend to take for granted until we are unable to perform it ourselves. Much criticism has been aimed at the level of priority given to such a basic need when caring for people with profound disabilities (Griffiths & Boyle 1993). Access to dental services should be equitable, and most (if not all) health authority trusts offer a domiciliary dental health service to meet the needs of this client group. Dental hygiene routines may be difficult for carers to perform, perhaps because the individual has an exaggerated bite reflex, or simply does not enjoy the experience of having his or her teeth cleaned. A range of techniques can be employed to make teeth cleaning much easier, such as using desensitization techniques for the individual's face and mouth prior to attempting to brush the teeth, or the use of an electric tooth brush if tolerated. Plaque disclosing tablets may give the carer some reassurance regarding the effectiveness of the teeth cleaning. Where possible, the avoidance of high sugar-content food and drinks may also be worth considering.

Some specific issues that should be considered by carers are:

- the impact of medication, particularly some anticonvulsants, on oral health
- the particular problems that the individual with Down syndrome may have
- general feeding difficulties.

The impact of medication

High sugar-content versions of medications, especially if they have to be taken on a regular basis, should be avoided where possible, and sugar-free alternatives considered. For example, if an individual has paracetamol in an elixir form, there is a sugar-free option available.

Another issue regarding medication relates to a frequently used group of drugs, the anticonvulsants (drugs taken orally for various forms of epilepsy). The most common problems here concern phenytoin, which is linked to a condition known as gingival hyperplasia, in which the gums become tender and sensitive and may bleed. Gingival hypertrophy is also a problem. The important care issue here is not to stop the phenytoin but to implement good oral hygiene strategies and to make sure that the dentist is aware of any medication being taken.

Down syndrome

There are two main issues that carers should be aware of in people with Down syndrome: any underlying cardiac condition, which is considered to be a significant problem for people with Down syndrome (Burns & Gunn 1993), and atlantoaxial instability (a form of cervical spine instability).

• **Underlying cardiac condition** Oral antibiotic cover is essential before and after dental surgery, including routine procedures such as descaling. The rationale for this is to prevent endocarditis caused by bacteria present in the mouth entering the blood stream.

• **Atlantoaxial instability** The Department of Health (DoH 1995) recently issued guidelines to reaffirm the need to avoid subluxation in an individual with Down syndrome. This is a problem that is considered rare, yet difficult to exclude. The Department of Health has acknowledged that previous advice, which supported the use of neck X-rays to identify individuals at risk, could not be relied upon. This supports a 5-year study by Morton et al (1995), which considered this problem in particular. The condition should always alert healthcare professionals to act with caution.

Feeding difficulties

An individual with severe cerebral palsy may have a range of feeding problems, including exaggerated bite reflex, malocclusion and swallowing difficulties. The exaggerated reflex can pose problems for carers trying to clean the individual's teeth; also, if the individual has particular difficulty in chewing and swallowing, there could be a build-up of food in the mouth. This can be a particular problem if the person has to be fed by a carer who is not experienced in assisting someone with such needs. Again, it is important to reiterate the need for good regular oral hygiene care for the individual.

RESPIRATORY PROBLEMS

People with multiple disabilities often have respiratory problems. There are many reasons for this: for example poor swallowing and/or gag reflex, poor cough reflex, immobility, inability to be in the upright position, as well as common problems such as asthma and colds. The reason for including respiratory problems in this chap-

Activity 11.5

Consider the following.

Given that attitudes towards people with profound and multiple disabilities still focus upon the 'tragedy model', and that although attitudes may be professed to be positive, unconscious attitudes of 'I'm glad it's not me' still prevail, one needs to give some attention to the image that the general public have of such individuals. What has this to do with oral health? Dribbling and mouth breathing, and hence halitosis, can be a major problem for the individual and should not be marginalized. Carers need to spend time with the individual considering ways in which to minimize the impact of the dribbling, e.g. using age-appropriate scarves rather than bibs, and considering medication such as scopolamine skin patches. The problem of halitosis can be increased if the individual is unable to tolerate oral food and fluids, and so oral hygiene is very important. In such cases carers should seek advice from the individual's general practitioner, as there may be a need for additional saliva (Glandosane) to minimize the discomfort of a dry mouth.

ter is that because of their existing problems individuals with profound and multiple disabilities may have more difficulties with ailments such as colds. Some conditions associated with varying degrees of learning disability are also linked with various respiratory disorders, in Down syndrome, Goldenhar syndrome, chromosome 4 problems and CHARGE association problems for example, as well as conditions that are life limiting and associated with learning disabilities, such as Batten's disease and other metabolic conditions. There are also links between extreme prematurity of neonates with learning disabilities and with additional respiratory problems. For example, bronchopulmonary dysplasia is linked with immature lung function as a result of prematurity, and with the treatment such neonates require.

The main aims of caring for this client group in relation to respiratory function are:

- to maintain the individual's health
- to promote ways in which respiratory function can be enhanced
- promotion of awareness in carers, both formal and informal, of the risks associated with feeding, in terms of aspiration and potential aspiration pneumonia
- to ensure that any respiratory infections or difficulties are promptly identified
- to ensure that the range of treatment options for respiratory conditions meets the needs of the individual.

Prevention/minimization

It is important that carers work closely with the physiotherapist in considering ways in which an individual's respiratory health can be promoted. This can include daily chest physiotherapy, including postural drainage to prevent the build-up of excess secretions, especially if the individual is relatively immobile. Oral and nasal suction techniques may be necessary to assist in clearing excess secretions, so that the individual can breathe without discomfort. Also, the removal of excess secretions helps reduce the incidence of respiratory infection.

Changing the individual's position at regular intervals, as well as maintaining comfort and helping prevent pressure sores, is useful in maximizing respiratory function.

Promoting good respiratory function need not be expensive or time consuming for carers: simple things that may help include the way in which pillows are positioned while the person is in bed; and making use of times when an individual is perhaps lying over a wedge to encourage head control, to facilitate drainage of excess secretions.

CONTINENCE CARE

Continence care can be a major issue for people with profound and multiple disabilities. In childhood particularly, it is important to ensure that there are no underlying factors that could be exacerbating the continence difficulties, but the primary cause is likely to be in relation to the degree of learning and physical disability. Certainly the problem can be exacerbated by a urinary tract infection and renal abnormalities, which need to be treated.

Incontinence can be urinary and/or faecal, and there are a number of strategies that carers should be aware of, particularly concerning the individual who is relatively immobile.

Continence aids will be required to meet the individual's needs. These are available through local health authority trusts, many of which have a nurse practitioner who is a designated continence advisor, and who works closely with the professionals involved in supporting clients and carers. It is important to consider the impact of incontinence on the individual in terms of body image, comfort (some continence aids can be very bulky to wear), and skin care, in terms of prompt skin care regimens and the use of appropriate barrier creams.

Care issues

The most common form of incontinence is urinary, and a range of continence aids is available. Intermittent or long-term catheterization may be an option and can be very successful for people with neurological conditions, such as spina bifida, or paraplegia-related difficulties. There are a number of points that carers should be aware of in catheter care management to ensure the individual's comfort and prevent problems. For example, if long-term catheters are being used then the choice of type is important: silicone catheters are more comfortable and less likely to be associated with problems of urinary crystallization. Monitoring the pH of the urine may seem 'over the top', but can be useful to assist in the early identification of a urinary tract infection, and thus ensure prompt treatment. The consumption of up to 400 ml of cranberry juice daily is currently suggested as being beneficial in minimizing the incidence of urinary tract infections (Nazarko 1995). A good fluid intake generally is very beneficial, especially in this client group, because urinary stasis and the potential problem of urinary tract infection are exacerbated by immobility.

Faecal incontinence is particularly distressing, and carers need to consider ways in which, for example, the odour can be minimized. The most effective strategy is simply prompt skin care after defecation and the effective use of the appropriate continence aids. However, faecal incontinence does not mean that an individual should have to endure diarrhoea or constipation. Constipation is a problem considered to be associated with immobility, and it is therefore important for the individual to have a well balanced diet that is high in fibre (unless medically contraindicated) and an adequate fluid intake, as well as opportunities for mobilization, both passive and active. Medication is often prescribed to aid defecation, e.g. stool softeners and aperients, but the use of medication for constipation should be minimal and only under the guidance of a person's general practitioner.

EPILEPSY

Epilepsy is a condition often associated with profound and multiple disabilities (Kay et al 1995a). Before all the aspects of this subject are explored in relation to the client group being considered in this chapter, the reader is advised to turn to Activity 11.6.

What is meant by the term epilepsy?

Activity 11.6

- What do you understand by the term epilepsy?
- How do you envisage that epilepsy can affect the life of the individual with profound and multiple disabilities?
- What information do you think carers may want as regards caring for someone with profound and multiple disabilities who also has epilepsy?
- How would you access that information?

McMenamin and Bird (1993) define epilepsy as 'recurrent, episodic, uncontrolled electrical discharge from the brain. Epilepsy is the term for recurrent, unprovoked seizures or convulsions.'

Epilepsy is a condition that produces a range of images for both professionals and the general public, and it is important that readers examine their attitudes, beliefs and values regarding this condition. It is essential that professionals have a significant understanding of epilepsy, given the incidence of epilepsy in this client group. However, it is important to stress that having epilepsy does not equate with learning disability, and this must not be assumed. A number of studies have attempted to identify the factors that would signify a link between learning disability and epilepsy. Certainly epilepsy within the first year of life is seen as a significant (although not definite) related factor with learning disability (Curatolo et al 1995, Willie et al 1989), but it should be emphasized that there are a number of reasons why this may be so, such as prenatal malformations within the brain, and all the other linked pre- and postnatal conditions that are associated with learning disabilities. Indeed a case-control study by Curatolo et al (1995) highlighted the multitude of factors that can influence the development of learning disability alongside epilepsy, and also cerebral palsy.

If carers suspect that the individual has epilepsy, how is it diagnosed? Epilepsy is not usually diagnosed as a result of a single seizure, but rather if and when a second seizure occurs. The reason for this is that that we all have the potential for a single isolated seizure. However, this does not mean that medical advice should not be sought when a seizure occurs, as it may be a sign of an underlying medical condition that requires investigation and treatment. It is important that carers maintain a diary of an individual's seizures before and after formal diagnosis, as this will help ensure that the treatment prescribed is appropriate and meets the individual's needs.

Diagnosis is made primarily on the clinical history and using diagnostic tools such as EEG (electroencephalogram) and CT (computed tomography); both are non-invasive procedures. The medical practitioner will wish to exclude any underlying medical condition, and a blood sample may be taken for analysis.

Types of epilepsy and medications used

Epilepsy can manifest itself in many forms, although most people tend to be aware of the more common types: tonic–clonic seizures (often referred to as *grand mal* seizures, a term now disregarded owing to the limitations of its meaning) and absence seizures (again often referred to by the traditional term *petit mal*). All areas of the brain can be affected, although the frontal, parietal and temporal lobes of the cortex are most often linked with epilepsy.

- **Simple partial seizures** This is when symptoms affect only one side of the body. Consciousness is not affected and the person often experiences unusual feelings. Simple partial seizures often occur while the person is asleep.

- **Complex partial seizures** This form of seizure is often difficult to describe, and the value of maintaining a thorough diary will help in assessing whether seizures are of this type. The temporal lobe of the brain is associated with this type of seizure, and the individual is often said to be unaware of their surroundings, as consciousness is affected to a degree. The person may experience what is termed as an aura beforehand, e.g. an unusual smell. Automatisms – i.e. the term used to describe repetitive behavioural responses such as 'finger flapping' – can be evident. Partial seizures are often treated with carbamazepine (Tegretol), phenytoin (Epanutin), lamotrigine (Lamictal) or vigabatrin (Sabril).

- **Absence seizures** 'A brief loss of awareness, without any obvious jerking or falling down' (McMenamin & Bird 1993). These can occur frequently throughout the day, and again the carer's diary may indicate that a review of medication to limit the frequency of such episodes is required. It is sometimes possible to take steps to minimize recurrent episodes by ensuring that the individual is not over-tired or under undue stress, and that blood sugar levels are not low. As with all forms of epilepsy, medication prescribed to control the seizures must never be stopped except on medical advice. Absence seizures are usually treated with sodium valproate (Epilim) or ethosuximide (specifically for absence seizures) (Zarontin).

- **Generalized tonic–clonic seizures** As stated earlier, this type of seizure is the best-known form of epilepsy, and carers often refer to it as causing the greatest anxiety, because of its manifestations. It can be the primary form of epilepsy, but it can also occur as a secondary form following other types of seizures, such as complex partial seizures. The seizure involves two stages, tonic and clonic, although it may be difficult for onlookers to differentiate between them. The tonic stage involves loss of consciousness, and a person may look as though they have become rigid as the muscles go into extension. This is followed by a clonic period, which is typically seen as the muscles alternately rapidly contracting and relaxing. There may be urinary incontinence during the seizure and the person may also bite their tongue. After the convulsing has ceased a period known as the postictal phase follows, in which the person often is very drowsy yet rousable. They may wish to sleep for a time after the tonic–clonic phase has ended. It is important that carers are aware of the usual pattern of the individual's seizures so that any digression from that pattern can be investigated. Tonic–clonic seizures are usually treated with sodium valproate (Epilim), phenytoin (Epanutin), vigabatrin (Sabril) or lamotrigine (Lamictal).

There are other types of epilepsy that carers may need to be aware of, and professionals should always be aware of the number of ways in which epilepsy can manifest. These include myoclonic seizures, atonic seizures and seizures as a result of Lennox Gestaut syndrome. Carers and other professionals also need to be aware of the potential problem of what is termed status epilepticus, where a tonic–clonic seizure is prolonged (i.e. longer than usual for that individual) or the seizure is followed by another within a short time without the person regaining consciousness. This is classed as a medical emergency and requires prompt treatment in terms of immediate first aid and advanced management, and will almost certainly require medical treatment unless the problem is rectified by the administration (if prescribed) of diazepam in a specially prepared format for rectal administration (Stesolid).

Given the potential range of physical effects of epilepsy on the daily life of an individual with profound and multiple disabilities, it is a condition that cannot be ignored because of its psychosocial impact on the individual and their family. When the seizures are frequent and severe, the impact on everyday life may be phenomenal and the level of care required may seem insurmountable. Readers are advised to contact the British Epilepsy Association for more detailed information.

OTHER ISSUES IN THE CARE OF PEOPLE WITH PROFOUND AND MULTIPLE DISABILITIES

This section is by no means exhaustive and covers only few of the many aspects of care that could be explored. Because profoundly disabled people have unique needs, it is hoped that this chapter will act as a catalyst for the reader to develop a wider and more empathetic understanding of these needs. Thus this section will consider:

• aspects of pain management
• the impact of the life expectancy debate
• mental health issues
• age and ageing
• leisure
• support for carers.

Readers are advised to consult other chapters for more in-depth consideration of leisure needs, sexual identity and sexual health.

Pain management

There are many misconceptions regarding pain, its existence, manifestations and treatment. The purpose of this section is to direct the reader to challenge their beliefs, values and knowledge concerning pain. The inability to communicate verbally and the limited ability of some individuals with profound and multiple disabilities to communicate non-verbally could mean that they are marginalized in terms of pain management, as the assessment of pain is subjective. If the carer is not familiar with the means by which an individual communicates, the ways in which they express pain may be misinterpreted. The measure of someone's pain should not rely solely on verbal expression of its existence, and professionals should work with the client and their carers to ensure that pain relief is given where appropriate and its effectiveness monitored. It should not be assumed that by prescribing analgesia the pain will be relieved. Pain management tools should be adapted to enable the person's behaviour to be measured objectively.

Behavioural tools such as those used in paediatric nursing, for example the Children's Hospital of Eastern Ontario Pain Scale (CHEOPS) (McGrath et al 1985), may be extremely effective if adapted to be age appropriate, as adult pain relief scales depend on verbal communication and a significant level of cognitive understanding. However, as with all behaviour-based assessments, they are dependent on observable behaviour. Thus the carers who will use them must be aware of how the individual behaves when well, as well as when ill or in pain. There must be agreement as regards the subjective interpretation of an individual's behaviour to ensure a consistent and effective approach to pain management. Carers need to be aware that behavioural tools can only suggest, rather than represent an absolute indicator of pain (Carter 1994). Also, carers must be aware that the generally construed signs of pain, such as crying, do not have to be present, and pain may be felt even if the individual does not cry (Grunau et al 1990). This is an important factor, as some people have negative perceptions regarding the individual with profound and multiple disabilities and may assume that 'they can't feel anything anyway'; hence one of the benefits of pain assessment tools is to objectively demonstrate pain and pain control responses. They also have the added benefit of ensuring a consistent approach and enabling pain control strategies to be evaluated. There is a range of pain management strategies that may be particularly useful with this client group, in addition to the more traditional pharmacological methods. These include distraction, relaxation via touch and massage, aromatherapy, acupuncture and all the other complementary therapies. The use of TENS (transcutaneous electrical nerve stimulation) has already been described and could be given further consideration as it is effective, safe and non-invasive. Whatever is used, it is important that the strategy is tailored to the individual's needs. Inadequate and ineffective pain management is unacceptable.

Life expectancy

It is important to acknowledge that there are a number of health issues for this client group, but the expectation of morbidity should not be encouraged. The focus of work with this client group needs to be on the maintenance and promotion of health (Evans et al 1990). A study by Murphy et al (1995) highlighted that the care of adults with cerebral palsy with acute healthcare needs was satisfactory, but that a 'major concern was the lack of preventative health care' (Murphy et al 1995). Cerebral palsy does not necessarily equate with profound and multiple disabilities, but the need to provide adequate preventative healthcare is a global one.

Kudrajacev et al's (1985) study stated that severe learning disability was a factor that should be considered in relation to life expectancy, although this study is now over a decade old and the life expectancy of children with severe learning disabilities has increased considerably, with 90% of children with cerebral palsy now

reaching adulthood (Evans et al 1990). A study by Crichton et al (1995) highlighted some factors that are still considered as concerns, these being epilepsy, the degree of the learning disability, respiratory conditions and impaired mobility. These studies are particularly pertinent given the current medicolegal and ethical debates regarding infants and children and quality of life, and even the right to life itself. Hence the requests to discontinue medical care in relation to enteral feeding being debated as an extraordinary treatment for a young child with profound and multiple disabilities, and Re C (wardship: a minor) [1996], who was a ventilated premature infant with a prognosis of profound and multiple disabilities, are particularly poignant. Similar cases are Re B (wardship: a minor) [1981 All ER 927] in relation to an infant with Down syndrome, and Re J (wardship: a minor) [1990 All ER 930] in relation to a ventilated 27-week gestation infant (cited in Campbell & McHaffie 1995).

Readers are strongly advised to consult recent medical/legal/ethical journals regarding these debates, as well as biomedical ethics texts, and also to refer back to Chapter 5. It is likely that these debates will become more and more pertinent and frequent given the current climate within medicine. Readers should also be aware that there are a number of conditions associated with profound and multiple disabilities that are considered to be life limiting. Examples of these are Batten's disease and other metabolic conditions, degenerative conditions such as Tay–Sachs syndrome, and other inherited conditions, as well as the range of neurodegenerative conditions such as leukodystrophy and spinal muscular atrophy. Readers are advised to consult specific texts regarding the care of an individual with a life-limiting condition, as there is too much material to cover here. Some of these texts are included in the Reference list. It is important that both professionals and informal carers should seek to network with colleagues in the locality, as clients and their carers have a right to the full range of information and options regarding support. Support may include hospices, home care, short-term breaks and family-to-family support, as well as practical support and symptom control (such as pain management clinics).

Mental health

To state that this client group do not have mental health issues would be to deny feelings such as frustration, anger, sorrow and happiness, which are felt by all of us. What makes this subject more difficult is that it is difficult for the person with profound and multiple disabilities to voice their feelings and express them in the way that 'normal' people might.

The concept of mental health issues in this client group needs a great deal of further development (Naylor & Clifton 1993). However, it is acknowledged that it is difficult to know how an individual is feeling, even if we express genuine empathy. We can never be that person, and that person's needs, wishes and feelings are always interpreted by an able-bodied carer, particularly if they have limited non-verbal communication skills. Hence the need for a named worker or nurse when an individual is cared for in a formal setting, or even at home, so that they can become familiar with the person's means of expressing their feelings. Multiple carers do not equate with better understanding. Carers should remember that the individual is unique and may have many feelings regarding altered body image, stress or depression. Having a profound learning disability does not mean people do not have these feelings: it just means they are expressed differently, and this depends on the communication skills of the individual and their carers.

Age and ageing

Readers may be aware of the negative stereotypes associated with people who have learning disabilities. These include the 'Peter Pan syndrome' and the 'everlasting child', and this is particularly the case as regards individuals with profound and multiple disabilities. Consider the scenario described in Activity 11.7.

Adolescence is a time when identity synthesis is evolving. It is a time when the individual explores what 'I' and 'self' means to them and to their peers and family. In the United Kingdom and other western societies adolescence is seen as a time that leads to self-definition (Kroger 1996). However, this process of self-definition is often not fulfilled by adolescents with profound and multiple disabilities, because of the identity they have been 'given' since infancy, i.e. that of being profoundly disabled, and because of the belief of the 'eternal child' which can surround such an identity. It is thus important that carers (and professionals) are supported in re-evaluating their beliefs regarding adolescence in this client group (Baker 1991). It can be a time of great turmoil within the family, with questions such as:

- When does my son/daughter have to move from children's to adult services?
- Do I have a choice, does my son/daughter have a choice about when that should happen?
- I have known these professionals throughout my son/daughter's life; will the 'new' staff ever know him/her?
- What happens after school finishes?
- What centres are there, and will they allow my son/daughter to go every day?

It is a time that could poignantly remind the family of 'what might have been', as friends' children prepare for further education or work. At this time, parents often express concern about what will happen if they themselves become ill and are

Activity 11.7

You are a newly qualified nurse and for the past 6 months since qualifying have been assigned to the local community team for children with learning disabilities. You are visiting one of the special schools that you have been asked to liaise with. One of the teachers, while in general conversation with you, asks if you could "go and talk to one of her mums". She expresses concern that Zoe, one of the teenagers in the special care group, always seems to be dressed in clothes that are more suitable for a 5-year-old rather than a 15-year-old. The teacher then shrugs her shoulders and says that she feels that Zoe's mother 'might listen to you more as you are a nurse'.
What should you do?

unable to carry on caring, as it is a time when the individual can no longer truly be seen as a child. It also reminds the parents of their own age, adding to their concerns for their son or daughter's future.

Adulthood is a vast subject area, and so only one other major lifetime continuum event will be discussed – i.e. the older person with profound and multiple disabilities. This may appear a contentious subject, but readers are referred to the section earlier in this chapter regarding life expectancy and this client group, and asked to reflect upon recent papers which have completed longitudinal studies on this issue.

Before one can consider specific issues surrounding the care of the older person with profound and multiple disabilities, readers are asked to look at Activity 11.8.

It has been argued that individuals in this client group should be considered 'older' from the ages of 40–50 years, because of premature ageing and reduced life expectancy (Day 1985, Collacott 1987, Dalton & Wisviewski 1990). However the reader is asked to consider all the information available before accepting this as a definitive view, and to consider this subject on an individual basis.

It is acknowledged that people with Down syndrome have specific needs, as they are known to be more at risk of developing Alzheimer's disease in middle age (Mann 1988, Cooper & Collacott 1994). However, the papers that explore the links with learning disability and premature ageing tend not to include people with profound and multiple disabilities, and do tend to focus on people with mild learning disabilities as a client group with mental health needs and ageing con-

cerns (Cooper & Collacott 1994, Van Minnen et al 1994). It is therefore important that readers contemplate the issue of ageing and this client group further, particularly as regards leisure and health needs, such as osteoporosis and reduced joint flexibility, for example, and the right to access services designed to meet the needs of people in their 'third age'.

Leisure

Leisure and the occupational needs of this client group may appear to be a challenge to carers (see also Chapter 13). It is important that leisure needs are not disregarded, and facilities and activities should be age appropriate and wide ranging, so as to provide stimulation and pleasure as well as exercise.

There are a number of activities which can incorporate care needs while creating a leisure focus. Massage and multisensory activities can also incorporate some of the individual's physiotherapy needs, although it is important that there are times in the day that are purely for relaxation and leisure. Another important aspect in terms of leisure/stimulation is the need to experience different environments, as well as some time outdoors. If the individual is cared for in a formal unit, it is likely that all their care will be provided for in one building, and so there will be no specific need to go outdoors. This can also be the case even when the individual is cared for at home, as they may be taken to the designated day centre or other service via specialized transport, only experiencing being outdoors on transferring to and from the transport. This can inhibit the opportunity to experience wind, the sun or even rain.

Leisure needs must therefore be carefully integrated into lifelong planning as well as education/occupational needs. There is a wide variety of leisure experiences that the individual may enjoy, depending on personal preference. It is access in terms of transport, moving and handling and carer support for these leisure activities that can and does make the difference. Readers are advised to build upon their knowledge network regarding leisure facilities and the level of access available for this client group.

Activity 11.8

- What do we mean by the terms 'older person' and 'ageing'?
- Are these terms different when one is discussing the individual with profound and multiple disabilities?
- If so why, and if not why not?

Support for carers

It is important that carers are seen as equal partners with professionals. Consider the comment made by Madden (1995) regarding the parents of children with learning disabilities. It could be seen as a poignant statement on behalf of all carers:

Parents are at the start of a lifelong journey they did not bargain for. They need to know that professionals are going to be with them. Professionals need to learn to think and act collaboratively so that parents have fewer experiences of duplication, confusion or professional rivalries (Madden 1995).

Supporting the carers thus requires commitment from professionals, who can act as enablers and facilitators. It involves implicit recognition that it is the carers who are actually doing the caring, and this is a 24-hour, 7-days-a-week responsibility. Support involves recognizing the unique needs and coping strategies of each family. Some may wish for regular contact from professionals, and others would rather just have access to a 24-hour professional helpline. Professionals need to realize that the level of support required will vary over time.

Requests for information, advice, just listening for rather than to the carer, or even formal counselling may be services that the carer may require at some time or another. There are key times when it is recognized that perhaps additional support will be needed. These include:

- the birth/diagnosis of disability
- the care of the preschool child
- preformal education assessment and statementing
- educational statementing reviews
- before transition to adult services
- times when the individual is unwell
- ill health of the main carer
- general increasing care needs of the individual.

This list is endless and should never be seen as prescriptive. Professionals need to adopt the 'key worker' approach, as stated earlier in the chapter, and need to be able to offer a comprehensive range of services to carers. The reader should refer to Chapter 17, which describes a range of support services and agencies for parents and carers.

Short-term breaks

Access to such services is regarded by many families as an essential part of service provision. Professionals need to be aware of the range of short-term breaks available for this client group. It can be difficult to access family-based care for individuals with profound and multiple disabilities, owing to the level of care that may be required. This is especially so if the individual has additional complex health needs. It has been highlighted in a UK study by Robinson and Stalker (1990) that short-term break services for this client group are generally underresourced, despite being in demand. Robinson and Stalker (1990) argue that:

Parents generally placed a high value on respite services, often seeing them as a "life-line" and a means by which they managed to cope. Given the importance of services to parents and their cost-effectiveness compared to long term care, it is a matter of real concern. . . . If the policy of community care is to retain any credibility, this is a situation that must be rectified (Robinson & Stalker 1990).

Short-term breaks are not a 'panacea for all ills', but should be regarded as an integral part of service provision. The need to involve parents/main carers in service planning and review cannot be underestimated. Thus to conclude this chapter, 'people first' should be the final words: people in terms of the individual with profound and multiple disabilities, and people in relation to their main carers. It has to be the essence of any professional involvement.

REFERENCES

Baker P A 1991 The denial of adolescence for people with mental handicaps: an unwitting conspiracy? Mental Handicap 19(2): 61–65

Ball B 1991 cited by Bradley P, Darbyshire P Helping with mental handicap. In: Shanley E, Starrs T A (eds) (1993) Learning disabilities. A handbook of care, 2nd edn. Churchill Livingstone, Edinburgh

Black P D 1980 cited by Bradley P, Darbyshire P Helping with mental handicap. In: Shanley E, Starrs T A (eds) Learning disabilities. A handbook of care, 2nd edn. Churchill Livingstone, Edinburgh

Blair E, Ballentyne J, Horsman S, Chauvel P 1995 A study of dynamic, proximal stability splint in the management of children with cerebral palsy. Developmental Medicine and Child Neurology 37(6): 544–554

Bottos M, Paato M L, Vianello A, Facchin P 1995 Locomotion patterns in cerebral palsy syndromes. Developmental Medicine and Child Neurology 37(1): 883–899

British National Formulary No. 31. March 1996. British Medical Association and the Royal Pharmaceutical Society of Great Britain

Brown H, Smith H 1992 Normalisation. A reader for the nineties. Routledge, London

Burns Y, Gunn P (eds) 1993 Downs syndrome. Moving through life. Chapman & Hall, London

Campbell A G M, McHaffie H E 1995 Prolonging life and allowing death: infants. Journal of Medical Ethics 21: 339–344

Carter B 1994 Child and infant pain. Principles of nursing care and management. Chapman & Hall, London

Caudery A, Russell O 1995 Vitamin C status and dietary intake in a long stay unit for clients with learning disabilities: implications for community care. British Journal of Learning Disabilities 23: 70–73

Collacott RA 1987 Management of problems in Downs syndrome patients. Update 15 January: 195–201

Cooper S A, Collacott R A 1994 Relapse of depression in people with Down's syndrome. British Journal of Developmental Disabilities XL (1)(78): 32–37

Crichton J U, Mackinnon M, White C P 1995 The life expectancy of persons with cerebral palsy. Developmental Medicine and Child Neurology 37: 567–576

Curatolo P, Arpino C, Stazi M A, Medda E 1995 Risk factors for the co-occurrence of partial epilepsy, cerebral palsy and mental retardation. Developmental Medicine and Child Neurology 37: 776–782

Dalton A J, Wisviewski H M 1993 In: Roberto K A (ed) The elderly care giver. Caring for adults with developmental disabilities. Sage Publications, London

Day K A 1985 cited by Quinn F, Mathieson A Associated conditions. In: Shanley E, Starrs T A (eds) Learning disabilities. A handbook of care, 2nd edn. Churchill Livingstone, Edinburgh

DoH 1994 COMA. Report on nutritional aspects of cardiovascular disease. HMSO, London

DoH 1995 Standing Medical Committee (CMO (86) 9). Cervical spine instability in people with Downs Syndrome.

Doble D, Goldie C, Kewell C 1992 The White approach. Nursing Times 88(40): 36–37

Dodds A 1993 Rehabilitating blind and visually impaired people. Chapman & Hall, London

Dodds A G, Helawell D J, Lee M D 1991 Congenitally blind children with and without retrolental fibroplasia: do they perform differently? Journal of Visual Impairment and Blindness 85(7): 306–310

Evans P M, Evans S J W, Alberman E 1990 Cerebral palsy: why we must plan for survival. Archives of Disease in Childhood 65: 1329–1333

Gisel E G, Applegate-Ferrante T, Benson J E, Bosma J F 1995 Effect of oral sensori-motor treatment on measures of growth, eating efficiency and aspiration in the dysphagic child with cerebral palsy. Developmental Medicine and Child Neurology 37(6): 528–543

Grunau R V E, Johnston C C, Craig K D 1990 Neonatal facial and cry responses to invasive and non invasive procedures. Pain 42: 293–305

Griffiths J, Boyle S 1993 Colour guide to holistic oral care. A practical approach. Mosby Year Book, London

Griggs C A, Jones P M, Lee R E 1989 Videofluoroscopic investigation of disorders of children with multiple handicap. Developmental Medicine and Child Neurology 31: 303–308

Halpern L M, Jolley S G, Johnson D G 1991 Gastro-oesophageal reflux: a significant association with central nervous disease. Journal of Paediatric Surgery 26: 171–173

Harries D 1991 A sense of worth: a report on services for people with learning disabilities and sensory impairment. Committee on the Multi-handicapped Blind, London

Hatton C, Emerson E 1995 Services for adults with learning disabilities and sensory impairments. British Journal of Learning Disabilities 23: 11–17

Heine R G, Reddihough D S, Catho-Smith A G 1995 Gastro-oesophageal reflux and feeding problems after gastrostomy in children with severe neurological impairment. Developmental Medicine and Child Neurology 37: 320–329

Hoare P, Russell M 1995 The quality of life of children with chronic epilepsy and their families: preliminary findings with a new assessment measure. Developmental Medicine and Child Neurology 37: 689–696

Hotchkiss D 1989 Demographic aspects of hearing impairment: questions and answers 2nd edn. Galludet University Press, Washington DC

Jolley S G, Smith E I, Tunnell W P 1985 Protective anti-reflux operation with feeding gastrostomy. Annals of Surgery 201: 736–739

Kay B, Rose S, Turnbull J 1995a Continuing the commitment. The report of the Learning Disability Nursing Project. Department of Health, London

Kay B, Rose S, Turnbull J 1995b Learning Disability Nursing Project Resource Package. Department of Health, London

Klemz A 1977 Blindness and partial sight. A guide for social workers and others concerned with the care and rehabilitation of the visually handicapped. Woodhead-Faulkner, Cambridge

Kroger J 1996 Identity in adolescence. The balance between self and other, 2nd edn. Routledge, London

Kudrajacev T, Schoenberg B S, Kurland L T, Groover R V 1985 Cerebral palsy: survival rates, associated handicaps and distribution by clinical subtype. Developmental Medicine and Child Neurology 35: 900–903

Lane D, Stratford B (eds) 1985 Current approaches to Downs syndrome. Holt, Rinehart and Winston, Sussex

Langer J C, Wesson D E, Ein S H et al 1988 Feeding gastrostomy in neurologically impaired children: is an anti reflux procedure necessary? Journal of Paediatric Gastroenterology and Nutrition 7: 837–841

Laurent S 1992 Atmospherics. Bulletin 90/9. British Institute for Learning Disabilities, Bristol

Madden P 1995 Why parents: how parents. A keynote review British Journal of Learning Disabilities 23: 90–93

Mann DMA 1988 Alzheimers disease and Downs syndrome. Histopathology 13: 125–137

McGrath P J, Johnson G, Goodman G T et al 1985 cited in Carter B 1994 Child and infant pain. Principles of nursing care and management. Chapman & Hall, London

McKinlay I, Holland J 1986 In: Gordon N, McKinlay I (eds) 1986 Neurologically handicapped children: treatment and management. Blackwell Scientific Publications, Oxford

McMenamin J, Bird M 1993 Epilepsy. A parents guide. Brainwave. (The Irish Epilepsy Association), Dublin

Mirrett P L, Riski J E, Glascott J, Johnson V 1994 Videofluoroscopic assessment of dysphagia in children with severe spastic cerebral palsy. Dysphagia 9(3): 174–179

Moller M A 1993 Working with visually impaired children and their families. Pediatric opthalmology. Pediatric Clinics of North America. 40(4): 881–890

Morton R E, Bonas R, Foune B, Minford J 1993 Videofluoroscopy in the assessment of feeding disorders of children with neurological problems. Developmental Medicine and Child Neurology 35(5): 388–395

Morton R E, Khan M A, Murray-Leslie C, Elliott S 1995 Atlantoaxial instability in Down's syndrome: a five year follow up study. Archives of Diseases in Childhood 72(2): 115–118

Murphy K P, Molnar G E, Lankasky K 1995 Medical and functional status of adults with cerebral palsy. Developmental Medicine and Child Neurology 37: 1075–1084

Naylor V, Clifton M 1993 People with learning disabilities – meeting complex needs. Health and Social Care in the Community 1(6): 343–353

Nazarko L 1995 The therapeutic uses of cranberry juice. Nursing Standard 9(34): 33–35

O'Grady R S, Grain L S, Kohn J 1995 The prediction of long term functional outcomes of children with cerebral palsy. Developmental Medicine and Child Neurology 37: 997–1005

Powell C A 1991 Choices for the deaf child. Maternal and Child Health. April: 106–110

Prasher V P, Robinson L, Krishnan V H R, Chung M C 1995 Podiatric disorders among children with Downs syndrome and learning disability. Developmental Medicine and Child Neurology 37: 131–134

Robinson C, Stalker K 1990 Respite care – the consumer's view. Norah Fry Research Centre, University of Bristol

Rogers B T, Arvendson J, Msall M, Demerath R R 1993 Hypoxaemia during oral feeding of children with severe cerebral palsy. Developmental Medicine and Child Neurology 35: 3–10

Silverman W A 1980 Retrolental fibroplasia. A modern parable. Grune & Stratton, New York

Thompson T, Mathias P 1992 Standards and mental handicap. Keys to competence. Baillière Tindall, London

Van Minnen A, Hoelsgens I, Hoogduin K 1994 Specialised treatment of mildly mentally retarded adults with psychiatric and/or behavioural disorders: inpatient or outreach service? British Journal of Developmental Disabilities. XL(1)(78): 24–31

Waterlow J 1992 The Waterlow Scale. Newlands, Curland, Taunton

Willie E, Rothner A D, Luders H E 1989 Partial seizures in children: clinical features in medical treatment and surgical considerations. Pediatric Clinics of North America 36: 343–364

Yeates S 1995 The incidence and importance of hearing loss in people with severe learning disability: the evaluation of a service. British Journal of Learning Disabilities 23: 79–84

Communication

R. Ferris-Taylor

INTRODUCTION

Communication is important to many of the things we do in our everyday lives. We communicate with one another for a wide range of reasons. Crystal (1992) summarizes the main functions of communication as the exchange of ideas and information, emotional expression, social interaction, control of reality, recording facts, thinking and expressing identity. In addition to speech we use a range of non-verbal means to communicate, for example gestures, tone of voice, eye contact, facial expression and body posture. These vary culturally.

Communication is a two-way process, involving at least two people who alternate in sending and receiving messages.

The focus of this chapter is communication as a whole, not just speech and verbal communication. It takes the approach that all human beings use a variety of means of communication, and that all of these have a place, no one means being inherently superior. In working with people with learning disabilities we need to be prepared to learn to recognize a wide range of behaviours as possible communication, and to use a variety of methods in communicating back. Carers and professionals have an influential role in interacting with people with learning disabilities and seeking to reduce the impact of any communication difficulties. This is linked to the overall approach in this chapter, of utilizing a social rather than a medical model of disability.

In recent years there has been lively debate about ways of defining and understanding disability (Oliver 1990, Morris 1991, Reiser & Mason 1992). The social model of disability emphasizes a holistic approach, taking into account the person's views, that is, disability is not a question of a fixed impairment, but rather varies according to the environment. For example, someone who uses a wheelchair in central London is likely to be significantly restricted by the environmental barriers involved in using public transport, gaining access to buildings etc. Someone using a wheelchair in Milton Keynes is likely to be less restricted in moving about the town, owing to its layout. In relation to communication, someone who uses sign language as their first language will experience significant difficulties if others do not understand, use and value it, whereas in an environment where everyone uses sign language, non-sign users will be disadvantaged. Sacks (1990) described just such a situation in Martha's Vineyard in the USA.

Recent legislation, such as the Children Act 1989 and the NHS and Community Care Act 1990, emphasizes the importance of involving disabled adults and children in their own assessments of need, planning for their own futures and taking account of their views about the services they receive. In particular, the Children Act asserts that 'Even children with severe learning disabilities or very limited expressive language can communicate preferences if they are asked in the right way by people who understand their needs and have the relevant skills to listen to them'. This should not be dependent on age or mode of communication, and challenges professionals to find creative ways to enable this to take place. For example, Minkes et al (1994) describe the development of a range of tools, such as simplified questionnaires, photographs and pictures, to obtain the views of disabled children about the respite care they received. Millner et al (1991) describe creative approaches to involve adults with learning disabilities in quality action groups.

In recent years, methods of speech and language therapy have begun to concentrate more on interaction with others and less on individual work away from real-life settings. Other important changes have been the development of approaches which take account of both intentional and non-intentional communication, so that it is possible to work with people with severe and multiple disabilities, rather than waiting for prerequisites to spoken language to develop. The growth in our understanding and use of alternative and supplementary means of communication, such as Makaton, has also brought about positive results for many people with learning disabilities.

The incidence of communication difficulties among people with learning disabilities is high. Depending upon definitions and the population involved (e.g. hospital or community), it has variously been estimated as 40–50% (Mansell 1992). This has led some to suggest that there is an almost open-ended need for speech and language therapy. Certainly, communication will be a key consideration for all who come into contact with people with learning disabilities, especially those who do so on a regular basis.

It is important to remember, however, that the range of people described as having learning disabilities is very wide, from those with profound and multiple disabilities to those with only mild difficulties. Correspondingly, and given the complexity of communication, the nature of communication difficulties can be very diverse. Accordingly, this chapter will discuss and put forward general principles (and there are always likely to be exceptions). It is important that people with learning disabilities and their carers have access to individual assessment and advice by speech and language therapists, in order to maximize their communication.

THE NATURE OF COMMUNICATION

Communication involves the transmission of meaning from one person to another, irrespective of the method. Thinking broadly, it may involve dance, music, Braille, pictures, telephones, the Internet and sexual activity! Yet we generally tend to think mostly in terms of speech and language as our prime means of communication.

Using language to communicate involves understanding and producing the rules of grammar and word order (syntax), and formulating meaning (semantics) in a way that someone else can understand (pragmatics). This is complex because there is no reason why particular words should stand for particular objects or ideas. Whether the word *dog*, *Kalb* (Arabic) or *chien* (French) is used, there is no relationship between the chosen sound formation and the animal it represents. It is by convention that we learn to associate sound sequences in our first language with their referents. In addition, many words cannot be taught by easy reference to an object or event. For example, a word such as 'in' can be demonstrated by placing objects in boxes, drawers, cups etc. However, 'in the swimming pool' may be a little harder to understand, and other meanings of the same word, such as 'in time', 'in the first place', cannot be demonstrated so readily.

Consider the complexity of grammatical rules and word order. For example, 'The dog chases the cat' has the same meaning as 'The cat is being chased by the dog'. Also, although there are various grammatical rules, many of these have exceptions. For example, English noun plurals are often formed by adding 's' to the end of the word, but some plurals, such as 'geese' and 'mice', are formed differently. Similarly, the past tense of verbs is often formed by adding '-ed' to the root of the verb, but there are exceptions, e.g. 'went', 'brought'.

Pragmatics is also a complex area. For example, language varies according to the social context, so that the spoken and body language used with friends is different from the more formal approach used at a job interview.

In addition, non-verbal communication, which can be conscious or unconscious, adds to the meaning of what we say, either to reinforce it or to give a contradictory message. Abercrombie (1968) suggests that 'We speak with our vocal organs but we converse with our whole bodies'. Morris (1987) contends that as much as 50% of our communication is accomplished non-verbally.

Argyle (1977) suggests that non-verbal communication has three main functions:

1. **Communicating interpersonal attitudes and emotions** We tend to judge whether someone likes or dislikes us by subtle features of their non-verbal communication (although dislike is often deliberately concealed). In fact, when there is a mismatch between the verbal message and the non-verbal communication, the non-verbal communication often assumes more significance. For instance, a friendly message delivered in an unfriendly tone of voice and facial expression will usually be interpreted as unfriendly.

2. **Supporting verbal communication** The way something is said – the timing, pitch and stress patterns – provides punctuation and may change the meaning. Compare 'I *can't* wait for you' with 'I can't wait for *you*'. Gestures may also add to the meaning, for example pointing. Turn-taking in conversation is regulated by a variety of non-verbal signals, such as gaze shifts, head nods and grunts. Non-verbal communication also enables us to obtain feedback about how others are responding to us. Are they in agreement, disagreement, bored, surprised etc? This information is obtained chiefly from looking at others' faces, particularly the eyebrows and month. Attentiveness tends to be signalled by looking at the other person more when listening than when talking.

3. **Replacing speech** This may occur, for example, in a noisy environment such as a cafe or racecourse, or during a rescue action by the fire brigade. It may also be used where verbal communication is difficult because different languages are in use, e.g. the hand talk systems developed by native Indian peoples in America. It can also be a first language, as used by deaf people, such as the British Sign Language or Cantonese Sign Language.

 Activity 12.1

Which methods of communication do you use most in your daily life? Which do you feel most at east with and why? Many adults will have a preferred sensory modality, e.g. vision, hearing, touch: which is yours? How does this relate to people with learning disabilities whom you know?

DEVELOPMENT OF COMMUNICATION

Many studies have examined the fascinating process of how communication develops before speech (see, for example, Crystal (1984) for a general overview and Hewitt & Ephraim (1994) for a very detailed description of one mother–infant interaction and a framework for observations). In this section the aim is to highlight some of the crucial processes involved, rather than give a stage-by-stage account.

Babies' communication usually develops as a result of using all their senses and mental processes to make sense of environmental stimuli, and in the context of appropriate interaction with carers. The baby plays a very active role in this two-way process, to some extent controlling the interaction. To begin with, the baby's messages to his or her carers are unintentional, i.e. the result of physiological changes such as pain, hunger, boredom etc., but not deliberately intended to convey a given message. However, carers tend to respond as if the baby's cries or changes in facial expression do have a deliberate meaning. Gradually the baby learns that different behaviours result in different responses from the carers, and repeats them in anticipation of these responses. The baby is now beginning to send intentional messages, and to understand the nature of cause and effect and the sense of being a powerful and influential person. For instance, at around 9 months of age many babies begin to point to objects in order to draw attention to items and request them. This has an enormous impact on communication. Previously, carers could only guess at what the baby wanted, perhaps following his or her direction of gaze and trying to infer from that. Now, the baby is able to convey the object of intention very clearly and deliberately, and will often experiment by doing so repeatedly and imperiously! In many instances of early communication there is two-way turntaking, with the carer pausing to give the baby the opportunity to vocalize or gesture and being responsive to the baby, taking his or her lead and framing conversation around the baby's actions.

Non-verbal communication develops alongside and before the development of speech and language. It has been observed that newborn infants move in synchrony with the voices of people around them (Trevarthen 1977). These minute movements may not be readily observable or obvious to those around, but have been demonstrated by analysis of filmed sequences of interaction. Linked to this is the probability that hearing is the first sense to develop in utero, so that the baby is able to hear the sound of his or her mother's voice and environmental sounds, perhaps even before birth.

Young children continue to develop synchronous movements to their own speech and that of others, and this is particularly the case with hand movements. For example, first words are often accompanied by gestures, e.g. raised hand, palm facing upwards, accompanied by the word 'where?'.

Before speech develops an infant hears thousands and thousands of words a day, becoming very familiar with the sounds and speech patterns of his or her first language. Gradually, through familiar routines and activities, the infant begins to build up an understanding of familiar words in context; for example, he or she may appear to understand the word 'bath', but only in the context of the time of day, hearing and seeing the bathwater running, smelling the soap etc.

Understanding of words and concepts will continue to develop throughout the early years. Even when a child has developed a purely linguistic understanding of words independent of the overall context, there will be some situations where he or she will be continuing to work out the multiple meanings that words can have (for example the difference between a 'plug' in an electrical socket in the wall, as compared to the one in the sink). What appears to be a rapid acquisition of a first language is, in fact, underpinned by years of daily experience of being constantly exposed to that language before becoming a fully competent speaker.

These processes demonstrate the importance of two-way interaction in the development of communication, with each person being influenced by and taking their cues from the other. They are useful in considering how to facilitate communication with people with learning disabilities, although this should always be done in an age-appropriate way.

COMMUNICATING WITH PEOPLE WITH LEARNING DISABILITIES

This section highlights some of the general issues which are significant when devising strategies to communicate with people with learning disabilities.

Active involvement with others and the development of relationships

As outlined above, communication usually develops as part of a pleasurable, reciprocal, social process. For some people with learning disabilities, communication may not be enjoyable because they are ignored, bored or cannot see the value of or any results of their attempts to communicate. The process may also be too effortful or threatening: in some instances, for example, for some autistic people social interaction may be positively fear inducing.

Despite service aspirations towards community integration, most children and adults with learning disabilities are still segregated in special schools, day centres, special clubs and other organizations. Their experience of non-disabled people is usually in relation to receiving help and support, which can reinforce a sense of helplessness and power imbalance. Community participation is perhaps one of the most difficult of O'Brien's (1986) five service accomplishments to achieve.

A feature of many institutional settings is that service users may see themselves in a less active, powerful role. For example, a study of non-disabled children in nurseries (Tizard et al 1972) found that staff speech to the children tended to be predominantly controlling (i.e. designed to begin, control or terminate activities) rather than conversational (designed to explain, give or ask for information). In a further study by Tizard and Hughes (1984), it was noticeable that young chil-

dren used a less complex language at school than at home. This seems to be related to the demands of a task-orientated situation (for example, utterances such as 'Where's the glue?' were typical at school, compared to more complex questioning at home, e.g. 'Why is the grass green?').

This preponderance of 'controlling speech' as compared to 'conversational speech' has similarly been demonstrated in settings for adults with learning disabilities (see, for example, Van der Gaag & Dormandy 1993).

Where children and adults are using sign or symbol systems to communicate, a repeated finding is that the non-disabled person tends to dominate the communication, initiating more frequently and taking more turns in the interaction (Williams & Grove 1989, Basil 1992).

For a person who is dependent on others to meet their basic needs, routines may take over, so that there are few opportunities to communicate. Bruce (1993) gives examples of children with physical disabilities whose lack of opportunities for free-flow play contributed to reduced opportunities to learn and to communicate.

People with learning disabilities may inherently make fewer demands, either sending fewer messages or else messages which are not in a form carers can easily recognize, such as ambiguous gestures, unintelligible sounds or words. If these attempts at communication meet with little success, they may decrease. The carer may attempt to compensate by speaking more, thus giving the person even less opportunity to communicate. This can become a vicious circle, with adverse effects on the person's motivation, confidence and use of skills. The effect on their self-esteem is thus likely to be very detrimental. This links to Wolfensberger's second core theme of normalization: role expectancy and role circularity, that is, low expectations tend to be self-fulfilling (see Chapter 4 for a fuller description and discussion).

In summary, in the reciprocal process of communication carers may dominate owing to the demands of the task, in an attempt to overcome communication difficulties or through devaluing the potential role of a person with learning disabilities in active communication. The person with learning disabilities may not behave in ways that are interesting to the carer, or readily understood. If communication is too fast (our average rate of speaking is around 250 words per minute) and there is insufficient time to respond, the person may give up. For example, if Leslie needs 80 seconds or so to begin to reply, but her carers typically repeat, rephrase or answer the question themselves after around 20 seconds, she will eventually conclude that there is little point in bothering.

So, what can be done? Some general principles are:

● Learn to take the person's lead. This may involve noticing small signals they make and acting upon them, e.g. eye movements in the direction of a desired item. Or it may involve picking up on what the person wants to talk about and finds important and interesting, such as a bereavement, someone else's epileptic fits, or aspects of family relationships.

● Monitor the amount of speech you use, compared to that of the children or adults you are communicating with. Do you dominate the conversation? Can the other person get a word in edgeways? The use of audiotape or video cassettes can be very helpful in encouraging you to be more objective about this, although sometimes painful to watch!

● Consider carefully the type of speech you use. Where does it come along the dimension 'control' as compared to 'conversational'? Once again, video or audio cassettes can be revealing. Try to make more use of comments that convey genuine information. Questions can be useful, particularly open-ended ones, if the person can understand them. Be aware, though, that too many questions can be controlling or confusing.

● Adapt the pace of your communication to suit the other person. Allow sufficient time for them to respond. This may feel uncomfortable if their pace is much slower than your own. However, it is possible to learn to do so and this method has been used to good effect in a structured way in 'expectant time delay' (see Kozleski 1991 for a fuller explanation).

● Try to create opportunities for the person to

have contact with positive role models of other disabled people with communication difficulties, for example deaf people using sign language, images of Stephen Hawking, the book and film 'Annie's Coming Out' (Crossley & McDonald 1982), members of self-advocacy groups, videos/ performances by theatre groups such as Strathcona, or the pop group Heart 'n' Soul, who are all people with learning disabilities.

Influencing the environment by exercising choice and being listened to

The range and type of daily choices, both large and small, is likely to be restricted for people with learning disabilities compared to others of a similar age. Given that a primary motivation to communicate is to make choices and influence what happens next, it is important to recognize nevertheless that exercising choice is a complex process. It involves the following:

● Awareness that choices are possible and available.

● The opportunity to make choices – this is easy to pre-empt because when someone has communication difficulties it may often be easier or quicker to choose for them, or to anticipate what they want. Halle et al (1981) described three levels of pre-empting:

    1. Environmental: the desired item or activity is physically present or readily available, so there is no need to communicate in order to obtain it.

    2. Non-verbal: the person's need is anticipated by others, who offer or provide it.

    3. Verbal: that is, others notice the individual's likely need and verbally initiate or offer it before the person has a chance to express it themselves.

● Awareness or experience of what choice means. For instance, someone who has never been horse-riding or received a massage before may not be able to choose between the two, and is likely to need to experience the activities first.

● Understanding the consequences of choice, i.e. that if you make a choice, you may not like what you have chosen. For instance, if you choose 'four seasons' pizza in a restaurant, you're stuck with that choice, even if you don't like it! This element of learning by mistakes is important, and one that people with learning disabilities are often protected from.

• The constraints inherent in financial contributions or the impact of our choice on others. Given that people with learning disabilities are likely to be among the poorest people in society, their choices may be unduly constrained. Similarly, living in group settings with others may mean there are more rules and more compromises to be made.

• Assertiveness to carry through your choice and 'stick to your guns', even if others disagree with or dislike the choice you have made. This may be particularly difficult if choices are being suggested by a member of staff the person wants to please, and therefore they think they have to find the 'right' answer. This can also link to fluctuations in decision making.

• Having a means of expression to convey your choice. The person needs to have spoken, signed or symbol vocabulary which is understood by others and acted upon. With use of sign and symbol systems it is particularly important to try to select and teach initial vocabulary which corresponds to the individual's preferences. It can be very difficult to divorce yourself from your role in the person's life and to consider what they might want to communicate about, rather than what would be helpful or convenient to you.

• Choosing from a range of alternatives that is within the person's memory and understanding, for example two or more concrete items which are physically present, rather than items or activities which are not present, or are more abstract.

Some strategies to facilitate choice making include:

• Consideration of the range and type of choices available: are there ways to extend this?

• Ensuring that the environment does not pre-empt the making of choices. The Intecom communication package developed by Jones (1990) provides an assessment and observation check-list together with a framework for planning to widen opportunities. It also provides useful suggestions to avoid pre-empting, based on the three levels mentioned by Halle (1981).

• Providing the person with spoken, signed or symbol vocabulary which is potentially reflective of their choices.

• Providing opportunities to develop assertiveness skills. This may be as basic as the opportunity to learn to use a sign or symbol for 'No', or it may be the chance to develop these skills through attendance at an assertiveness or self-advocacy group (see Holland & Ward 1990, Downes 1996, Crawley 1988 for examples of relevant approaches).

Knowing the person's current level of communication and starting from there

Careful observation will show that most people do communicate in some way, even if this is unintentional and their signals or messages are not readily understood by others. A key principle is to recognize that a person with learning and communication difficulties is often making his or her own best efforts to communicate, and to treat all behaviour as if meaningful.

For example, if the person enjoys flicking or twiddling string, one approach would be to sit some distance away and do similarly. Eventually the person may allow you to sit nearer and a possible dialogue may develop, with the pace, rhythm and timing of string flicking being influenced by one another. This is a type of mirroring, which is a key component of intensive interaction or augmented mothering (Hewitt & Ephraim 1994).

Another example is in a group movement to music activity, where each person is asked to contribute a movement for the others to copy. Someone who does not seem to understand or deliberately suggest a movement may make one inadvertently, e.g. a knee jerk. This can then be copied by the others as if it was a genuine suggestion. Attention can also be drawn to what the individual has done and the fact that everyone is copying, so that over time the person may begin to gain more sense of cause and effect. Explicitly referring to what the person has done (e.g. 'Well done Kamal, you moved your knee') may be more useful in promoting this concept than generalized praise ('good, well done').

In situations where someone's behaviour is very ambiguous, it can be useful for carers to share their different perceptions about how the person is communicating. It may emerge that carers have very different views about a particular aspect of behaviour. For example, one may think a particular head movement indicates 'more', whereas another thinks it means 'no'. Viewed from the perspective of that person, the results can be very confusing because they are likely to experience different and potentially conflicting responses. In this example, one carer is likely to give more food in response to this head movement, whereas the other is likely to remove it altogether.

As discussed earlier, given that communication usually develops intentionally through relatively consistent relationships and interaction with carers where consistent meaning is assigned to actions, it is important to try to establish this. If, in the absence of clear evidence of a particular meaning to a given signal, carers decide to treat it consistently as if it has one meaning, e.g. 'more', then over time it is possible that a degree of intentional communication may result. In effect, this method involves systematically overinterpreting the person's communication (Campbell & Wilcox 1986, Baumgart et al 1990).

It is important to consider that even difficult or challenging behaviour has a communicative function. There is a high incidence of communication difficulties among people regarded as having challenging behaviour (Mansell 1992). Challenging behaviour may be an attempt to communicate messages such as 'I'm hungry', 'I'd like a coke', 'My skin is itchy', 'I'm in pain', 'I don't want to do this'. The difficulty is that the form of the message may be very unclear, or it occurs in a form which is unacceptable or conflicts with the behaviour/tasks required in the context. Take, for example, Jyoti, who has no speech and does not use signs or symbols to communicate with. In the middle of a relaxation session she gets up and goes to the door. A member of staff walks after her, blocking the door and bringing her back to the main part of the room. Jyoti again gets up, this time grabbing the staff member's hand and putting it on the door handle. The staff member explains that it is time to relax and brings Jyoti back to her chair. This is repeated several times, until Jyoti scratches the worker's hand and slaps her on the side of the face. Jyoti's behaviour is now recorded in her file as being challenging and uncooperative in relaxation sessions. In fact, Jyoti might enjoy music but, because she has no way of drawing others' attention to anything other than items which are physically present in the room, she has few means to indicate her needs. Her behaviour may be her best attempt to get her needs met, rather than a deliberate attempt to disrupt the relaxation session.

An alternative approach would be to allow Jyoti out of the room, accompanying her to see what she wants. For instance, she might want to go to the toilet, to get a drink or simply for a walk up and down the corridor. The member of staff could then show Jyoti a sign for the desired object/activity, modelling it and prompting her to copy, if amenable. In this way, Jyoti might gradually begin to develop a small signed vocabulary for her everyday needs. Pictures or written symbols might facilitate this, as these rely on recognition rather than recall and so may be easier on the memory. Remember, in describing language development, how much repetition may be needed before someone can use a word or sign themselves. So, bear in mind that Jyoti will probably need to see the signs or symbols being used for quite some time before she can use them meaningfully herself.

Challenging behaviour may also be related to difficulties in understanding others' speech, and being confused by picking up only part of a message (see later in the chapter).

Importance of culture and race

It is easy to overlook the cultural and racial background of someone with learning disabilities when it differs from that of the professionals involved.

There are likely to be misunderstandings and inaccuracies involved in assessing someone's speech and language in anything other than their first language. Assessments may use materials which are unfamiliar or offensive to someone on account of their religious or cultural background. The involvement of an interpreter and careful planning for how to work together is crucial to effective assessment. Although family members are frequently involved in this way, it is preferable to avoid this as there may be difficulties owing to family roles, status and conflicting interests. For instance, Amira was thought to have a severe communication difficulty. However, once an appropriate interpreter was found it emerged that she had much greater fluency in her first language and that the issue was more one of difficulty in learning a second language. She was also able to express strong ideas about the day and residential services she was receiving, in particular those aspects which conflicted with her religious and cultural views.

Some children and adults will have merged language development, that is, through moving regularly between different cultures and communication systems, components from two languages may be used. For example, English words may be incorporated into Punjabi sentences. Or the person may have some degree of fluency in both languages but the vocabulary in each may not overlap readily, so that interpretation or translation from one to the other is difficult. This is sometimes known as semilingualism.

It is both useful and courteous to learn to use a few words that occur frequently in the person's first language, and to encourage their peers to do so. Also, remember that non-verbal communication is linked to language and culture, and there may be different rules, for example about eye contact, and conventions about bodily proximity and touch. Gestures may have different meanings in different cultures. For instance, whereas in British culture a 'thumbs up' gesture is interpreted as having a positive meaning, for some Bengali-speaking people it may be interpreted as being quite rude.

Baxter et al (1990) have described in detail some issues connected to double discrimination for black people with learning disabilities, on account of both race and learning disability. They also provide some striking examples of some of the issues relating to communication.

General good practice guidelines:

- Use materials which are appropriate to the person's culture, in both assessment and any subsequent work.
- Ensure that the environment contains a range of images which include people of different races in a variety of roles (this should be the case irrespective of the racial background of people using the service); this can encourage relaxed and relevant conversation.
- Learn some key words in the person's first language; encourage other colleagues and peers to do so.
- Use an interpreter for an assessment or other important meetings or appointments.
- Ensure that you understand some of the cultural and non-verbal rules of the person's first language, to minimize misunderstandings. Avoid making assumptions about the person's preferences and customs based purely on culture. Find out from the person and their family, where possible.

Importance of sensory information

Information from all five senses is important in developing and maintaining communication skills. However, the main sensory channels related to communication are the distance senses of hearing and vision. Many people with learning disabilities have additional difficulties in communicating because of sensory disabilities. Clarke-Kehoe (1992) estimates that as many as

Activity 12.2

Imagine that you used a sign to convey something you wanted. You knew what it meant but no-one responded. How would you feel? How might you show these feelings?

45% of people with severe and profound learning disabilities may have some kind of visual or hearing impairment. Sensory disabilities are also more common in elderly people. Approximately 34% of people aged over 60 have a significant hearing loss, which rises to approximately 74% in those aged over 70 (RNID 1990).

Screening tests of hearing among groups of people with learning disabilities reveal substantial underestimates by carers of hearing loss (Yeates 1995). So, there is a need generally to be aware of possible signs of hearing or visual impairment, and also to recognize that, as for the rest of the population, sensory disabilities may be more prevalent in people with learning disabilities as they age.

However, when someone has a learning disability, any other difficulties they experience can often be attributed by carers to the disability, rather than any additional impairments. Heider (1958), in his attribution theory, describes how we tend to explain people's behaviour in terms of one cause rather than multiple causes. If someone is described as having a learning disability, this will often take precedence over any other explanations of unusual behaviours or problems. For example, someone's lack of attention and concentration may be attributed to their learning disability rather than that they also have a hearing difficulty, or that they are becoming bored or irritable during mainly visual tasks because of a visual impairment. A person who seems to be able to hear in some situations but not others may be labelled as stubborn or uncooperative ('can hear when they want to'), but fluctuating hearing levels can be characteristic of some types of hearing loss. Someone who leans down to the table to eat may be regarded as having an unusual mannerism or poor posture, rather than a possible visual impairment.

In addition, some people with learning disabilities may spontaneously begin to compensate in ways which make a sensory disability less obvious to carers. For instance, someone with a hearing loss may attend more to the facial expressions, lip patterns and gestures of others. This may only become apparent if someone turns away or speaks to them from the next room.

Someone with a visual impairment may avoid tasks involving small details, and may explore things more by touch.

Often, no allowances are made for sensory disability unless it has actually been diagnosed. This may mean that unrealistic expectations are placed on people. It is important not to assume that people with learning disabilities have good vision or hearing. Some conditions related to learning disabilities are so closely associated with sensory disability that extra vigilance is recommended on these grounds alone, for example, a great many people with Down syndrome have hearing loss, and there are strong links between rubella damage and hearing or visual loss, or both. It is important that nurses be aware of and vigilant for possible signs of sensory disability. (The Royal National Institute for Blind People produces very detailed fact sheets, containing checklists with possible signs to consider: see also Boxes 12.1 and 12.2).

Thorough professional assessment is needed where there is any suspicion of sensory disability. Audiological or ophthalmological services for

---

Box 12.1   Behaviour or features which may indicate a hearing impairment

- Pulling, poking or rubbing the ears
- Watching the speaker's face and lips constantly
- Tilting the head to one side, towards the speaker or source of sound
- Appearing to hear on some occasions but not others (this may be due to a fluctuating hearing loss, or the fact that some voices may be easier to hear than others; some acoustic conditions are also more favourable than others)
- Speaking very loudly (typical of a sensorineural hearing loss, where the person raises their voice so it is audible to themselves)
- Speaking very softly (typical of a conductive hearing loss, where the person may match their own voice to the level at which they hear others' voices)
- Dislike of loud sounds (this may be due to recruitment, where the person has a reduced range between the point where they can just hear sounds and the point where sound is perceived as unbearably loud)
- Appearing startled when someone approaches
- Visible signs of discharge from the ears, or excessive wax

Box 12.2 Behaviour or features which may indicate a visual impairment

- Poking or rubbing the eyes
- Exploring items by touch
- Not appearing to notice people or things unless they are very close; needing to examine things at close quarters
- Reluctance to move around, especially when in new places
- Reluctance to look for/search for things visually
- Appearing startled when someone approaches
- Dislike of predominantly visual tasks/reluctance to engage in such tasks
- Visible signs of eye pathology, e.g. inflammation, swelling

children are available through GPs or the school medical service. However, there are often difficulties in obtaining adequate assessment for adults. Staff in audiological or ophthalmological services for adults may not feel sufficiently skilled in assessing people with learning disabilities, or be reluctant to see them at all, regarding the process as too time consuming or not beneficial for someone with learning disabilities. However, the learning disability makes it even more important to obtain an accurate idea about a person's sensory abilities. As mentioned earlier, some people with learning disabilities may spontaneously attempt to compensate by using their other senses more fully. However, others may have great difficulty in adapting and learning new skills, and so extra help is vital. In such situations, it may be that one of the roles of the nurse, social worker or other professional is to persist in asking for hearing or visual assessment, acting as an advocate on the person's behalf.

Most methods of visual and hearing assessment require a degree of cooperation, understanding and response from the individual. However, if materials are presented at an appropriate level and pace, many people with learning disabilities can respond reliably. Again, there is a role for someone who knows the person to give support by attending the appointment, reassuring the person and working with specialists in the clinic to ensure that the person understands what is required.

The effects of such impairment on the person will vary according to:

- Age of onset: if the person has had the experience of seeing and hearing this will have helped them learn to communicate. An acquired sensory loss means the person has to adjust to taking in information in new ways.
- Severity of impairment: in general, the more severe the impairment the more marked the probable impact on the person.
- The type of visual or hearing loss: Sensory impairments are not an all-or-nothing matter. Most people described as 'blind' or 'deaf' will have some usable vision (e.g. for light or dark perception) or hearing (e.g. for some sounds, for example bass tones). Some types of hearing loss, e.g. conductive (arising in the outer or middle ear) involve general distortion and loss of volume. Sensorineural hearing loss (arising in the cochlea or auditory nerve) involves distortion of particular pitches of sound.
- Whether one or both senses are involved: it will be more difficult to make sense of the world and to communicate if both vision and hearing are affected.
- The person's ability to compensate: this may be partly related to their level of cognitive ability. The more severe the learning disability, the more difficult it may be to adapt to learning new skills.

 Activity 12.3

Consider how many of the people with learning disabilities you know have a visual or hearing impairment. If the numbers are very low and do not correspond to those mentioned in this chapter, could this be due to lack of assessment/awareness of possible signs of impaired hearing or vision? Are you aware of possible indicators of sensory impairment? What facilities exist in your locality for assessment?

Can you build up positive links with staff in audiological and ophthalmological services to facilitate cooperative working?

Assisting people with hearing impairment

If someone has had an audiological assessment and a hearing aid is recommended, nurses and carers will have a vital role to play in helping the person to use it. Unfortunately, a hearing aid does not restore hearing to 'normal', and so it may take a long time for the person to adjust to it. The hearing aid will amplify sounds non-selectively, not just speech, and all sounds may appear particularly distorted in noisy places, such as on public transport, in the canteen or in the street.

It is important to introduce the hearing aid to the person gradually and, in order to do this, nurses and carers themselves need to be familiar with the components of the aid, how it works and basic maintenance.

There are three main types of hearing aid:

- Body worn
- Behind the ear, or postaural
- All in the ear.

Generally, body-worn hearing aids are used by people with severe hearing loss who need more powerful amplification. They are sometimes used by disabled or elderly people with arthritis, who may find the control switches of a behind-the-ear aid difficult to operate. All-in-the-ear aids are predominantly used by people with very mild hearing loss. The most frequently used are behind-the-ear aids (Figure 12.1).

The main components of a hearing aid are:

- The microphone: this picks up the sound and therefore needs to be kept free from dirt or other debris.
- The control switch: this usually has three settings: O = off; T = transduction loop; M = microphone; this is the 'on' switch. The transduction loop setting can be used in environments which have an induction loop. By using this switch, the person will be able to hear the important sounds by radio link, without the interference of background noise. Induction loops are available in some public buildings, such as theatres, cinemas or churches. They can also be fitted in an individual's home, to assist with hearing the television.

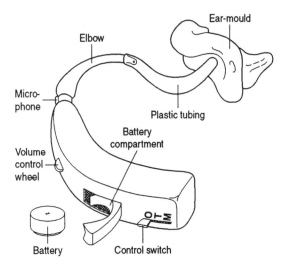

Figure 12.1 Behind-the-ear hearing aid.

- Volume control wheel: this will need to be adjusted to the optimum level for the person, as advised by the audiologist. However, it is likely to need adjusting in different circumstances, for example turned down in a noisy environment. Some volume control wheels are numbered, others are not, and it can be useful to mark the optimum level with a spot of Tippex for easy reference.
- Battery compartment: this flicks open to allow easy changing of the batteries. It is essential that the battery is inserted the right way round, with the '+' side on the battery aligned with the '+' mark on the battery compartment. Batteries last a variable time, depending on the amount of use. They should be retained and returned for exchange to the audiology department or, in some cases, local health clinics maintain battery supplies.
- Plastic tubing: amplified sound is relayed from the aid to the earmould via this tube. It needs to be cleaned regularly and replaced if distorted or cracked.
- Earmould: relays sound to the person's ear and is individually made for him or her. Again, this needs to be cleaned regularly (after disconnection from the hearing aid) and inspected for obvious signs of damage. It is important that it is a good fit.

The person will need to be introduced to the aid gradually, as it may be difficult to explain the potential benefits beforehand. It may be useful to prepare the person for having something in or around their ears by using sunglasses or personal stereo earphones for a while. Initially the aid should be worn for short periods in a quiet room with good acoustics, preferably during an enjoyable activity. Tolerance to wearing the aid for longer periods and in a variety of settings can be developed gradually. It can be helpful to teach the person, early on, how to take the aid out, so that they have some feeling of control (Ferris-Taylor & Pinney 1994).

Tips for communication Irrespective of whether the person uses a hearing aid or not, the following points are important to remember when talking to someone with a hearing loss.

- Ensure that you have the person's attention and that they are looking at you before you start talking, so that they can make use of lipreading and your facial expression.
- Allow the person to see your face clearly. If possible, face the window so the light is shining on your face and not in their eyes.
- Slow your speech – this generally makes it clearer.
- Use reasonable volume but do not shout.
- Avoid exaggerating your lip patterns – this will distort the natural rhythms and visible patterns of speech.
- As far as possible, cut out any background noise such as TV, running water etc.
- Get reasonably close to the person. If they use a hearing aid, the optimum distance apart is approximately 3 feet; beyond that, background noise will sound as loud as speech.
- Be aware that group settings will be more difficult for the person, particularly where there are rapid changes of topic or speaker.
- Ensure that the person has had a recent opthalmological assessment; if they have a hearing impairment it is all the more important to know about their visual acuity. Encourage the use of spectacles, where appropriate.

- Use your facial expression, body language, gestures and signs from the Makaton vocabulary to back up what you say.

Assisting people with visual impairment

As with hearing impairment, it is important to establish the degree and type of visual impairment. For instance, very few blind people have no useful vision at all. Types of visual impairment vary, for instance tunnel vision compared to peripheral vision. It is important to be aware that the nature of the visual impairment may mean that the person behaves in ways which can easily be misunderstood. For instance, if the person has some peripheral vision they may turn their head to one side in order to maximize the vision they have. This can easily be incorrectly interpreted as ignoring or avoiding the other person. It may also, for similar reasons, be difficult to establish eye contact with the person.

It is crucial to help the person make best use of whatever vision they have. If they wear spectacles these need to be cleaned regularly and checked for comfort, for example, do they rub the bridge of the nose or behind the ears? Lighting needs consideration, and the source should be from behind the person so that glare is avoided. Magnifying aids may be useful; advice may be obtained from the social services visual impairment team regarding such equipment and aids for the home, such as talking clocks.

There is a need to use more verbal cues to alert the person to what is happening and to explain what and who is present. The person will need more time to explore objects by touch. For example, a sighted person is able to gather information quickly by rapid visual scanning. A blind or partially sighted person will need much more time to become familiar with the location of objects in the room, and to explore them by touch. For a person with severe learning disabilities, understanding of everyday objects and the words used to denote them may be very difficult. Items such as cups may have very different properties, such as size, texture, shape, or the presence or absence of handles. Sighted people will have seen many, many examples of different cups, but a blind person will only have experience of the ones he or she has actually touched. Some items may be very difficult to comprehend as a whole by touch: for example, Rudyard Kipling wrote a poem about three blind men each touching different parts of an elephant, and each having a completely different idea of what the animal was.

It is not automatically the case that a blind or partially sighted person will make maximum use of their other senses. Some people may be tactile defensive, that is, fearful of touch and liable to avoid or withdraw from it. Tolerance will need to be built up gradually in predictable situations. The use of massage can be helpful and enjoyable, and the interactive massage sequence (Sanderson & Harrison 1992) can be used as a guide to progress, working from passive to more interactive communication.

Smells can be used systematically to alert the person to different activities and events in the day. Consistent use of the same toiletries can also help the person to identify different nurses or carers. Similarly, a tactile reference, such as encouraging the person to feel your ring, bracelet, watch or wristband, can assist with this.

Tips for communication General points for communicating with a blind or partially sighted person include the following:

• Use your speech to supplement for non-verbal cues which the person will be missing out on. For example, when speaking to the person use his or her name, especially when first beginning to talk. Indicate that you are listening by saying 'Yes', 'Mmmm', 'I agree' etc., rather as you do during a telephone conversation. In a group, encourage people to say who they are each time they talk. If others are pointing to something or using facial expressions which are particularly important, then describe what is happening. Tell the person who is coming into the room or leaving, or what is about to happen, e.g. 'I'm going to get your dinner'.

• Use language carefully where directional words are concerned, for example 'It's over there' is not very helpful, whereas 'The box is next to the table' may be. Words such as 'look' or 'see' do not necessarily need to be avoided, as the person may have residual vision, but it may be more appropriate to use alternatives such as 'touch' or 'find'.

• Try to help the person understand the meaning of what you are saying by encouraging him or her to feel the object, or by demonstrating the appropriate action.

• If it is appropriate to use signs or symbols as a means of communication, these will need to be adapted. For example, signs which are made out in space in front of the person's body will not be perceived or understood, but can be adapted so that they give more contact and feedback to the person. 'Hands-on' approaches to teaching signing are often used, that is, taking the person's hand and physically guiding them through the sign. Symbols will need to be enlarged, presented in bold colour contrasts or using raised materials (Best 1987, Bradley & Snow, undated).

• Additional tactile means of conveying information should be considered if appropriate, for example, Braille or Moon.

Braille represents letters of the alphabet by a matrix of six raised dots, each composed in different configurations. It therefore requires good language and tactile skills. Moon is simpler, consisting of raised letters based on the written alphabet. For both systems the person will need existing literacy skills or the ability to develop them. Advice can be obtained from local services for blind and visually impaired people. Carers will need to learn the system too.

Dual sensory losses

Where the person has a dual sensory impairment, or a profound and multiple disability accompanied by visual or hearing impairment, then specialist advice should be sought from organizations such as Sense, the national deaf–blind organization (see also Chapter 11).

SPECIFIC ISSUES REGARDING INDIVIDUAL COMMUNICATION

Gaining an accurate idea of the person's comprehension of language

It can be difficult to work out how much someone with learning disabilities can understand of what we say. Although in many instances we tend to assume that understanding and expression are on roughly equivalent levels, this is not always the case.

If you judge someone's understanding by their ability to express themselves, you may jump to false conclusions. They may have relatively good understanding but little or no speech. This could lead you to underestimate their understanding (think of any experiences you have had of learning another language and being at the stage where you can understand more than you are able to say). Conversely, some people with learning disabilities appear to be able to express themselves fairly well. This may lead you to overestimate their understanding. (Once again, think of yourself learning a new skill, such as computing, where you may have begun to use some of the jargon but do not fully understand it.)

Sometimes it may be very obvious when the person has not understood what we say. However, often they may understand the total situation rather than what is actually said, and so respond appropriately. To take a simple example, you might say 'Go and get your dinner', but an appropriate response might be caused by a variety of factors, other than understanding the language used. Consider the other cues in the situation: the person may know from routine that it is dinnertime (and may be hungry), and sees others going towards the dining room. Possibly you are gesturing and propelling her towards the dining room, and maybe she can smell the food. On a verbal level, she only really has to grasp one word, 'dinner'. So she is getting a variety of cues – time related, visual and olfactory – and the verbal message is only one part of the situation. The person may need all these additional cues, but lack of clarity about how much language is understood may lead to unrealistic expectations and instructions later on.

It is important to try to find out how much language the person understands, independently of other cues, in order to consider:

• how to talk to the person appropriately in

general conversation, when communicating important information and when teaching new skills;

• whether the person needs additional cues, such as signs, pictures or symbols, to help them understand others' communication. (Pictures, symbols or signs are not just a means for the person to express themselves, but can also be aids to understanding, since they often have a more obvious link to the underlying idea than do words. For example, the sign for 'tea' or a drawing of it has a more obvious link to this drink than the spoken word.);

• why any inappropriate responses or challenging behaviour are occurring. Is it because the person is bored, uncooperative etc., or is it because they have been unable to understand what is required of them?

There are various methods which speech and language therapists can use to assess a person's understanding of speech. What most of these involve is structured ways to experiment with the amount of non-verbal cues used, and setting up situations that involve purely linguistic understanding. The Derbyshire Language Scheme provides a useful framework for assessing the number of information-carrying words a person can understand at a time. The assessment methods and suggested development activities can be adapted for use with adults.

Factors which may make language difficult to understand include:

• Vocabulary: there are many different words which can be used to say the same thing, for example the same drink could be referred to by various people as squash, pop, fizz, juice or a brand name. Tidying up could be referred to as clearing things up, cleaning up, or sorting out the mess! Conversely, some words may have a range of different meanings, for example 'my hand', compared to 'give me a hand' or 'hand me a cup'. Words may also be used metaphorically, in a way which may be confusing or taken literally by people with learning disabilities, for example, 'skating on thin ice' or 'Don't fly off the handle!'

Understanding of words may be linked to particular contexts or experiences. For instance, one disabled child who was asked if she would like to go to the theatre declined the offer and appeared quite fearful. It emerged that her main experience of the theatre was the operating theatre, because of a persistent illness.

Crystal (1987) discusses how vocabulary is acquired according to its relevance to the individual. For example, it might be assumed that a child would learn vocabulary related to bodily parts in a fairly predictable sequence. However, if a child has had unusual experiences or illness, he or she may have acquired some surprisingly complex or detailed vocabulary. Similarly, an adult with learning disabilities may have acquired some complex vocabulary in relation to the rest of his or her communication, owing to experiences such as blood transfusions.

• Complexity of ideas: for example, words connected to time may be difficult to understand because the underlying concept is very abstract, e.g. tomorrow, yesterday, next week. This can lead to the person repeatedly asking the same question, such as 'When's my sister coming?' Ways to make this clearer might revolve around having a diary, simple filofax or chart, where the keyworker can draw pictures or symbols to indicate when things will be happening. It can be helpful for this to be compiled with the person on a daily basis, or to have see-through pockets or Velcro on the back of the symbols or pictures. In this way it is possible to remove any items or activities which will not be happening on that particular day, and so avoid potential confusion.

• Sentence construction: some features of sentence construction can be especially difficult. For example, negatives can be embedded in sentences in a variety of ways: 'There's no bread'; 'There isn't any bread'; 'There's no more bread'. These can be easily missed so that the person thinks the sentence has the opposite meaning to that intended by the speaker. This can lead to confusion, where, for example, the person repeatedly hears the word bread but still does not receive any. In the case of an instruction the person may appear deliberately to do the opposite, having misunderstood what was said.

• Sentence length: the person may understand the individual components of the sentence but have difficulty assimilating the whole: 'Please may I borrow your knife to cut my orange?' is a polite, reasonable and explanatory request, but the person may repeatedly proffer the orange, since it is the last-named thing.

Tips to ensure you are understood

• Address the person by name and ensure you have their attention, visually if you are using signs or symbols to communicate.

• Aim to be consistent in the vocabulary you use yourself, and also check to see if this is the same vocabulary used by the other carers involved with the person. Note important points in the care plan to assist with this.

• Use short, simple sentences, making sure that these are still age appropriate in style.

• Ensure that you talk to the person frequently – language is learnt through repetition. Even where the person is unable to respond verbally, he or she may understand what is said or, if not, be generally responsive to tones of voice.

• Do not overwhelm the person with too much at a time. Where an instruction has several parts, break it down into several sentences as necessary, for example, instead of 'Go and bring the eggs, butter and flour and put them in a bowl', the request could be broken down as follows: 'Bring the eggs' 'Now bring the butter; great' 'Bring the flour' 'Please put them in the bowl'.

• Avoid complex sentence structures such as negatives and complex time dimensions.

• Judge pace carefully. Speak slowly and give the person time to respond, as necessary.

• Supplement what you say with gestures and other cues. Be aware that some people find apparently simple gestures difficult to understand: for example, pointing may be ambiguous. Head nods and shakes may be difficult for some people to distinguish, and do not always have the same meanings across cultures.

Alternative and augmentative communication systems

When someone has no speech, speech which is difficult to understand and/or finds it difficult to understand other people's speech, it may be helpful to use an alternative or augmentative communication system. 'Alternative' refers to the possibility that it may be used by the person as an alternative to speech; 'augmentative' means it may be used to support (or augment) any existing speech or other means of communication. This is likely to involve either signs or symbols, or a combination of both.

Systems which use signs are sometimes referred to as manual or unaided systems, since they involve using the hands and no other equipment. Systems which use symbols are sometimes referred to as graphic or aided systems, since they involve drawing or writing, which may be displayed on a chart, book or computer VDU. Regardless of the system, the overall aim is to help the person communicate in everyday circumstances, and for those in contact with the person to be able to communicate back.

The Makaton vocabulary

One of the most commonly used methods for people with learning disabilities is the Makaton Vocabulary Language Programme, which involves the use of signs, symbols and speech. It was originally designed to meet the needs of people with learning disabilities who also had a hearing loss and were living in a hospital. It was designed by Margaret Walker in the early 1970s. Now, it is used with both adults and children with learning disabilities whose communication difficulties may be related to a variety of factors, not just hearing loss. It has also been used with some people who have communication problems unrelated to learning difficulties, e.g. after a 'stroke' (see Grove & Walker 1990 for a full description).

Makaton consists of a core vocabulary of 350 words, signs and symbols, with an additional resource vocabulary of approximately 7000. The signs are derived from British Sign Language (BSL) for deaf people, but have been standardized, that is, the dialectical variations in signs which are a striking feature of BSL have been eliminated to avoid possible confusion for people with learning disabilities and their carers. The symbols have been designed by the Makaton Vocabulary Development Project and are linked to Rebus (originally a reading scheme using symbols, now also used as a primary means of communication).

The Makaton core vocabulary is grouped into eight stages, designed as a guideline for teaching everyday essential vocabulary in a meaningful sequence and progressing from simple to more abstract concepts. For example, in Stage 1 everyday ideas such as 'bus', 'cup', 'I', 'you', 'where' and 'what' occur, while in Stage 7 more abstract ideas, such as 'late', 'early', 'how much' and 'how many' are included. However, an important feature is personalization of the vocabulary to suit individual needs, that is, at each stage vocabulary should be selected which is relevant to the individual in terms of their interests, daily activities and environment. This can be very convenient for nurses and other carers because it means that it is possible to learn a variety of useful signs and then adapt the precise selection according to the needs of the individual. It is important that everyone who knows the person is kept updated about the signs they use.

One of the important features of Makaton is economy of use, that is, building up from teaching a small selection of important everyday concepts and expanding where necessary. Normal grammatical speech should be used by nurses and other carers, although generally only key words are signed. The additional resource vocabulary, which is grouped into topic areas (e.g. sexuality, emotions and relationships, the early attainment targets of the national curriculum, fire and its hazards), contains concepts which can be introduced as necessary. The national curriculum resource also contains many grammatical items which can be introduced if needed.

Another key aspect is that Makaton offers the

opportunity for multimodal communication. Symbols can be used in the following ways:

- As a basic means of communication for learning-disabled people who have an additional physical disability. They can be mounted on a chart or in a book so that the person can indicate choices.
- To assist with learning language. Since symbols provide a more permanent message than either speech or signs, they may help those with memory difficulties. They can be used to help build up language structure.
- To help with understanding of the written word (by being paired with it) or as a means in itself of 'writing' notes, shopping lists, instructions, postcards etc. The symbols are designed to be simple and quick to draw by hand.
- As an additional means of communication, to give flexibility so that the person can select their preferred mode or vary the mode according to circumstances (in the same way that we do in our own communication). Autistic people may prefer symbols because of their concrete nature, which allows repeated examination over time and the likelihood that using symbols involves less intense interaction with others (Mirenda & Schuler 1988).

British Sign Language (BSL)

This is a language in its own right and is used mainly by children and adults who are born deaf. It cannot therefore be accurately described as an alternative or augmentative communication system. It has its own structure and word order, which differ from that of spoken English, and is not generally used with speech (see Miles 1988 for a description). Some profoundly deaf people with mild learning disabilities may use BSL. If so, it is important that others learn to use it and that the person has contact with other BSL users via the deaf community.

Signed English

This was developed as a means of encouraging reading, writing and spoken English among deaf children, and based on signs from British Sign Language. For this reason, it is used with speech and follows English word order and structure. Every word in a sentence is signed, and additional signs are devised to convey the grammatical elements of spoken English. Signed English may be used by people with learning disabilities.

Paget–Gorman Sign System

This was devised to represent all the elements of spoken English. As in Signed English, all the words in the sentence are signed. There are precise rules about how to produce the signs, which require very fine coordination. Although in the past the Paget–Gorman Sign System was used with people with learning disabilities, it is now used chiefly with children with specific language disorders.

Blissymbols

These were originally devised in the 1940s by Charles Bliss, with the intention of being an international graphic language. During the 1970s they were adapted for use as a communication system for non-speaking people with cerebral palsy. The symbols are composed of nine abstract geometric shapes of differing sizes and orientation, which represent different meanings when combined. The written word is always used with the symbol. Because of their complexity, both visually and conceptually, they are often thought to be too complicated for people with learning disabilities.

Picture charts

These can be developed on an ad hoc basis, according to the needs of the individual. Pictures or photographs can be used, based on things within the person's experience. Although these have the advantage of being easy to understand, provided the person has sufficient symbolic understanding to comprehend pictures, there is the disadvantage that it is difficult to convey abstract ideas.

Tangible symbols

These are manipulable symbols with raised, tactile features which bear a close perceptual relationship to the item they represent. They can be very useful for people who are not able to understand abstract symbol systems. They will need to be individually developed for each person who needs them (Rowland & Schweigert 1989, Clark-Kehoe 1992).

Objects of reference

These are similar to tangible symbols and may be very useful to help orientate a person with severe learning disabilities and additional sensory impairments. Objects are used in a systematic way to help the person understand and begin to anticipate what is happening next, for example a swimming costume and towel to indicate swimming, or a spoon to indicate kitchen. Gradually, once the person has understood this link, the object could be made more symbolic, for example a small piece of towel instead of the whole towel. The person could also be encouraged to use the items to communicate their own wishes.

Rebus

These simple symbols were originally derived from a reading scheme (the Peabody Rebus Scheme) and adapted for use as a communication tool. The original reading scheme contained many verbal puns (e.g. a picture of a tin can to represent the verb 'can'). Although these are amusing for children learning to read, they may be very confusing to people with learning disabilities. These puns have been deleted from the use of Rebus symbols as a communication system. The symbols are arranged alphabetically in a dictionary, so that they can easily be selected by professionals and carers (Devereux & Van Oosterum, 1985).

Facilitated communication

This method was originally used with people with physical and communication disabilities, but has also been used with people with autism. Specially trained facilitators use emotional and physical support to enable the person to use communication boards. Although there have been enthusiastic reports of success (e.g. Scrivener 1993), many of the claims have not been upheld by objective research (see Howlin 1994 for a summary).

Why might signs and symbols facilitate communication?

Possible reasons include:

- The nature of signs and symbols: words are very fleeting, whereas signs can be held still long enough for the individual to process them. Symbols are even more permanent.
- The visual nature of signs and symbols: many people with learning disabilities show a preference for visuospatial information. Therefore, this information may be easier for some people to process than spoken language, which relies on auditory vocal processing.
- The iconic nature of some signs and symbols may assist in learning the sign and, ultimately, the corresponding word. 'Iconicity' means the strength of association between the sign and the idea it represents. For example, the sign for 'cup' gives more links to the corresponding idea than the word, which is arbitrary.

Important considerations

- **Choice of system** It is important to obtain a thorough assessment of the individual's communication skills and professional advice about the most appropriate method to use. There are various guidelines which include issues to consider in system selection (Allen 1989, Walker & Ferris-Taylor 1991).
- **Individual preferences** Owing to the nature of the person's communication difficulty it may not be possible to involve them in choosing the system. This makes it important to take into account any apparent preferences (e.g. like or dislike of using gesture or pictorial materials), both at the outset and once the system is in use.
- **Training** It is important that everyone who

uses the system on a regular basis feels confident about using it. Some methods, such as Makaton, offer a range of formal and informal courses tailored to meet different needs.

• **Real-life use** The success of any method of communication depends upon the extent to which it is used, by the person concerned and everyone else. Often, practice is sufficient to enable carers to feel comfortable using it, both indoors and outdoors.

Although training is crucial, everyday use may be facilitated by memory joggers and sufficient repetition, so that use becomes automatic rather than consciously thought out. Some establishments have adopted a 'signs of the week' approach, where the emphasis is on gradual practice/relearning of a few signs each week, with one staff member taking responsibility for teaching others a small number of signs as selected and prioritized by the staff group (Spragale & Micucci 1990).

Real-life use can also be encouraged by the extent to which signs and symbols are available in everyday settings. For example, Makaton symbols have recently been used in some community settings such as shops, libraries, the

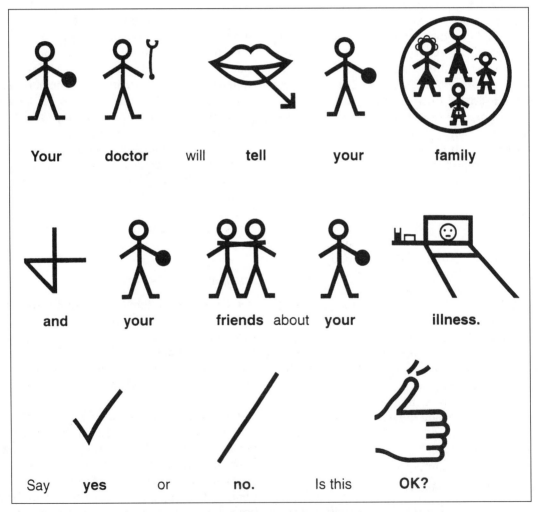

Figure 12.2 Examples of Makaton symbols from the Hull and Holderness NHS Trust Patient's Charter (with permission from the Makaton Vocabulary Development Project).

Hull and Holderness NHS Trust *Patient's Charter*, and Benefits Agency leaflets (see Fig. 12.2).

Given the wide range of carers who may come into contact with those with learning difficulties, it is important to have convenient and effective ways to pass on information about their method of communication. Personal 'passports' have been used with deaf–blind people and their carers. Caldwell et al (1995) describe these as 'a booklet which described in a human way everything a carer needed to know about the person and, in particular, his or her unique style of communicating with others'.

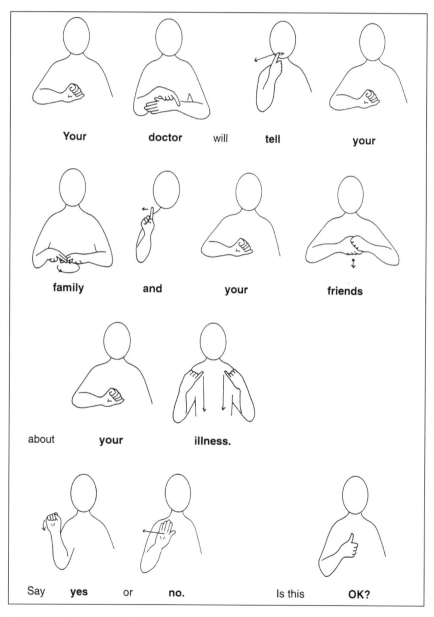

Figure 12.3   Examples of Makaton signs from Hull and Holderness NHS Trust Patient's Charter, corresponding to symbols in Figure 12.2 (with permission from the Makaton Vocabulary Development Project).

• **Individualized use** The person's coordination, vision or visual perception may mean that they use symbols or signs in ways which carers need to 'tune in to'. For example, someone using a communication board or chart may access the board in a variety of ways, such as pointing with their finger, fist or eye pointing. Particularly where eye pointing is concerned, carers will need to take time to adjust and respond.

Many people with learning disabilities will produce Makaton signs which are very unlike the standardized versions taught in workshops and reproduced in booklets. This may be due to factors outlined above. However, it may also be a component of learning signs, analogous to the phonological processes involved in learning speech (Dunn-Klein 1988). It is useful to analyse the person's sign production, looking for patterns or themes rather than just thinking it is 'wrong'.

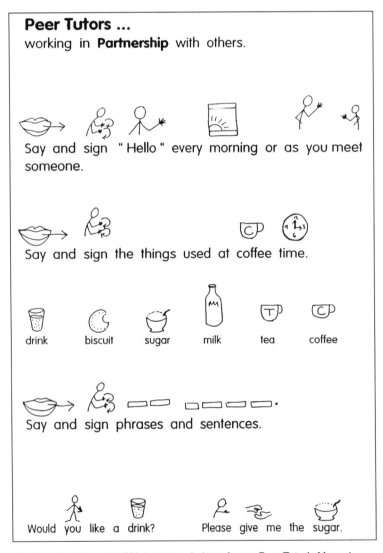

Figure 12.4 Example of Makaton symbol use from a Peer Tutor's Manual (Hooper and Newnham 1994) (with permission from Helen Hooper and the Makaton Vocabulary Development Project).

Makaton can be adapted for one-handed use. It has also been used with people with visual impairments, once again with adaptations to maximize the use of kinaesthetic and tactile features of signs (Mountain 1984). The symbols can be adapted in size or made tangible for students with visual disabilities.

• **Making best use of a system** Using a sign or symbol system will not, in itself, automatically solve all communication difficulties. It is important to bear in mind the principles of positive communication contained throughout this chapter. The following points are particularly important:

• Help the person understand and use the system: they may not automatically understand the meaning of the signs and symbols without clear links being made. They also may not understand the principle that the signs or symbols can con-

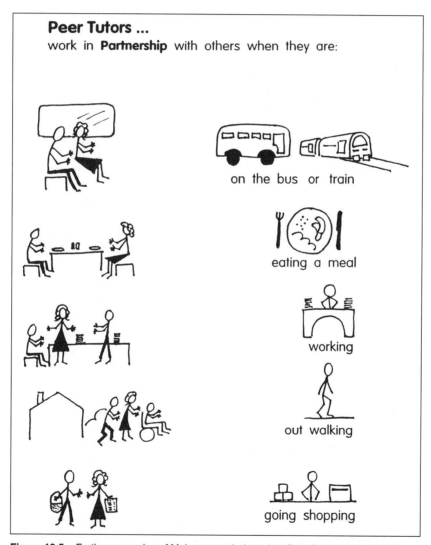

Figure 12.5 Further examples of Makaton symbol use in a Peer Tutor's Manual (Hooper and Newnham 1994) (with permission from Helen Hooper and the Makaton Vocabulary Development Project).

help them to express their wishes. ... to be demonstrated.

- Provide reasons to communicate and opportunities to do so, in the context of pleasurable social activities. If it is difficult to ascertain the person's preferred activities then it is important to spend more time observing and noting preferences and, where necessary, providing the opportunity for a wider range of activities.

- Use the system in everyday life yourself. The person will need to see others communicating with signs or symbols in order to recognize that this is an acceptable and valued means of communication. Also, in order to extend skills, he or she needs to see a model of sign or symbol use which is a little beyond his or her own capacity. Some research has suggested that individuals tend to use signs most in the presence of interactors who use them too (Grove & McDougall 1988, 1989).

Encourage friends and peers to use the signs and symbols. Effective Makaton peer tutoring courses have been developed, where people with learning disabilities can learn to teach others to use Makaton. There have been exciting developments in the use of peer tutoring, which can involve social and linguistic gains for both tutors and their peers (Hooper & Bowler 1991, Hooper & Newnham 1994) (see Fig. 12.3).

Expression

Speech

Speech is the spoken output of the language system. It involves the movements we make with our lips, tongue, jaws, teeth and hard and soft palates. The energy source comes from air via the lungs activating the vocal folds in the larynx.

Speech involves the fastest movements and the finest coordination of any part of our body. As an example, think of what you are doing when you produce an 's' sound. Your tongue is raised to the roof of your mouth, with the tongue tip usually positioned just behind the teeth. The sides of the tongue are raised and touching the sides of the hard palate, and the tongue is grooved all the way along the centre. The vocal folds are close together but not touching, so that air from the lungs passes through the larynx on an outward breath without causing the vocal folds to vibrate. The soft palate is raised so that the uvula touches the back wall of the pharynx. This means that air is channelled through the mouth, rather than entering the nasal cavity. The air is channelled continuously along the groove along the middle of the tongue, creating friction. And all this for one sound! (See Nolan & Warner 1984 for a fuller description of speech production.)

Owing to this complexity, it follows that there are many factors which can make it difficult for someone to produce clear speech. Some examples are:

- Dysarthria: a difficulty in speaking due to neurological damage affecting coordination of the muscles of the mouth, tongue, throat etc. Severity may vary, so that the person's speech may be so mildly affected that only a few speech sounds are distorted, or it may be so severe that speech is completely unintelligible or absent.

- Dyspraxia: a difficulty in voluntary programming affecting the functional use of a group of muscles. The person has no visible paralysis. Dyspraxia affects the motor programming of speech, making it difficult for the person to produce and sequence sounds within a word. On some occasions the person may be able to make some sounds/words clearly and effortlessly. This may particularly be the case with emotional words, such as swear words. Dyspraxia may also occur in the limbs, and may therefore give rise to difficulty in producing signs.

- Hearing impairment: we use our hearing to learn language, but also to maintain our communication by tuning in to the sound of our own speech. Therefore, a hearing loss may make it difficult for someone to develop speech and produce all sounds clearly. For example, if someone has a high-frequency hearing loss they will find it difficult to hear high-pitched speech sounds such as 's', 'p', 't' and 'k', and therefore these sounds may be distorted in their own speech. Someone developing a hearing loss in later life may gradually show signs of deterioration in their speech, depending on the level of the loss.

- Phonological difficulties: phonology is the rules for combining speech sounds together. The person may be able to produce a range of speech sounds in isolation but may have difficulty in organizing them into the required sequence within words. For example:
  - Clusters of sounds may be simplified, e.g. 'blue' may be produced as 'bu'.
  - Unstressed syllables may be deleted, e.g. 'tomato' may be produced as 'mato'.
  - One sound may replace another, e.g. 'car' may be produced as 'ta'.
  - One sound in a word may affect the production of another e.g. 'dog' may be produced as 'gog' or 'dod'.

It may be that these processes simplify the complexity of speech production or are related to the way the person perceives speech.

- Difficulties with fluency of speech, such as stammering (or stuttering, which is the same). This is a pattern of speech which involves hesitations, repetitions of syllables or words and silent blocks (getting stuck on a sound). Difficulty in speaking may be accompanied by altered breathing patterns and physical gestures. The person may avoid feared sounds, words or situations, so that the actual stammering may appear mild or infrequent to others, but it can come to dominate the person's choice of words and social situations. The causes of stammering are not known.

There is considerable debate about whether 'stammering' in adults with learning disabilities is, in fact, stammering, or is part of a person's overall communication development, (that is, analogous to children, who often pass through a period where their speech is non-fluent owing to underdeveloped control over speech musculature and speech patterns), rather than being perceived as a difficulty. Defining factors would involve the degree of awareness and anticipation of difficulty and struggle in the actual production of speech. Although speech modification techniques, such as prolonged speech (which tries to shape speech towards fluency) can be intro-

duced, these can be difficult for anyone to monitor and maintain in everyday life. It can be helpful to analyse when the difficulties occur, i.e. with particular people, or in particular situations. The difficulties of these situations and the emotions involved can then be discussed. Perhaps the most productive approach is to consider your own communication. In particular:

- Maintain an unhurried pace of communication yourself and do not rush the person.
- Allow the person to finish what they were going to say – do not finish it for them (you may get it wrong).
- Keep eye contact with the person.
- Do not 'put the person on the spot' by making them speak in front of others, unless they have indicated that they wish to do so.
- Communicate with the person's family, if applicable, so that they avoid pressuring the person to 'speak normally'.

Helping someone to improve the clarity of their speech will probably be a very slow process, if it is appropriate at all within the context of their overall strengths and difficulties in communicating. There are likely to be severe limits to the changes which can be made by adulthood.

It is important that a full assessment is made by a speech and language therapist. This will look at the sounds someone can produce, those which are omitted and distorted, and how this differs in different sequences within words and connected speech. For example, someone may be able to produce the sound 's' in isolation, and in the word 'sun', but omit it in the word 'spider'. Another person may produce fairly intelligible single words but become difficult to understand in connected speech.

The speech and language therapist would also consider the range, speed and accuracy of movements the person can make and, combined with analysing the speech patterns, attempt to make a differential diagnosis. This is important, because depending on the cause, a different approach might be appropriate. For example, if the cause is dyspraxia, a carefully structured approach involving much repetition and building up to practice of sequences of sounds may be adopted. Dyspraxia is now being much more frequently identified in childhood, among children both with and without learning disabilities. Comprehensive programmes, such as the Nuffield Dyspraxia Programme, have been developed.

If the speech difficulty is related to hearing loss, then assistance in using a hearing aid may be beneficial. Some individuals may adjust their speech spontaneously when using their hearing aid, because they can hear themselves more clearly.

From the assessment it may be possible to devise a realistic programme, working from what the person can do and gradually building up, so that confidence is developed and maintained. Motivation is also a crucial factor here: the person needs to have sufficient awareness and the wish to change their speech patterns. Practice will need to be done little and often, so that although the therapist would devise and supervise the programme, he or she will be unlikely to carry it out in its entirety. The active involvement of nurses, social workers, family members and others concerned with the person on a daily basis is crucial.

It must be borne in mind that the cause of the speech difficulty may be a combination of factors: for example, someone with cerebral palsy may have dysarthria and a hearing loss. In addition, the person's level of learning disability will have an overall impact on their speech and language development. If the person has a small vocabulary it may be easier to differentiate the words they are trying to say, and more important to extend this vocabulary, than to attempt to improve actual speech production.

It may be helpful, in the first instance, to try to 'tune in' to what the person is saying and for the carers to develop a shared 'glossary' of the words/meanings the person is trying to get across. This may be more helpful, and reduce frustration for both parties, than immediately trying to improve the person's speech. It may be that peers, through their familiarity, can understand one another more readily. This was most strikingly exemplified by Joseph Deacon (1974),

in his book *Tongue Tied*, a testimony to communication between people with learning disabilities.

Other pragmatic approaches include building up a list of target words which the individual needs to use more frequently, or which are particularly important. This may be done by accompanying the person in everyday situations, noting the words they use or attempt to use, and drawing up a priority list. The person can then be helped to practise producing these words more clearly, supplemented by facial expressions and gestures to get the meaning across. Such practice can include role play of the relevant situation, progressing to the actual situation.

If the person's speech is particularly unclear or absent altogether, it can be helpful to use a supplementary means of communication, such as Makaton. This may be used to get meaning across to the listener and so reduce frustration. There are many anecdotal suggestions among speech and language therapists that the use of such systems can reduce the pressure on being understood by using speech, and some suggestions from research that the person's speech may spontaneously improve without specific work on speech production being undertaken (Reid et al 1983).

Earlier in this chapter there was a discussion of the close links between speech and gesture in communication development. From a neurological point of view, speech movements are represented in the brain in the precentral gyrus, adjacent to the area responsible for the control of hand and arm movements. It is possible that encouraging communication through signs may stimulate the adjacent areas of the brain, thereby stimulating speech development. When Makaton is used with children with learning disabilities, the aim is always to develop speech where possible and fade out the use of signs when they are no longer needed. We would not realistically expect this in adults, where it may be a means of communication in itself. Nevertheless, it is important also to encourage any concurrent vocalization or speech.

Use of language

Many adults with learning disabilities may have

difficulty in using the syntax of spoken language and produce sentences which are telegram-like in form. One of the most helpful approaches can be to ensure that the person hears an expanded version of what he or she says, for example if the person says 'Kevin's eating', you could respond with 'Yes, Kevin's eating a cake'.

Games involving modelling use of the target language structure and encouraging the person to copy, in a variety of contexts, can be used (see Warner & McCartney 1984 for useful ideas). However, it may not always be considered necessary or appropriate to try to do this.

Other individuals can appear to express themselves reasonably clearly, but sometimes closer acquaintance shows that their use of language masks underlying problems of understanding. Two particularly striking features to look out for are echoed speech and perseveration.

Echoed speech

This is the repetition of words or sentences spoken by other people. For instance, if you ask the person 'Where are you going?', he or she may echo the last word, 'going', or perhaps the whole sentence. This may indicate that the person has not understood and it may be beneficial to simplify the level of language. However, it can be easy to overlook this in everyday circumstances. For instance, a person might always choose coffee because when they are offered 'tea or coffee', this is always the last-named thing.

Some people will use echoed speech in a delayed way, so that the echo is not obvious, and these phrases may be used over and over again. Alternatively, they may be related to particular circumstances. For example, one woman used the phrase 'Give me a twirl' whenever she had her hair done, because this phrase had been used once when she had shown others her new hair-do. She remembered, associated and used it within that situation, but when its origin was not apparent to new people its use was very puzzling. Although she remembered the phrase and had no difficulty in producing it clearly, she did not really understand it, and she could not use the individual words outside this fixed phrase or

situation. Nevertheless, it was helpful to her carers to understand its origin.

Many autistic people echo phrases in this way, often remembering and reproducing very elaborate conversation. However, we should not be misled by this into developing very high expectations of the person's expressive language. Aarons and Gittens (1992) have produced a useful checklist for assessing in detail the subtle and often very confusing aspects of autistic people's communication, with suggestions for development. Bebko (1990) has argued that mitigation in echolalia (i.e. a change in some feature of the utterance being repeated, rather than a verbatim repetition) is a crucial characteristic, because it implies a degree of voluntary control and symbolic functioning. By contrast, exact repetition implies little evidence of the ability to understand or use speech meaningfully. This argument is developed to suggest that those with no speech or unmitigated echolalia may fare best with a sign or symbol system, whereas those with mitigated echolalia may have a more positive prognosis for developing speech. However, this model is derived from studies of existing research and is a theoretical one which so far has been untested.

Perseveration

Perseveration means the continuation of speech or activity which was appropriate in one context but is now no longer appropriate. For example, the person may continue to repeat the same word, phrase or sign even when others have responded. This may also be more evident in more general conversation, where the person may find switches from one topic to another confusing. Factors such as the pace of conversation, or the person's hearing acuity, can make it difficult to keep up with topic changes in a group setting. It may be neurologically based, that is, a difficulty in initiating and terminating responses, or it can be habitual or, once again, related to a lack of understanding of what others have said. Perseveration may also occur in a broader sense. The person may keep on entering into a dialogue about the same event or theme, and this may go on for weeks, months or even years. Once again, the reasons may be very diverse. For example, such conversation may be the person's sole focus of interest (e.g. the royal family, or a particular TV programme). It may be their way of trying to come to terms with a particularly significant or distressing event (for example, if we are upset by a divorce or bereavement, we may wish to discuss it repeatedly with different friends, or a counsellor. However, because of our language skills we have a wider range of possible things to say about it). It may be related to limited appreciation of time and the words used to express various timescales. In elderly people with learning disabilities it may be that the long-term memory is better than the short-term, so that it is easier to refer to events remembered from the more distant past. Such repetitive and insistent speech can be very irritating, difficult and puzzling for those in daily contact with the person. This should not be underestimated, particularly where it persists, relatively unchanged, for very long periods. The approach will vary, depending on the cause. However, in general it is helpful to be aware of the person's level of understanding of language and tailor your own speech accordingly. It is also important to be aware of changes in either the form or the tone of voice used, in order to cue in to the person's emotions.

Finally, where someone has relatively good understanding of speech but little or no speech themselves, full assessment may be helpful to determine whether they have a specific speech or language disorder.

CONCLUSION

There is a range of factors specific to the individual which may adversely affect his or her communication. However, in seeking to minimize communication difficulties, it may often be more appropriate and hopeful to focus on environmental factors and the impact of our own communication on the dialogue.

The importance of communication is crucial. As Anne McDonald says, 'Communication falls into the same category as food, drink and shelter: it is essential for life. Without it life becomes worthless.'

Acknowledgements

The author is grateful to the Makaton Vocabulary Development Project for kind permission to reproduce examples of signs and symbols from the Makaton Vocabulary, and to Tom Reid, for helpful discussions during preparation of this chapter.

REFERENCES

Aarons M, Gittens T 1992 The autistic continuum: an assessment and intervention schedule. NFER-Nelson, Windsor
Abercrombie K 1968 Paralanguage. British Journal of Disorders of Communication
Allen J 1989 Augmentative communication: more than just words. ACE Centre, Oxford
Argyle M 1977 The psychology of interpersonal behaviour. Pelican, Harmondsworth
Basil C 1992 Social interaction and learned helplessness in severely disabled children. Augmentative and Alternative Communication Journal 8: 361–368
Baumgart D, Johnson J, Helmstether E 1990 Augmentative and alternative communication systems for persons with moderate and severe disabilities. Paul H Brookes, Baltimore
Baxter C, Poonia K, Ward L, Nadirshaw Z 1990 Double discrimination – issues and services for people with learning disabilities from black and ethnic minority communities. Kings Fund Centre, London

Bebko J M 1990 Echolalia, mitigation and autism: indicators from child characteristics for the use of sign language and other augmentative systems. Sign Language Studies 66: 78–88
Best A B 1987 Steps to independence. BIMH, Kidderminster
Bradley J, Snow B (undated) Making sense of the world sense. National Deaf Blind and Rubella Organisation, London
Bruce T 1993 Time to play in early childhood education. Hodder and Stoughton, London
Caldwell M, Calder J, Aitken S, Millar S 1995 Use of personal passports with deaf–blind people. Talking Sense 43(3): 9–12
Campbell P, Wilcox J 1986 Communication effectiveness of movement patterns used by non-verbal children with severe handicaps. Abstracts from the 4th International ISAAC Conference, St David's Hall, Cardiff 1986
Clarke-Kehoe A 1992 Towards effective communication. In: Brown H, Benson S (eds) A practical guide to working

with people with learning disabilities. Care Concern/ Hawker Publications, London

Crawley B 1988 Learning about self advocacy. Values Into Action, London

Crossley A, McDonald R 1982 Annie's coming out. Pelican, Harmondsworth

Crystal D 1984 Listen to your child. Penguin, Harmondsworth

Crystal D 1987 Teaching vocabulary: the case for a semantic curriculum. Child Language Teaching and Therapy 3(1): p 40–56

Crystal D 1992 The Cambridge encyclopaedia of language. Cambridge University Press, Cambridge

Deacon J 1974 Tongue tied. Mencap, London

Devereux K, VanOosterum J 1985 Learning with rebuses glossary. EARO/LDA, Ely

Downes R 1996 Know your rights. Greater London Association of Disabled People, London

Dunn-Klein M 1988 Pre-sign language motor skills. Communication Skill Builders, Texas, Arizona

Ellis D (ed) 1986 Sensory impairments in mentally handicapped people. Croom-Helm, London

Ferris-Taylor R, Pinney S 1994 How to help with hearing loss. Hexagon, New Malden, Surrey

Grove N, McDougall S 1988, 1989 An exploration of the communication skills of Makaton students: Part I: The Children (1988); Part II: Interviews with Teachers and Speech Therapists (1989). Report to the Leverhulme Trust, St George's Hospital Medical School, London

Grove N, Walker M 1990 The Makaton vocabulary: using manual signs and graphic symbols to develop interpersonal communication. Augmentative and Alternative Communication 6(1): 15–28

Halle J W, Baer D M, Spradlin J E 1981 Teachers' generalised use of delay as a stimulus control procedure to increase language use in handicapped children. Journal of Applied Behaviour Analysis 14(4): 389–409

Heider F 1958 The psychology of interpersonal relations. Wiley, New York

Hewitt D, Ephraim G 1994 Access to communication: developing the basics of communication with people with severe learning difficulties through intensive interaction. David Fulton, London

Holland S, Ward C 1990 Assertiveness: a practical approach. Winslow Press, Bicester, Oxon

Hooper H, Bowler D M 1991 Peer tutoring of manual signs by adults with mental handicaps. Mental Handicap Research 4(2): 207–215

Hooper H, Newnham C and M V D P 1994 Peer tutor manual. Makaton Vocabulary Development Project, Camberley, Surrey

Howlin P 1994 Recent research into facilitated communication. Abstracts from Forum on Learning Disability – Communication and Learning Disability: A Briefing and Update on Recent Developments. Royal Society of Medicine, London

Jones SE 1990 Intecom. NFER, Windsor

Kozleski E B 1991 Expectant delay procedure for teaching requests. Alternative and Augmentative Communication 7(1): 112–131

Mansell J L 1992 Services for people with learning disabilities and challenging behaviour or mental health needs. HMSO, London

Miles D 1988 British Sign Language – a beginner's guide. BBC Publications, London

Millner L, Ash A, Ritchie P 1991 Quality in action – a resource pack for improving services for people with learning difficulties. Norah Fry Research Centre, Bristol

Minkes J, Robinson C, Weston C 1994 Consulting the children: interviews with children using residential respite care services. Disability and Society 9(1): 47–57

Mirenda P, Schuler A L 1988 Augmenting communication for persons with autism: issues and strategies. Topics in Language Disorders 9(1)

Morris D 1987 Manwatching – a field guide to human behaviour. Grafton Books, London

Morris J 1991 Pride before prejudice. Women's Press, London

Mountain M 1984 Signing with the visually and mentally handicapped non-communicating child. College of Speech Therapists Bulletin 386: 12

Noland M, Warner J 1984 Hearing and speech: the structure and function of the ear and speech organs. In: McCartney E (ed) Helping ATC students to communicate. BIMH, Kidderminister

O'Brien J 1986 A guide to personal futures planning. In: Bellamy G G, Wilcox B (eds) A comprehensive guide to the activities catalog: an alternative curriculum for youth and adults with severe disabilities. Paul H Brookes, Baltimore, Maryland

Oliver M 1990 The politics of disablement. Macmillan, London

Reid B, Jones L, Kiernan C 1983 Signs and symbols: the 1982 survey of use. Special Education, Forward Trends 10: 27–28

Reiser R, Mason M 1992 The medical model and the social model of disability. In: Reiser R, Mason M (eds) Disability equality in the classroom: a human rights issue. Disability Equality in Education, London

Rowland C, Schweigert P 1989 Tangible symbols: symbolic communication for individuals with multisensory impairments. Augmentative and Alternative Communication 5(4): 226–234

Royal National Institute for the Deaf/Coast Project 1990 Hearing matters! A Training Pack on Hearing Loss and Older People. RNID, London

Sacks O 1990 Seeing voices. Picador, London

Sanderson H, Harrison J 1992 Aromatherapy and massage for people with learning difficulties. Hands On Publishing/John Abbott Ltd, Leicestershire

Scrivener T 1993 Somebody inside with something to say. Community Living 6(4): 10

Spragale D, Micucci D 1990 Signs of the week: a functional approach to manual sign training. Alternative and Augmentative Communication: 96–104

Tizard B, Hughes M 1984 Young children learning. Fontana, London

Tizard B, Cooperman O, Tizard J 1972 Environmental effects on language development: a study of young children in long stay residential nurseries. Child Development 43: 337–358

Trevarthen C 1977 Descriptive analysis of infant communicative behaviour: theory and method sign language studies 21: 317–352

Van der Gaag A, Dormandy K 1993 Communication and adults with learning difficulties. Whurr Publishers, London

Walker M, Ferris-Taylor R 1991 Guidelines for selection of children and adults with communication difficulties for a Makaton vocabulary programme. Makaton Vocabulary Development Project, Camberley, Surrey

Warner J, McCartney E 1984 Teaching language forms: phonology and syntax. In: McCartney E (ed) Helping ATC students to communicate. BIMH, Kidderminister

Williams M, Grove N 1989 Getting to grips with aided communication: an overview of the literature. British Journal of Special Education, 16(2): Research Supplement: 63–68

Yeates S 1995 The incidence and importance of hearing loss in people with severe learning disability: the evaluation of a service. British Journal of Learning Disabilities 23:79–84

USEFUL ADDRESSES

Blissymbolics Communication Resource Centre (UK)
South Glamorgan Institute for Higher Education
Western Avenue
Llandaff
Cardiff
CF5 2YB
Tel: 01222 537770

British Association for the Hard of Hearing (BAHOH)
7 Armstrong Road
London
W3 7JL
Tel: 0181 7431110

British Deaf Association (BDA)
Head Office
38 Victoria Place
Carlisle
CA1 1HU
Tel: 01228 48844

Learning Development Aids (LDA)
Duke Street
Wisbech
Cambridge
PE13 2AB
Tel: 01945 63441

Makaton Vocabulary Development Project
31 Firwood Drive
Camberley, Surrey
GU15 2QD
Tel: 01276 61390

Multilingual Matters Ltd
The Bank House
8a Hill Road
Clevedon
Avon
BS21 7HH

Paget–Gorman Sign System
3 Gipsey Lane
Headington
Oxford
OX3 7PT

Royal Association in Aid of Deaf People
27 Old Oak Road
Acton
London
W3 6HN
Tel: 0181 7436187

Royal National Institute for the Blind (RNIB)
224 Great Portland Street
London
W1N 6AA
Tel: 0171 3881266

Royal National Institute for the Deaf (RNID)
105 Gower Street
London
WC1E 6AH
Tel: 0171 3878033

The National Deaf Blind and Rubella Association – SENSE
311 Grays Inn Road
London
WC1X 8PT
Tel: 0171 2781005

13

Leisure

D. R. Lewis   J. Phillips

INTRODUCTION

Obtaining a good quality of life for all people
regardless of disability has become an important
objective. Although work retains its role as a
major function in life, an increasing number of
people now seem to have more time and
resources to undertake pursuits of a non-voca-
tional nature.

A greater understanding has emerged of the
benefits that can be derived from leisure activities, to such an extent that a huge emphasis is
placed upon leisure provision in most western
societies.

The meaningful and constructive use of leisure time
is emerging as an important life goal for a growing
number of persons in our society (Bender et al 1984).

For people with learning disabilities who are
unlikely to acquire a full-time vocation in life,
there is an even greater sense of importance
attached to the development of leisure and recreational skills.

Bender et al (1984) proposed that leisure could
be conceptually divided into three categories:

• First, it appears to constitute a persons' own
time when not working, and when viewed in this
way the less it is seen as work and toil, the more
likely it is to provide pleasure and satisfaction.
Because it is a period carrying no obligations
towards others, it is, unfortunately, seen by professionals as less important in the development
of disabled people, almost appearing to be the
responsibility of the disabled person themselves,
and an area where choice can be freely exercised

without it compromising the aims of the care providers.

• Secondly, leisure is seen in relation to the concepts that underpin leisure activities, such as the knowledge and awareness of leisure and the skills used in activities, and in particular interaction skills, which also reflect values and attitudes, and the ability to choose and make decisions.

• Thirdly, leisure is seen as an integral part of an individual's functioning, enabling self-fulfilment through freedom of choice, and with this aspect in mind it can be seen that the provision of leisure activities is both meaningful and essential to an individual's quality of life.

It is the authors' intention to focus upon these last two categories, where leisure is recognized as being important to an individual's self-actualization and integral to their functioning.

Atkinson and Williams (1990) emphasize the ability to demonstrate creativity and imagination as enabling the formation of a bridge between one's personal identity and a much-needed social identity. Although many leisure pursuits involve others and are of a social nature, often the vehicle chosen for self-expression involves thought and fantasy, which are solitary pursuits. It is unlikely that one will be able to spend all one's time with others, although being a recipient of care often means one has little personal time. Also, there are often misconceptions as to the learning-disabled person's ability to conceptualize. Atkinson and Williams (1990) support this misconception in referring to the poems of Sandy Marshall which, when read out at the centre to the people he spends his time with, caused surprise that 'this man who kept himself to himself could produce such articulate ideas and feelings' (Atkinson & Williams 1990).

The importance of leisure

If an individual is to reach their maximum potential leisure must be integral to this process, for it represents a learning domain where fun and enjoyment are sought-after outcomes. Alan Marshall (1990) illustrates this in his dictated précis entitled 'The happiest time'.

We went on holiday, mum, dad and me, same place in Cornwall in a caravan near the pubs. I packed my case, put all my clean things ready, and got ready to go out on the booze. After we went to that place we got pie and chips.

I was happy because me, mum, dad and my sister and her husband Alan, my brother in law, went out to buy me a ring. After we came back, we went out on a boat trip, fishing. There were lots of shops in the town everywhere, which made me happy.

I got a date with some girls on holiday and that made me happy. I feel happy when I go to see my girlfriend Ellen. I play tapes when I'm happy. I have a can of beer with my dad. I like football. I like Bristol City. I stay at home and help my mum and dad vacuum-cleaning.

I feel happy, I feel like singing. (Reproduced in entirety from *Know me as I am*, edited by D Atkinson and F Williams (1990).

The words of Alan Marshall reflect the simple enjoyment found in everyday life, and he demonstrates how he gains pleasure from a range of activities, none of which are complex, yet all of which are rich in learning opportunities and easily accessible within appropriate educational settings or a family atmosphere. Wherever people care for each other and warm to each other's strengths and weaknesses, there is an excellent climate for learning, and the most beneficial way to learn is to participate in something you enjoy.

Brudenell (1987), when describing the therapeutic role of the carer, recognized that 'Teaching must be "normal", teaching must be in context' (cited in Parish 1987) yet at no time in the entire publication is the carer directed toward using leisure as a means of achieving independence. Possibly this reflects the lack of importance given to this area, which constitutes a considerable part of everyone's life. This also applies to later publications that have presented models for care delivery.

Publications that have focused on contributions from learning-disabled people themselves, or their direct carers, illustrate more definitively the importance of leisure as a central medium for learning (Brandon & Brandon 1988), whereas publications aimed at professionals more often lose sight of 'ordinariness', despite claiming 'ordinary living principles' as a basis for their content. Thus the image of non-ability so readily associated with disabled people is perpetuated.

Historical influences

Historically this image of 'non-ability' not only served to physically segregate those unable to adopt a 'productive' role in society, it also isolated them in terms of opportunity and recognition of their personhood. Many early pioneers in the education of the disabled concentrated primarily on the teaching of self-help and communication skills, through systematically applied educational processes. Jacob Redgrives Pereire (1715–1780), Jean Marc Gaspard Itard (1774–1838) and Edouard Onestitues Seguin (1812–1880) were examples of those who demonstrated some degree of success with persons previously deemed 'ineducable' (Kanner 1967).

However, Johann Jakob Guggenbuhl (1816–1863) may have been the first to truly consider the environment as being crucial to the quality of life for disabled people. He came to the conclusion that 'residential care in a suitable environment was an indispensable necessity' (Kanner 1967).

As with many pioneers he was subjected to much criticism, for anything that appears to challenge the traditional discourse of professionals seems to promote a hostile response. The initial support that he received waned and disappeared once 'faults' had been exposed, and his ideas and methods were discredited, to such an extent that even today the emphasis Guggenbuhl placed upon aesthetic beauty and the curative power of nature is given no credence in care delivery for the disabled.

Unfortunately, 'Abendberg', the institution founded to provide this care for 'cretins', with whom Guggenbuhl chose to work, became the model for the many institutions which were built following his death. Kanner (1967) states, 'But Guggenbuhl must be acknowledged as the indisputable originator of the idea and practice of the institutional care for feeble minded individuals. The hundreds of institutions now in existence derive in direct line from the Abendberg'. Guggenbuhl's ideas as to the siting of such homes were ignored in favour of his ideas about the structure itself, which would surely have been determined by the financial support available to him.

The negative imagery associated with retardation led in time to a service which ignored the potential of leisure as a medium for learning, and as the institutions expanded so too did the idea of the sheltered workshop. The importance of occupying the disabled people paved the way for their exploitation in simple industrial and farm work.

It is no real surprise that, as professionals have led care services for disabled people for over 100 years, their knowledge and authority has become a difficult area to challenge. Even today, the range of leisure provision available to the disabled has been initiated by voluntary organizations and charities dependent upon unpaid input; the facilities used by normal people have only really been opened up since the creation of legislation to ensure equal access for disabled people.

Current thinking

Many care organizations developed leisure services, but these were seen as satisfying critics and relatives, rather than being of major importance to care delivery. With the integration of learning-disabled people into community settings they once again became dependent on voluntarily run entertainments such as those run by the National Federation of Gateway Clubs. The services did little to develop leisure provision, relying on the philosophy that the disabled person should access the facilities that are available to the general public. They failed to recognize that leisure can be expensive and that disabled people would almost certainly be inhibited by lack of finance.

It is encouraging to see that leisure and recreation skills are included in most assessments for care provision today, but there is still a failure to perceive the part leisure can play in relation to learning. Bender et al (1984), in their leisure learning units, give an integrative learning chart that illustrates the relationship between a particular leisure activity and other major learning areas. They also consider the activity in terms of lead-up and follow-up strategies, and demonstrate how one activity can fulfil a wide range of learning needs.

When this is coupled with the obvious plea-

Activity 13.1

Select an activity, such as having a barbecue. Identify short-term objectives in relation to it, the 'lead-up' and 'follow-up' strategies you could use, and consider the activity in relation to other areas of learning. For example:

Maths
- Read food advertisements and compare prices
- Consider the cost of meals
- Handle money efficiently when purchasing food and supplies

sure and enjoyment that can be derived from undertaking the activity itself, then its significance as an area of intervention must surely be recognized.

LEISURE AS A LEARNING MEDIUM

It is evident that care providers should plan leisure activities in such a way that they are fulfilling for the person; they may perhaps increase their employability, but more importantly they can create a socially valued individual capable of both solitary and social activity.

Benefits

The emphasis on the occupational benefits of leisure should be reduced, and greater recognition given to the more obvious and achievable benefits, such as independent functioning, decision making and cooperating with others.

The activities considered must take account of success and failure, achievement and non-achievement as acceptable outcomes, and although praise and reinforcement can initially be good motivators, the long-term objective should be that of self-motivation, which is essential to autonomy in a world where rewards are more impersonal and of a monetary nature, and do not consist of constant praise.

It thus becomes apparent that leisure pursuits need to be reinforcing in themselves, supported by physical environments that stimulate, motivate and are aesthetically pleasing.

Role of the care provider

The role of the carer is clearly facilitative in nature, and the control so often apparent in the organizations that provide recreation needs to be shifted so that it lies with the person the activities are meant to benefit.

If the carer needs clarification as to how they might best participate, the foremost characteristic to be considered is attitude; in that there must be enthusiasm coupled with a positive valuing of all people, regardless of their abilities. There must also be acceptance that success and failure are equally valid outcomes, for either can be the result of having tried. It is therefore the attempt itself which is the objective, and if the person makes the attempt the objective has been achieved.

The only undesirable outcome is that of not having made the attempt. Unfortunately, professionals place far too much emphasis on success, and although non-competitiveness is not being advocated, there does need to be greater recognition of the individual who has given something of themselves.

One must also remember that when a person tries, it may not always be their best. People can and do improve, and performances will fluctuate depending upon a number of factors, both mental and physical. Carers must not expect that the learning-disabled person will comply and 'do as they are told' simply because they are asked!

It would be better for the carer to avoid a professional approach when facilitating leisure activities, but at the same time the activity should not be devalued by failure to demonstrate a degree of expertise so that its benefits cannot be appreciated. Effort and enthusiasm are needed both by client and carer, and satisfaction can be derived from the endeavours of both parties.

Carers with specialist skills

It is disappointing that far too often the qualified carer seems satisfied that all that is needed to be able to facilitate quite complex leisure activities is the original qualification of 'teacher', 'social worker' or 'registered nurse in learning disability'. This also applies to the unqualified carer, who has only their experience of learning disability as a background.

It would be far better if those involved in this area had a degree of expertise, either in the leisure activity itself or in leisure education, rather than relying upon a qualification that does not necessarily generate the required enthusiasm. There is a lack of specialized courses in this area, which may reflect the general failure to emphasize this essential part of a person's life.

Care managers do not generally evaluate providers as to whether they can adopt this specialized facilitative role, and therefore opportunities are missed which might reveal staff strengths and weaknesses in this area. Rarely are the wide range of leisure courses available at local further education colleges used to develop the recreational and leisure skills of care staff. Social education centres have frequently sent teams to events such as the Special Olympics led by well-meaning but totally unqualified staff. In the centre of North London, an ex-professional footballer whose experience of people with learning disability was negligible, was employed to cover leisure and recreational skills. This is an example of a serious failure to understand the therapeutic role of leisure and recreation. The 'Human Horizon' series of books, developed during the 1980s to promote a range of issues with disabled people, adopted a very positive stance towards disability, yet even here carers were often seen as 'just carers'. This is illustrated by Mike Cotton (1993), who suggests that highly specialized activities such as rock climbing, caving or mountaineering require precise staff skills, yet suggests that many other activities do not need any specialist skill from the carer. He goes on to suggest that the role of support can be undertaken by someone else, who may well be unfamiliar with the complex needs of people with learning disabilities, teaching only the activity and not understanding its relationship with other learning needs.

Because of their disabilities, people with learning difficulties tend to experience lifestyles dominated by extensive periods of inactivity. If leisure and recreation facilities are not provided, this will most certainly reduce the potential of such individuals and affect their overall quality of life.

The right environment, the right atmosphere, the right results

What type of environment should an organization consider when providing for their disabled clients' needs?

Often staff attending [an activity programme] with their handicapped trainees or pupils, would say how successful the educational aspects of a course had been even if they had travelled originally to follow a more active based programme; and that their mentally retarded youngsters had seemed to learn more in a week than they had over many previous years (Cotton 1983, 1).

Cotton goes on to state 'the right environment, the right atmosphere, the right results!'.

Successful outcomes can be transferred to other aspects of life, aiding the development of an autonomous individual capable of independent living, a goal that care providers seem to have lost sight of. The richest learning environment we have, our own local environment, is often sadly overlooked. It is both inexpensive and easily accessible, providing many learning opportunities and activities particularly relevant to the person with a learning disability. Too often, the opportunity to create a fun activity from everyday activities is lost, because of carers' lack of imagination and enthusiasm.

- What 'collector' does not relish the idea of the Sunday morning car boot sale, looking forward to the opportunity to mix with others, barter, negotiate, find a bargain and arrive home with their prize.
- Any playing field on a Sunday can provide the sports enthusiast with a huge choice of free sporting entertainment, as millions of sports people take to the greens to play purely for the love of the game.
- Every day the newspapers and television can provide the stimulus for talk, discussions and fantasy, if used appropriately by a carer with imagination and planning ability.
- Local stations meet the needs of the train enthusiast, local museums provide insight into local history and cultural development, and a wide range of public footpaths can take the indi-

vidual on a cultural and social journey rich in experience and pleasure.

The emerging person

Leisure should be a self-motivating/self-reinforcing activity, providing the opportunity to develop an individual's 'personhood'. Their imagination can be cultivated and extended beyond the confines of purely functional cognition, which may lead to that person having dreams and aspirations in life. These may or may not be achieved, but can help others to recognize the person's true individuality and uniqueness.

Being able to make decisions and being a free thinker unafraid to voice an opinion, can be the outcome for a self-determining individual who participates in a range of enjoyable activities where they have been empowered to make decisions through choice, rather than leaving everything to the care provider.

CASE STUDIES

In order to illustrate these points, three case studies of environments are described, each different in both setting and client group, the aim being to offer the reader greater awareness and insight into how these needs are approached and met. They do not offer an ideal, they merely illustrate the opportunities available and how they are exploited.

Negative imagery

One common factor is suggested as being an area that requires greater consideration. Each of the case studies described tends not to use those environments and organizations which are established primarily for people with learning disabil-

Activity 13.2

Compile a list of the benefits derived from leisure and recreational activities that would enable the person with a learning disability to have an active social life.

ities, and which serve to perpetuate the negative labels and images associated with learning disability through continued segregation, the control exerted over the client group, and the emphasis upon 'special needs' which tends to inhibit risk-taking with other activities. The major strength of the three environments is that their leisure and recreation provision is integrative, related to the person's overall needs and allowing an interaction with the community in which they live. The result is a stronger individual with greater self-esteem who shares the same activities and therefore the same human values as all other community members. All of the settings are residential, providing a therapeutic home environment, but their client groups and the reasons for living there are very different.

The first is a residential home for young people aged between 11 and 17, sited in a very rural setting at Dolgellau, mid Wales. The background of such young people is often full of trauma and devalorization, and their failure to mix appropriately and often consequential criminal behaviour results in very low self-esteem.

The second is a small house providing a home for four young men with severe learning disabilities who present a range of problematic behaviours of an antisocial nature, and who previously lived in a large hospital for people with learning disabilities run by the National Health Service.

Thirdly, a hospital setting, previously called a ward, illustrates the positiveness shown by carers in relation to a number of people inhibited by the care provision and negative imagery.

Summary

It is apparent from these three Case studies that where leisure is integrated into care planning as an essential feature, its benefits will be greater. Too often assessment formats tend to rely upon single statements, often completed in isolation from other activities, to determine the competence of an individual as regards leisure skills. This leads to many leisure opportunities being overlooked and haphazard approaches to leisure provision that rely on the moods of both clients and staff, the initiatives of the manager and the

Case study 13.1

Residential educational setting in Dolgellau
Sited on a hill between the mountains of Snowdonia is a large stone building set in eight acres of natural beauty. It was built in the 17th century and was once a coach house; it now provides a residential and educational setting for 10 young people with special needs, whose problems prior to admission ranged from extreme family trauma to drug and alcohol abuse, and for whom other placements have been unable to alter their patterns of behaviour.

The whole programme of care is centred around the individual needs of each young person, and leisure and recreational activities feature highly within the programmes developed.

Living and learning on the same site requires a flexible approach and considerable planning is needed on a daily basis in order to adapt to the climatic and seasonal changes, and to the moods and attitudes of the young people themselves.

Weekdays are given over to an educational programme run by a highly experienced and well-qualified head teacher. The programme allows for a balance between formal education and informal learning opportunities, and the facilities allow for this, with two classrooms, one designed to teach in a formal way and the other laid out in a completely informal manner. Added to this is a craft workshop, fully equipped to develop skills that not only fulfil personal leisure needs but enable the young person to develop those skills necessary for self-maintenance and even possible employment.

The residential setting is homely and full of opportunities, both to learn and to relax. Each person has their own room and there is adequate provision for mixed or solitary activities.

The resources include not only an educational library, but books of a kind to meet an individual's personal interests; the library also includes a music and video section, developed to extend the cultural awareness of a young person and not just to occupy periods of inactivity.

The setting is rich in opportunity, with places of historic interest, museums, coastal resorts, nature walks and rivers, and these are included in the care programme.

Activities include canoeing and orienteering, supported by experienced staff qualified not only in care, but also in particular leisure areas too.

Unlike in many independent settings, where only managers and their deputies tend to hold nationally recognized qualifications, almost all of the core staff hold appropriate qualifications and the few that do not, utilize the local college to acquire them. The reason for this is that in order to meet the complex demands of individuals with special needs and problematic behaviour, it is felt that willingness and a healthy attitude are insufficient, and perpetuate the 'dependency factor'. The main aim of the staff is to facilitate independence through utilizing every opportunity and being able to

Case study 13.1 *(cont'd)*

transfer learning in order to acquire new and more complex skills.

Each day is rich in experience, and as the site is supported by farm animals and agricultural activities there is always something that needs to be done. The young people are encouraged to take on personal responsibility for some aspect of site care, and thus a greater sense of belonging develops.

Living and working together in itself has results:

Informality and involvement of living together almost always ensures that barriers are broken down and façades lifted. For better or worse, most individuals will come out of their shell and find the strength to be themselves (Lewis & Bedford 1996).

The argument that rural settings become segregated may be unfounded, as many non-disabled people elect to move away from urban life to adopt a more tranquil and therapeutic existence in an aesthetically pleasing setting; and some rural settings today are able to access urban facilities through adequate transport provision.

Sadly, it seems that those with learning disabilities often find themselves in the heart of a town, which inhibits their personal freedom and maintains the need for observation and support in accessing their chosen facilities for leisure and recreation.

Rural settings pose less risks than built-up environments, and hence increase the individual's personal mobility and independent action. 'Life in the fast lane', where speed of thought and action are considered essential in coping with community expectations, has obvious detrimental effects on people with learning disabilities. The reduced pressure of life in a rural setting creates less stress, increases the enjoyment of activities and allows for 'slowness' in a far more acceptable way. As life in the country is generally recognized as being slower, the person with a learning disability is far more likely to be accepted, as expectations differ. The 'handicaps' found so frequently within urban environments, often apply to everyone in rural settings, and this allows for individuals to adopt a valued social role. The result is 'the emergence of people with the confidence to stand up and be counted without feeling ashamed of their handicap' (Gates & Lewis 1987).

resources and finances available, which in many cases are insufficient to be able to fully enjoy recreational facilities in the community.

Leisure activities need to be perceived as essential to the care programme, for they are likely to be the learning medium enjoyed most by the clients, and as a consequence the area where success is most likely. Sheridan (1989) provides

Case study 13.2

Residential home, Pinner, Middlesex
The integration of people with learning disabilities into normal everyday housing has been a policy for many years: however, the placing of people with additional problematic behaviours represents a major challenge for all concerned. This residential home in the centre of a middle-class urban development has achieved a measure of success in providing a home for four young men with severe learning disabilities, and reflects the need for further development with this particular client group. Their previous home was a large purpose-built ward in a long-stay hospital, shared with a great number of people.

Life in a hospital is often referred to as 'poverty of experience', but this statement does not truly reflect the activities experienced, the care provided and the expertise available. More often it is used as an excuse to compensate for clients' lack of progress in their present settings, e.g. a community home which, as previously mentioned, can often be just as inhibiting. However, there is no disputing that the lifestyles of people in hospital are considerably different from those living in ordinary houses.

Several features of their previous lifestyle have had an adverse effect upon the functioning of this client group:

● The opportunities now offered are different from those previously available, and the clients' lack of understanding and reluctance to change often results in a negative response to newly introduced activities.
● The negative imagery associated with being hospitalized is reflected in the response of the local community to their presence. The semi-coldness experienced causes discomfort to both staff and clients, and hinders true integration.
● Behaviours developed as a result of previous poor staffing ratios mean that staff must develop strategies to prevent self-injury or damage. A one-to-one ratio is often necessary.

However, the staff have introduced a wide range of leisure activities that are carried out either regularly or whenever the opportunity arises.

The house is managed by a qualified practitioner but unfortunately, as with many homes in the private sector, the majority of support staff, including the deputy manager, lack appropriate qualifications. This is likely to result in activities being carried out for the activities' sakes alone, and reflects the caretaker approach rather than the facilitation that is necessary for activities to have a therapeutic value.

In order to provide the necessary one-to-one ratio for this client group there needs to be large number of staff, which presents a further problem in that staff turnover is high, and quite often activities are curtailed either by a lack of staff, or by the staff being new and inexperienced.

The client group's day care is met by a vocational

Case study 13.2 (cont'd)

service established several miles away in Edgware, which is also highly staffed. Here a number of activities are provided which can more appropriately be described as recreational rather than vocational. They include swimming, hiking, gardening, woodwork, art and crafts, walks and DIY. Specialists are brought in to provide relaxation and massage.

The residential unit provides similar activities, some of which are segregated owing to the nature of the activity, such as sailing and water sports. Within the house there are opportunities for crafts and cooking, but these seem to depend on the client's mood, rather than being integrated into a care programme.

The staff use the local community to provide experience of public houses and shops, but this too is dependent upon staffing levels.

Video nights are provided, and it is encouraging to note that videos are carefully selected so as to be of value rather than being randomly chosen.

The client group's behaviour is the single factor that determines whether these activities are undertaken, and this often prevents them experiencing these varied activities.

One must also consider the true value of some of the activities. The manager recognizes that a few seem to be undertaken in order to create a good impression, rather than because of their therapeutic value. They are more likely to impress care purchasers than to provide beneficial everyday learning opportunities.

Activity 13.3

Try to imagine yourself living in a hospital ward for people with learning disabilities.

● Describe your social life, friendships, activities and community interactions.
● Draw up a list of possible leisure activities available to you and highlight their benefits and pitfalls in terms of accessing them.

an insight when he states: 'You have to look not at people's disabilities but at their abilities and see their potential' (cited in Gaze 1989).

It must be recognized that for an environment to meet all of a person's needs, being near to facilities is not enough: activities need to be included and integrated into the philosophy of care, and play a substantial part in clients' daily lives.

Case study 13.3

Hospital setting, Hertfordshire
The hospital presents a daunting sight. Its immense size, ageing brickwork and apparently barred windows conjure up images of Bedlam and other such old asylums. Yet inside great efforts have been made to provide as normal a home setting as possible. Decorations and furniture are individual and modern, and very often well coordinated even if they are not always the clients' actual choice.

Sheer numbers tend to prevent a true feeling of homeliness, and despite the efforts of nursing staff it is very hard to lose the 'clinical' atmosphere that affects the place.

The individual, whether client or staff, tends to get lost in any large organizational set-up, and this is the case with leisure and recreation in the hospital environment. Often a service has to be provided which adequately meets the needs of all the clients, and hence 'departments' are established and 'centres' evolve, which become places to congregate when not attending day care services. These recreational centres tend to be minimally staffed and rarely get support from the residential environments, resulting in a situation where clients receive little input as to their leisure and recreational needs.

The emphasis on leisure has increased in recent years and, with improved environments and staff ratios, opportunities have evolved along similar lines to residential homes within the community.

The particular unit selected as an example caters for six residents who have been in hospital for many years and whose backgrounds warranted long-term hospitalization. They live in a converted staff residence that has been decorated and resourced like an ordinary home, and their daily life is similar to that of an ordinary family. Two staff are on duty each shift, one a qualified nurse (RNMH) and one an unqualified care assistant. As with most places, a list of facilities can be supplied which includes visits to the pub, cinema, leisure centre and shopping, the frequency of their use depending on finance, transport and the mood of the clients.

No-one is forced to participate, but the effect of many years receiving care has diminished the residents' capacity not only to initiate activities but even to participate in them, and they more often prefer aimless television watching, which can often take up entire evenings. One noticeable inhibiting factor is the lack of positive social interaction between the clients themselves, often the only interaction being an argument or disagreement.

The staff work hard to motivate the clients in all aspects of their daily life, but are having to combat the effects of a system that exerted considerable control in years gone by.

The qualified staff demonstrate considerable skill as a result of their intensive training, which has equipped them well to meet the needs of people with learning disabilities, and they receive considerable support

 Case study 13.3 (cont'd)

from the organization which manages them. Unfortunately, being part of a larger organization often necessitates compliance with inhibitory bureaucratic policies, and this certainly applies to any activities where a degree of cost is involved. Money has to be ordered in advance, and support, permission and staff cover planned beforehand, which affects spontaneity. The weather, often unpredictable, can disrupt activities planned in advance, and the clients have often changed their minds by the time the actual day of the activity arrives. This is frustrating for both staff and clients, and will only change when the responsibility for money lies with the clients and the unit, rather than being centralized within the organization.

As the hospital is sited in Hertfordshire, in the heart of suburbia, access to services and facilities is relatively easy, yet there is still a feeling of isolation. Although they are in the community, the hospital's origins appear to prevent integration, the local community seeming still to perceive it as an asylum built to segregate. Volunteers are hard to find, and there is a paucity of evening entertainment, resulting in special evening clubs being arranged and staffed by nurses, which tends to conflict with the informality needed to pursue leisure activities. The clients may well feel constantly observed.

As the hospital population decreases as a result of the NHS and Community Care Act (1990) those left suffer from inadequate provision outside their residential settings, leisure tending to be one of the first money-saving cutbacks, and the staff find themselves stretched in order to meet leisure needs when staff levels are at a minimum already.

SPECIALIST PROVISION

Many arguments persist as to the value of specialist services in fulfilling the leisure needs of people with learning disabilities, in particular that of segregation and its effect on the image of learning disability. However, one must remember the origins of these organizations in order to fully appreciate their past contributions, and to consider how they can play a positive role today.

The lack of leisure provision and the isolated existence of people with learning disabilities resulted in a severe deficiency of personal activity from the individual. Unable to either choose or initiate preferences, and shunned by mainstream society, the person with a learning disability fell into a state of apathy that not only perpetuated their dependency but also created an opportunity for others to exert control.

Organized primarily by parents, voluntary provision developed, designed to provide their offspring with the same kinds of opportunities available to normal children. The parents created an 'advocate' system, which they controlled and through which they exerted influence as collective organizations. Because they were able to access media outlets, they were able to implement change and influence policy-making and legislation.

Over the years these have developed from being voluntary groups in isolation, to solid organizations providing independently run homes and related services. Unfortunately, the tendency has been to maintain control, and despite the obvious vested interest in the person with a learning disability, this has not always been in that individual's best interest.

Many private organizations exist to provide a range of services, yet many seem to perpetuate the dependency culture and few, if any, are truly independent of non-disabled people in terms of control.

As long as clubs are still run specifically for people with learning disabilities, then segregation will occur, and from this evolves negative imagery and attitudes. In the past these clubs had 'negative' names, such as 'Peter Pan' club, and the activities offered and behaviours exhibited reflected this image. Even today it is not unusual to see an evening club totally controlled by non-disabled people, often parents and young volunteers, all nobly supplying their own time but still *providing* for their disabled clientèle.

Even with the emergence of self-advocacy for disabled people, one can find a number of non-disabled facilitators, usually professional people skillful in their handling of the group.

'Letting go'

One of the most difficult aspects for carers, either voluntary or paid, is the notion of the person with a learning disability being able to manage on their own. It is possible to find a hundred reasons why the ultimate power cannot lie with that person, and yet impossible to provide even one to justify their being in control.

With this in mind one must return to an earlier point, that of success and failure both being acceptable 'outcomes'. If an athlete trains for 4 years in order to compete in the Olympic Games, and fails to win a gold medal, should this be regarded as a waste of time and investment? It is the effort and the attempt that is laudable, and this should be accepted for people with learning disabilities and their activities. One is constantly reminded of the quote from Ray Loomis from Nebraska, in the USA, who despite his learning disability set about developing 'People First' and establishing his personhood: 'If you think you are handicapped you might as well stay indoors. If you think you're a person come out and tell the world' (Williams & Shoultz 1982).

A new direction

It would be wrong to persistently denigrate organizations specifically designed to meet the needs of people with learning disabilities, for within these many meaningful relationships exist and many people of all ages give up their time for others. They exist because of the failure of our society to provide integrated services which accept and value disabled people; yet in their continued existence they inhibit appropriate developments and changes from occurring. It is essential that the person with a learning disability gets the opportunity to achieve, participate, represent, enjoy and share through the activities on offer within specialist provision, if nothing else exists. Meyers (1979) states that the person with a learning disability will continue to be thought of as incapable when they are not offered real-life experience and when the expectations of their abilities are kept so low. He goes on to offer the notion of a 'citizen advocate', a person who will 'guide' or 'help', as would any good friend or neighbour, and yet today even this concept has undergone 'professional' development 'to such an extent that the "advocate" almost represents an extension of the professional discourse which maintains control over the field of learning disability.'

Whitehead (1992) identified an advocacy model as replacing a treatment model, and said, 'There has been a real shift in the balance of power as a direct result of normalisation' (cited in Brown & Smith 1992).

Society must begin to focus on the ability of the learning-disabled person and accept their fallibility as individuals. Fallibility is not only permissible but expected; it is part of being human.

No longer should carers have to ask in advance whether their clients can attend a leisure facility or visit a restaurant. They have a right to attend, a need to attend, and the public should be allowed and expected to assist them.

Individualism not standardization

The desire for learning, for culture and for knowledge of a person with a learning disability should not be underestimated. Our leisure interests and recreational activities are shaped by our families, friends and environment, and what emerges is a unique combination, on occasions quite diverse and unrelated, yet still personal and pleasurable.

The aim should be to encourage this combination in the person with a learning disability and to establish a network of leisure and recreational activities, at the same time recognizing their contribution to every other aspect of life. It is not sufficient merely to accept the standardization offered with the application of normalization principles, for this implies the acceptance of values belonging to the dominant majority, rather than, as Whitehead (1992) considers, people being able to live their lives in different ways as individuals.

Dalley (1992) makes reference to a quotation by Lukes (1973):

Individualism offers a private existence within a public world, an area within which the individual is or should be left alone by others and able to do and think whatever he/she chooses. (Cited in Brown & Smith 1992).

Individuals with no hobbies/leisure interests (or no way of following their interests without help) can become isolated, and more restricted in their social contact (Peck & Hong 1988).

An example of specialism: Special Olympics

Many organizations exist to provide specialized leisure facilities for people with learning disabilities, each with their own way of functioning and operating but most quite similar in their overall set-up. In selecting one to discuss there is no suggestion that it is any better or worse than the others, but it would require several books to discuss them fully, and information is readily supplied by each of them. A number of addresses are given at the end of this chapter that will enable the reader to find out more about any specific organization.

The Special Olympic organization was first established in the United Kingdom in 1968, and is affiliated to Special Olympics International Incorporated, which is a worldwide programme of sports training and athletic competition open to individuals with learning disabilities regardless of their abilities. Its mission is to provide year-round competition in a variety of Olympic-type sports for people with learning disabilities over the age of 8, providing opportunities for physical fitness, experiencing joy, the demonstration of courage and sharing of gifts, skills and friendship with their peers, families and the community.

The organization has a sound philosophy and has achieved public recognition and solid media coverage in recent years, culminating in one person with a learning disability recently receiving an MBE for contributions to sport. In the United Kingdom it is divided into a number of regions, each of which has a committee and a paid membership, and is accountable to a central office in London.

The committee is made up of volunteer representatives from each group belonging to the region. They are, however, generally non-disabled people, and despite their good intentions, this tends to reflect the high degree of control the non-disabled exert over the sports people themselves.

National games are organized every 2 years, and these are enjoyed immensely by the participants, who for a change are the centre of attention when performing and receiving their awards.

Categories exist to give everyone an equal opportunity and, although this differs from the actual Olympics, where for each event there will be only one gold medal awarded, it does reflect the way sport is organized throughout the country at different levels. This may mean, for example, four gold medal winners for the 100 metres, each winning gold within a different banding, but it does not detract from the courage and effort demonstrated by all the participants.

The argument that it segregates is a fair one, but for those who have experienced the actual event it does not seem important, for many heroic moments occur which overshadow such issues. Once again, it seems to be the professionals who dispute its value, and too little is heard from the actual people who take part. The media interviews with the clients themselves reflect joy and satisfaction and certainly no desire to exclude themselves.

Medals are given out freely for the many events organized throughout the year, but these are significant to a group of people who may have achieved very little throughout their lives; for some, they may represent their only achievements.

Sport is a universally recognized medium for development, essential in every school's curriculum and very much part of everyday life. For people with a learning disability it is particularly beneficial, in that employment is often unlikely and the emphasis is very much upon their developing through their recreational activities. 'Sport is the medium through which we help people with mental handicap to improve their health, enjoy their leisure, develop their skills, achieve success and express themselves more fully' (Lewis 1996).

Without doubt individuals grow in stature, their self-esteem greatly enriched (Lewis 1996), and if this results in an individual enjoying his life and developing a greater sense of self-awareness, then the benefits outweigh the deficits. However, as suggested earlier, those helping and those organizing could help even more by including people with learning disabilities in other ways, particularly on committees and in organizing other aspects.

One must also recognize that a number of the participants achieve high standards and fast times in their events, and could participate in ordinary athletic groups and other sporting groups with non-disabled people, thus demonstrating an ability to participate at a higher level. This should be actively supported and encouraged, relinquishing a degree of control and allowing these people to integrate as individuals.

CONCLUSION

The person with a learning disability has a right and a need to enjoy leisure and recreation in the same way as others do, free to exercise choice and create their own combination of interests, hobbies and activities. This is highly personal and could be in conflict with the aims and targets of the organizations within which they live and work, yet is essential in establishing their own uniqueness and personal identity.

Care providers need to see the value of leisure and recreational activities in relation to other aspects of learning, and would do well to see that they too have a need to develop specialist skills that will positively support the facilitation of such activities.

Underestimation of ability and fear of risk have culminated in unimaginative leisure programmes often being applied to the entire client group, which are too often repetitive and not needs based.

Greater emphasis on this particular learning medium is required within both assessment formats and care plans, with recognition of its value and pleasure for the individual concerned. It is perhaps one of the few areas where mixing with others, being in a teamwork situation and 'push-

Activity 13.4

Discuss with a person with a learning disability who is known to you their feelings about specialist clubs and organizations, e.g. Special Olympics, Gateway Clubs. Judge the value of these organizations in relation to quality of life for people with learning disabilities.

ing oneself to the limits' actually occurs, for most other skills tend to be learnt and developed independent of others, and if the aim is to develop a socially minded, integrated individual then this is the area that would be of most benefit.

It is strange that some organizations spend money freely on accessing employment services for their clients, yet appear reluctant to use those funds to purchase meaningful leisure activities. This reflects an ignorance of the value of leisure as a medium for learning, and suggests that service providers should review their total care provision in meeting an individual's needs.

REFERENCES

Atkinson D, Williams F (eds) 1990 Know me as I am. Hodder and Stoughton, London

Bender M, Brannan S, Verhoven P 1984 Leisure education for the handicapped. College Hill Press, San Diego, California

Brandon D, Brandon A 1988 Putting people first: good impressions. Hexagon Publishing, Surbiton

Brown H, Smith H (eds) 1992 Normalisation – a reader for the nineties. Routledge, London

Cotton M 1983 Outdoor adventure for handicapped people. Human Horizon Series, Souvenir Press, London

Gates R, Lewis D 1987 Learning to speak. Senior Nurse 2: 21–22

Gaze H 1989 Glory days. Nursing Times 85 (39): 21

Kanner L 1967 A history of the care and study of the mentally retarded. Charles C Thomas, Springfield, Illinois

Lewis D, 1990 A sporting life. Nursing Times 86(45): 33–35

Lewis D, Bedford R 1996 A retreat – the benefits to nurse education. Professional Nurse 11 (5): 293–294

Meyers R 1979 Like normal people. Human Horizon Series, Souvenir Press, London

Parrish A (ed) 1987 Mental handicap. Essentials of Nursing Series, McMillan, Basingstoke

Peck C, Hong C S 1988 Living skills for mentally handicapped people. Croom Helm, Beckenham

Williams P, Shoultz B 1982 We can speak for ourselves. Human Horizon Series, Routledge, London

---

USEFUL ADDRESSES

Many addresses represent the secretaries of organizations: these may change, so the address may need to be checked.

Arts Council
105 Piccadilly,
London W1V OAU

Arts for Disabled People In Wales
Channel View Leisure Centre,
Jim Driscoll Way,
The Marl,
Grangetown,
Cardiff CF1 7NF

British Canoe Union
Flexel House,
45–47 High Street,
Addlestone,
Weybridge,
Surrey KT15 1JV

British Mountaineering Council
Cranford House,
Booth Street East,
Manchester M13 9RZ

British Orienteering Federation
Lea Green,
Nr Matlock,
Derbyshire DE4 5GJ

British Sports Association for the Disabled
Wayward House,
1 Barnard Crescent,
Aylesbury,
Bucks HP21 9PP

Camping Club of Great Britain & Ireland
11 Lower Grosvenor Place,
London SW1W OEY

Central Council for the Disabled
34 Eccleston Square,
London SW1V 1PE

CP–ISRA (Cerebral Palsy International Sports and Recreation Association)
Secretary General, Dr A.A. Van Schawren,
c/o Heijenoordseweg 5, 6813 GG,
Arnhem,
The Netherlands

Disabled Living Foundation
380–384 Harrow Road,
London W9 2HU

Duke of Edinburgh Award Scheme
5 Prince of Wales Terrace,
London W8 5PG

HAPA (Handicapped Adventure Playground Association)
HAPA Office,
Fulham Palace,
Bishop's Avenue,
London SW6 6EA

MENCAP (Royal Society for Mentally Handicapped
Children and Adults)
MENCAP Centre,
123 Golden Lane,
London EC1Y ORJ

National Anglers Council,
Committee for Disabled Anglers
Cowgate,
Peterborough

National Association of Disabled Writers
18 Spring Grove,
Harrogate,
North Yorkshire HG1 2HS

National Association of Swimming Clubs for the
Handicapped
63 Dunvegan Road,
Eltham,
London SE9

National Caving Association
Sec: Mr Judson,
Bethnal Green,
Calderbrook Road,
Littleborough,
Lancashire

National Federation of Gateway Clubs
117–123 Golden Lane,
London EC1Y ORT

National Ski Federation of Great Britain
118 Eaton Square,
London SW1 W9AF

National Trust
42 Queen Annes Gate,
London SW1

Northern Ireland Information Service for the Disabled
2 Annadale Avenue,
Belfast BT7 3JH
Northern Ireland

Outward Bound Trust
Avon House,
360 Oxford Street,
London W1

PHAB (Physically Handicapped & Abled Bodied)
Tavistock House North,
Tavistock Square,
London WC1 H9HX

Ramblers Association
Crawford Mews,
York Street,
London W1H 1PT

Riding for the Disabled Association
Avenue R,
National Agricultural Centre,
Stoneleigh,
Kenilworth,
Warwickshire CV8 2LY

Royal Association for Disability and Rehabilitation
25 Mortimer Street,
London W1N 8AB

Scottish Sports Association for the Disabled
The Administrator,
Fife Sports Institute,
Viewfield Road,
Glenrothes,
Fife KY6 2RA

Scottish Sports Council
1 St Colm Street,
Edinburgh EH3 6AA
Scotland

Special Olympics UK Head Office,
Wellingboro Place,
London

Sports Council
16 Upper Woburn Place,
London WC1H OQP

Trust Fund for the Training of Handicapped Children in Arts
& Crafts
94 Claremont Road,
Wallasey,
Merseyside 44S 6UE

United Kingdom Sports Association for People with Mental
Handicap
First Floor,
Unit 9,
Longlands Industrial Estate,
Milner Way,
Osset WFS 9JN

Wales Council for the Disabled
Crescent Road,
Caerphilly,
Mid Glamorgan CF8 1XL

Wales Sports Association for the Disabled
c/o Sports Council for Wales,
National Sports Centre for Wales,
Sophia Gardens,
Cardiff CF1 9SW

Wales Tourist Board
Welcome House,
Llandaff,
Cardiff

Water Sports Division,
British Sports Association for the Disabled
29 Ironlatch Avenue,
St Leonards-on-Sea,
East Sussex TN38 9JB

14

Representation

S.J. McNally

CHAPTER CONTENTS

INTRODUCTION

The principle of representation is fundamental in society. It is connected closely with the concept of citizenship, which centres on the relationship between the individual and the state. Marshall (1950) referred to citizenship as a status bestowed on those who are full members of a community. He described three elements of citizenship: civil, political and social. The civil element comprises the rights which are necessary for individual freedom. These include personal liberty, freedom of speech, thought and faith, and the right to own property and to conclude valid contracts. The right to justice – a significant civil right – is the legal right to defend all of one's rights on an equal basis by means of the legal process. The political element concerns participation in the exercise of political power at local or national level. Participation may be either as an elector or as a member of an elected body (local government, Parliament) which is invested with political authority.

Marshall's social element refers to the whole range from the right to a modicum of economic welfare and security to the right to a full share in the social heritage, and to live the life of a civilized being according to the standards prevailing in the society. Citizens require access to social resources, including health, education and social services, in order to further their own and other people's civil and political rights (Gould, 1988).

We assert our interests and express our views. Adults usually represent themselves by making various choices and decisions which affect their lives. We are aware that we have certain rights as citizens, and exercise these rights seeking to change things if we are dissatisfied. There may be occasions when we need to consult a specialist representative, such as a lawyer, but we tend to speak for ourselves. We uphold our interests and we express our ideas and feelings.

Recent community care legislation (NHS and Community Care Act, 1990) has emphasized the importance of representation for service users. A central policy aim of *Caring for People* (Department of Health, 1989) was to give people more say in the services they use. Local authorities which provide social services are required to consult with users and user organizations (Monach & Spriggs 1994). The voice of the consumer is crucial. This recognition is particularly significant for members of vulnerable groups.

WHY IS REPRESENTATION IMPORTANT?

Freedom of self-determination is considered to be the most fundamental and valuable human right (Gadow, 1979). Historically, people with a learning disability have not had much control over their lives (Wolfensberger, 1972). The stigma attached to 'mental retardation' has been powerful: the label denotes a complete lack of basic competence (Edgerton 1967).

Choices which have affected such people's lives in a very direct way have been in the hands of others, often family members or service workers, so that representation can be seen as a vital tool for members of devalued, disadvantaged groups. It could be argued that effective representation is more important for a person with a learning disability than for a non-disabled person, because the former is so far behind in terms of experience of speaking up and making choices, and awareness of their rights. Representation through membership of a self-advocacy group may bring benefits for the person at an individual level, e.g. developing confidence, improved listening and speaking skills, greater knowledge of rights. It could also have an impact on the ser-

vices they receive, so that increasing awareness and assertiveness might lead to paid employment or better housing.

Participation is an important component of representation. Individuals have a right to be involved in decisions which affect their lives. If they are not, there is a danger that the service may meet the needs of staff rather than users (Gathercole, 1988). A fundamental principle here is that people with a learning disability should be involved in the planning, operation and evaluation of services which affect them.

Collective action involving user organizations such as Mencap can be a valuable form of representation. The recent government Disability Discrimination Act (1996) was an attempt to establish some basic rights for disabled people, such as employment, access to public places, access to goods and services. It was a move forward but fell short of the stronger measures envisaged in the unsuccessful Civil Rights (Disabled Persons) Bill of 1994, which had the support of organizations representing the interests of people with disabilities (McNally, 1995b). Disappointment with the new legislation has been expressed by groups concerned with disability in two key areas: the Act's likely influence on discrimination in the spheres of education, training, housing and employment; and the failure to set up a Disabilities Commission, as opposed to an advisory council (George, 1996).

DEFINITIONS

- **Empowerment** Makes it possible for disadvantaged people to exercise power and have more control in their lives.
- **Self-advocacy** Enables people to speak for themselves and to make their views known at an individual or group level.
- **Citizen advocacy** Establishes independent partnerships between people with disabilities and non-disabled people. Advocates are volunteers who assist their partners by representing their interests in numerous practical ways (West Midlands Learning Disability Forum, 1994).

REPRESENTATION AND EMPOWERMENT

The concepts of empowerment and autonomy are closely linked. Empowerment has several dimensions, and there are questions concerning the extent to which it is about professionals sharing power with users. It has been suggested (Simons, 1995) that empowerment is concerned with users actively taking control.

Gibson (1991) defines empowerment as:

a social process of recognizing, promoting and enhancing people's abilities to meet their own problems and mobilise the necessary resources in order to feel in control of their own life.

The concept of empowerment for service users and carers can be characterized as both a process and a goal. It is concerned with people having greater power to express their needs and to decide how these should be met (Parsloe & Stevenson 1992). In its absence empowerment is easy to define (Rappaport, 1984): powerlessness, real or imagined; learned helplessness; alienation; loss of a sense of control over one's life. Individuals may never have achieved power in their lives.

Government policies in recent years have acknowledged that user representation and empowerment are crucial in the provision of community care (NHS and Community Care Act, 1990). The voice of the consumer is now regarded as important (Jowell, 1991). The process of representation for someone with a learning disability may happen through the medium of self-advocacy or through citizen advocacy. Both of these approaches have considerable potential to empower the service user. The thrust of advocacy is in securing a greater degree of autonomy for a person, which may mean making choices and decisions and expressing freedom. An important proviso here is that the relevant information and support are available to the person, according to the context.

Autonomy is an important issue for professionals: service workers who feel empowered will be in a stronger position to enable their clients to become empowered.

TYPES OF REPRESENTATION

There are four types of representation: by self, by an unpaid person (such as a friend, relative or citizen advocate), by a paid person (perhaps a community nurse or social worker) or by an organization (People First or Mencap, for example). It is important to be aware of the difference between representation of an individual's interests, and collective action by an organization, which is less pure and direct. The difference could be characterized as that between advocacy and user representation.

Advocacy

This can be defined as the process of speaking out or acting on behalf of another person who is unable to do so for himself. Upholding the rights and best interests of an individual is a crucial element of the advocate's role. Action should result from this representation (McNally, 1995a). It is important that advocates have a genuine commitment to represent the person's interests as though they were their own (Tyne, 1991). Advocacy is a process whereby service users, individually or in groups, make service providers aware of their views and interests (Monach & Spriggs 1994).

Self-advocacy

Self-advocacy is practised by many of us as individuals, but groups can provide a good setting for developing self-advocacy skills, particularly for people who are at risk of being devalued in society. Definitions of self-advocacy often include 'speaking up for yourself', but that is only part of the picture. Making decisions, taking action and *changing* things are significant components which a number of self-advocacy groups have identified. Self-advocacy has great potential to enhance the lives of people with a learning disability in that they become more aware of their rights, expressing needs and concerns and asserting interests.

The following self-advocacy skills have been identified (Clare 1990):

- Being able to express thoughts and feelings with assertiveness if necessary
- Being able to make choices and decisions
- Having a clear knowledge of rights
- Being able to make changes.

Other important components include **being independent**: doing things for yourself as much as you can without other people always doing things for you; a person can be independent and have support when they need it. **Taking responsibility for yourself** means looking after yourself; using your common sense; not always waiting for other people to get things done for you, because that is not having your own responsibilities. 'Get things going yourself' is the advice of People First. **Concern for other people** is also part of self-advocacy.

The Self Advocacy in Action Group (1994), a group of 16 people with learning difficulties and their advisers, have made the point that self-advocacy affects 'the whole of your life the whole of the time'.

Crawley (1988) sees self-advocacy as:

the act of making choices and decisions and bringing about desired change for oneself . . . Any activity that involves self-determination can be called self-advocacy.

This last point is crucial. Some people have tended to perceive self-advocacy as something which is only relevant for the 'more able', verbally skilled individuals who have a learning disability. The erroneous thinking which underlies this assumption can be seen clearly in the light of Crawley's definition above. People with a severe learning disability can be and are involved in self-advocacy. How many people do not communicate at all, or do not have the capacity to indicate a choice? I contend that the answer here is 'very few', if any. 'Everyone can take part in self-advocacy at some level regardless of the severity of their disabilities' (Crawley 1988).

The challenge which faces us as professionals is to find out how individuals communicate, and to open up the pathways – perhaps with augmented communication systems or intensive one-to-one work – which enable them to express their needs and wants.

Types of advocacy are not mutually exclusive. A person with a severe learning disability may be involved in a partnership with a citizen advocate, who helps him to uphold his rights and represent his views. However, the same person may also be developing his self-advocacy skills at an individual level by making choices and decisions. He might be a member of a self-advocacy group, in which his participation is supported by a service worker or citizen advocate.

Citizen advocacy

Citizen advocacy is the supportive partnership which results when a volunteer develops a relationship with a person who is vulnerable to being disadvantaged through illness, age or disability. It is important that the advocate is a 'valued person', i.e. not disadvantaged themselves. Advocates form a close personal relationship with their partners, helping them to make choices and decisions. The advocate works independently of services to uphold the rights of their partner as a citizen. A citizen advocate

… chooses one or several of many ways to understand, respond to, and represent that person's interests as if they were the advocate's own thus bringing their partner's gifts and concerns into the circles of ordinary life (O'Brien 1981).

More explicitly:

Citizen advocacy refers to the persuasive and supportive activities of trained, selected volunteers and co-ordinating staff working on behalf of those who are disabled / disadvantaged and not in a good position to exercise or defend their rights as citizens.
Citizen advocates are persons who are independent of those providing direct services to people with disabilities. Working on a one to one basis, they attempt to foster respect for the rights and dignity of those they represent. This may involve helping to express the individual's concerns and aspirations, obtaining day to day social, recreational, health and related services, and providing other practical and emotional support (Gathercole 1986, cited in Butler 1988).

The benefits of partnership with a citizen advocate fall into two broad categories according to the nature of the needs met: expressive (human

Table 14.1 Possible gains from citizen advocacy (Adapted from Sang 1984)

Expressive	Instrumental
Affection	Access to financial benefits
Attention	Access to services
Companionship	Accommodation
Communication	Leisure and recreation
Friendship	Transport
Identity	Training and education
Love	Citizenship rights, e.g. voting
Developing social	Access to facilities, e.g.
networks	shops, pubs
Warmth	

emotional and social needs) and instrumental (material needs), as shown in Table 14.1.

Collective advocacy

This approach is about user representation. There is an important difference between advocacy and user representation: a self-advocate represents his own interests; a citizen advocate upholds the rights of their partner. User organizations cannot represent each individual's views but they can promote the cause of minority groups, including people with a learning disability, by raising public awareness and lobbying policy makers on their behalf. Key organizations which help to further the cause of people with a learning disability include Mencap, People First, BILD (British Institute of Learning Disabilities), Values into Action (formerly Campaign for Mental Handicap) and Scope (formerly the Spastics Society).

ADVOCACY AND NURSING

Learning disability nursing is concerned with the empowerment of service users. A recent Department of Health project on learning disability nursing concluded that: 'nurses should place stronger emphasis on the support of initiatives that enable people with a learning disability to advocate for themselves', and that the DOH should 'continue to support initiatives which develop better information for managers and professional staff on advocacy and self-advocacy' (Department of Health 1995).

Nurses have great potential to identify and help meet the developing advocacy needs of their clients. Empowering clients through self-advocacy is the essence of effective nursing. This is supported by the Royal College of Nursing's (1995) paper which, in discussing nursing generally, asserts that a 'prime function of nursing is to empower the client to have more control over their life, the ideal being self advocacy'. According to Gadow (1980), 'the nurse is in the ideal position among health care providers to experience the patient as a unique human being with individual strengths and complexities – a precondition for advocacy'. Some writers are more circumspect about nurses as advocates but acknowledge that in certain circumstances it is desirable that they should take on this role (Gates 1995).

HELPING WITH INDIVIDUAL REPRESENTATION

To be in a position to help an individual to represent their rights and interests, one must first build a relationship with that person. This will involve getting to know and value the person, and to understand their style of communication. Rogers (1967), considering education, believed that the interpersonal relationship between facilitator and learner is the most significant factor governing the learner's experience.

It is crucial to give the person time to say what they want to say and to be aware of one's own communication, keeping vocabulary and pace of delivery at a level which the person can follow. Individuality is the key here: knowing the person, their use of language and their range of interests is paramount. The importance of *knowing* the person cannot be overemphasized. Goode (1984) has noted the dangers of clinical perspectives which highlight what the service user cannot do, and can give rise to a fault-finding approach. The 'etic' perspective is a definition constructed by outsiders (i.e. how professionals believe that the person experiences the world). Goode discusses the desirability of understanding the person's own actual experience of reality: this is the 'emic' perspective. Practitioners need to be aware of the relationship between identity, behaviour and social context. Someone with a severe learning disability, whose spoken and received vocabulary is limited in a formal assessment setting such as a clinic, may communicate effectively at home. He or she may feel more confident and be aware that others – family members or house mates – are better able to understand him. The crucial aspect is that of time spent with the individual.

It is well documented that people who have close, sustained contact with people with severe disabilities tend to have positive, accepting views of them. Four dimensions of the non-disabled person's perspective have been reported (Bogdan & Taylor 1989):

- Attributing thinking to the other
- Seeing individuality in the other
- Viewing the other as reciprocating
- Defining a social place for the other.

Carers of people with severe intellectual impairment and multiple disabilities maintain a valuing, human perception of the other.

A useful approach is to keep conversation relatively simple and as clear and jargon-free as possible. Another important precondition is to find out what *they* want, as opposed to what you think they should want, although these things may correspond in terms of achieving change in their lives.

INDIVIDUAL CARE PLANNING

Individual plans of care such as life plans and shared action plans can provide an important focus for the needs and wishes of the service user. Shared action planning has its origins in normalization/social role valorization theory (Wolfensberger 1972, 1983) and the advocacy movement (Williams & Shoultz 1982). It also derives from the individual programme plan approach (Chamberlain 1985), from which it represents a development.

Typically there would be a 12-monthly cycle, involving several important stages, including the annual SAP meeting and a 6-monthly evaluation of progress. The person concerned should be in control of the process – after all, it is about their life – and, with support, be guiding it. This will involve who is present at the meetings, what the objectives are, and identifying who will help in achieving these (Brechin & Swain 1987).

Shared action plans aim to put the user at the centre of the plan; a key part of the process is the meeting between client and link worker prior to the SAP meeting. (A link worker has regular contact with the client and is chosen by the client.) This pre-review meeting, which may also involve the key worker (a professional who has regular contact with the client and coordinates the SAP process), has some important functions. Previous objectives are reviewed and needs are identified, as are specific assessments required. The discussion also considers who will be invited to the SAP meeting and who will chair it. The SAP meeting involves the client, *if they wish*, link workers, key worker, chair and invited others, including relatives, friends and advocate. The tasks of the annual meeting are to present the person's individual needs and choices; to review past goals; to identify priorities for a new life plan; and to identify actions and who will be responsible for carrying these out. After the meeting, client, link worker and key worker formalize the action plan, completing and circulating the relevant documents. Referrals may be made to other agencies and professionals; key people who are needed to complete the action plan are identified. The process is overseen by a coordinator, who should have a good understanding of the SAP process and knowledge of local services. Usually, the coordinator would act as line manager to the key worker and be in a position to ensure that each client has a key worker. The coordinator supports the development of the key worker. Highlighting deficits in services is an important aspect of the coordinator's role.

There is a clear connection between the centrality of the service user to the shared action planning process and the user's actual control of their life. A key principle here is the separation of the housing and support needs of the individual.

Historically, services for people with a learning disability have required users to fit in to the service structure in a geographical area. Residential provision has typically been a ward or villa within a hospital campus, a 20+-bedded hostel, a 'community unit' or, in recent years, a staffed group home. Organizational needs have tended to take precedence over the needs of the person. Clients have been placed into houses where a vacancy exists because of the economic imperative of the provider organization, and often without due consideration of the implications for the dynamics of the group. The difficulty here (and the past is riddled with examples of this) is that service users' needs have been assessed on a collective basis. (There is a parallel with the tendency to see people with learning disabilities as somehow having uniform needs dictated by their intellectual impairment, and submerging all other aspects of their identity.)

'Supported living' has developed in the United States as a means of providing individualized support, and is now gaining ground in this country. The National Development Team has defined supported living according to the following principles (Kinsella 1994):

- Separating housing and support
- Focusing on one person at a time
- Full user choice and control
- Rejecting no-one
- Focusing on relationships and making full use of informal support and community resources.

Supported living does not provide a formula for universal application, but represents a process based on the person's needs and wishes for housing – where they want to live, whether they wish to live with someone else, how they want to live – and support. Its cornerstone is that users themselves are the best judges of what they want. Listening to people and having a committed approach to helping them maintain and develop support networks is crucial.

Shared action planning and supported living are approaches which link directly to the phenomenon of care management which, in the context of the puchaser – provider split, has been a major innovation in the practice of community care during the 1990s.

Care management, which tends to target users with long-term, multiple or complex needs, also has an emphasis on tailoring services to the individual. Some clients with a learning disability are allocated a care manager. The contribution of care (or case) management has been defined as 'a dedicated person (or team) who organises, coordinates and sustains a network of formal and informal supports and activities designed to optimise the functioning and well-being of people with multiple needs' (Moxley 1989, cited by Challis in Malin 1994).

The process of care management involves the following stages (Davies & Challis 1986, Wintersgill 1991):

- Selection: identifying clients
- Assessment: finding out what service users need and want
- Planning: devising a plan in consultation with the client
- Implementation: putting the agreed plan into action
- Monitoring/review: checking that the services provided are as agreed and that the plan continues to be relevant to the client's needs. The plan may need to be reformulated or the case closed.

COMMUNICATION

The value of good communication cannot be overemphasized: service users need to be confident that staff members understand the points they are making. A key skill that supporters require is the capacity to build a trusting relationship with the client, which creates a context for clear communication. It is imperative that information is provided in a clear and concise way (it will possibly need to be repeated). It should also be free of bias, because the person may simply acquiesce with the perceived choice of the staff member.

It is also crucial to have an understanding of augmented means of communication which the person may use, e.g. Makaton or Rebus (Phoenix

NHS Trust 1993a). These methods are used along with speech, and so it is an important ground rule to always use speech as well as signs, and to encourage the client to speak. Some clients may use electronic switches and computer-generated artificial voices to help them communicate.

Pictorial methods of representing text are increasingly used by organizations concerned with people with learning disabilities. There has been a growing recognition in recent years of the need to make meetings and documents accessible to service users who do not read, or whose reading is limited (e.g. Dawson & Palmer 1991). User-oriented organizations such as People First and the King's Fund produce text supplemented with illustrations designed to convey its meaning.

Some NHS Trusts have produced effective illustrated documents which have been designed with clients in mind. Phoenix NHS Trust's *Are You Happy With the Help You Get?* is a good example (Phoenix Trust 1993b).

People tend to enjoy photographs, not just as records of particular phases of their lives and holidays, but because they also act as a catalyst to conversation. Photographs can be an immensely valuable aid to communication for people with a learning disability. They might be used to help a person to make a choice between alternative items or activities, or to prepare for an event. Photographs can also be used to devise a timetable for a client, who may not be able to read but can see a clear sequence of activities (e.g. shower, breakfast, horse-riding, lunch, shopping etc.).

Listening has been identified by a group of service users in Oxfordshire as vitally important in the lives of clients and staff. They have produced a set of guidelines for new staff, which state clearly the standards users have a right to expect (Barton Empowerment Group 1994). The following are some the principles of listening that the group highlighted:

- Look at the person who is talking to you.
- Stand still when somebody is talking to you. It is not clear that you are listening if you keep moving around.

- Give people time to get their point across, especially if they have difficulty talking.
- Do not walk away: it is very difficult to talk to someone who is always moving around.
- Think about what you are doing. Sometimes it may be acceptable to continue what you are doing while the person speaks.
- Think about what the person is saying to you. They will realize if you keep nodding and saying 'yes' in the wrong places. Give them feedback. Let them know if you have not understood them; ask them to repeat it in their own time.
- Space for talking and listening is important. The person needs to be in a place where they feel comfortable. This may be at home, perhaps in their bedroom if they choose, or in another venue away from the house, e.g. a cafe or pub.
- People who use wheelchairs sometimes feel left out and not listened to. Listen to the person in the wheelchair. Get down and talk to them at the same level. You have probably heard of the 'Does he take sugar?' phenomenon, whereby people tend to address the supporter. Nurses and other workers can use their skills to encourage communication between the wheelchair user and others, e.g. the shopkeeper or barman. Ordering or paying for an item presents a very good opportunity for contact for the wheelchair user.
- Talking to the right person. Part of listening is talking back and giving the correct information. If someone is asking a question to which you do not have the answer, you should put them in touch with someone who does know, or ask the question on their behalf.
- Telephones are an important means of listening and talking. Some people need support to make phone calls and to be listened to on the phone. People need to have the time to speak and listen, and access to a private place for this because calls may be personal. A staff member might help in getting a number and then leave the room, so that the person has the privacy and space they need.
- Going to house meetings. The group suggested that everyone should have the opportunity to go to a regular house meeting because things come up which people need to discuss. Group members hoped that everybody who lives

Activity 14.1

Choice
Think about the choices you make in a typical day. These may seem very ordinary things, such as what to wear, what to eat, who you see or telephone, whether you go out in the evening and what you do. At certain times you might make a major decision, such as where to live.

Now consider a person with a learning disability. How would the number and quality of their choices compare with yours?

and works in a house would talk and listen to each other.

• Responding. Listening is about what people are saying to you; it is also about acting on the information.

ASSESSING AND SUPPORTING CLIENT CHOICE

One of the chief ways in which nurses can support individual representation is by helping the person to develop their self-advocacy skills. With very few exceptions, people are capable of making choices and decisions at some level. They are able to express individuality and personal freedom by exercising the right to choose. This potential for autonomy can be developed by providing supported opportunities for choice making. There is an onus on organizations providing human services to achieve this 'accomplishment' among others (O'Brien 1987). Choice has been defined as 'The act of an individual's selection of a preferred alternative from among several familiar options' (Shevin & Klein 1984).

For choice making to be meaningful, a number of conditions must be met (Wilson 1992):

• An awareness that a choice is needed
• An awareness that a choice is being offered
• An understanding of the choice concept
• A self-picture
• A choice to be offered
• Information about the options
• The capacity and time to respond to the choice offered

• An understanding of the consequences of the choice.

It is important to bear in mind that a whole range of factors affect choice making. A person who has had little opportunity to make choices, because they have always been made by carers in the past, may take some time to get used to making decisions. The skills will need to be practised and developed. Some people are more assertive than others, and may relish the chance to have more say in their lives. Of course, some choices are more significant than others. The consequences of choosing a meal are less far-reaching than deciding on a place to live or work. It seems relevant here to say that choice making is not a skill which people suddenly acquire as adults. Our parents, teachers and so on support us in developing this from childhood. For children and young people with a learning disability, opportunities to make choices in a supportive environment are even more crucial, because they may be slower in grasping the implications of choice. Therefore choice making and self-advocacy should be a significant part of the school and college curriculum.

Environment is an important factor in choice making. A valid, genuine choice may be more likely to be made in the person's home environment. This is especially pertinent for those with a severe learning disability.

From a methodological perspective, the use of pictures to supplement verbal interaction in research situations is important. Simple faces, usually arranged in a three-point scale and ranging from happy to indifferent to unhappy, can be very effective in ascertaining clients' feelings about an issue (Conroy & Bradley 1985).

In order to support choice making effectively, service workers need to have a positive approach towards their clients' autonomy. This involves:

• being prepared to accept that a choice made by a person with a learning disability is as valid as our own
• being prepared to accept and support choices made by a person with a learning disability
• being prepared to look for imaginative and challenging ways of encouraging the person

with a learning disability to make choices in their own environment

- being prepared to support bad choices (CMH 1987).

To the above could be added:

- being prepared for new, different choices to be made
- being prepared to support developing knowledge and social networks.

For some people, especially those with a severe learning disability, partnership with a citizen advocate could prove most valuable in enhancing their capacity for self-determination. Therefore, it is important for nurses working in NHS Trusts and in other statutory and independent sector settings to know about local advocacy initiatives.

There may be an independent advocacy organization locally. This could be an Advocacy Alliance or Advocacy Development Group (or other scheme) which is involved in the recruitment, training and support of citizen advocates. Such schemes provide advocates for various user groups, including older people, mental health service users and people with a physical disability. A suitable citizen advocate can play a crucial role in strengthening a client's identity and developing their social networks. The relationship would usually begin with a sensitively managed introduction, and develop through time spent together. Friendship is distinct from advocacy, but advocacy can occur as a progression. For various reasons, not everyone will want to join a self-advocacy group (the person may feel that they manage well on their own) but this is also an avenue for support of the individual.

GROUP REPRESENTATION

Another key aspect of representation is the potential of the group to nurture individual development. Self-advocacy groups for adults with a learning disability are becoming increasingly influential, and recent years have seen an upsurge in their growth. The person whom you support may benefit from membership of a self-

Activity 14.2

Citizen advocacy
Consider the following questions:

- What citizen advocacy schemes exist in your area?
- Do you know service users who might benefit from a partnership with a citizen advocate?
- How would you support the introduction/relationship?
- How would user, advocate and nurses work together (e.g. in shared action planning, individual plan)?

advocacy group. Confidence, growth, trust, information are some of the gains reported for members (Williams & Shoultz 1982).

Self-advocacy groups

There are different types of self-advocacy group. Opportunities for joining a group will vary according to the developments in a local area. Professionals need to be aware of the options for the clients whom they support.

Types of Group

The great majority of day centres have a self-advocacy group, which may have a title such as 'Anytown Centre Users' Committee', or 'Anytown Centre Students' Council'. Initially, many centre-based groups began with a specific emphasis on tackling day centre issues (e.g. access, meal and break time arrangements, smoking at the centre). A group which has discussed wheelchair access at a centre may have moved on to consider the wider implications for the local area. Many groups have evolved so that the issues have become wider and more significant for others confronted with similar issues. Lobbying against proposed cuts in local services, not necessarily just those for people with a learning disability, would be an example of such action.

Some groups are People First groups and these are affiliated to the national organization (People First England) or People First London. The organization originated in the USA and has an international network, which is supported by conferences. The third international People First conference took place during 1993 in Toronto, involving self-advocates from 32 countries.

Independent groups have begun to flourish in recent years, not linked to a particular local service or to People First. They meet at an independent venue, usually a mainstream community facility such as a community centre or church hall. In some cases they have their own office premises, and receive statutory funding and generate income, e.g. through staff training.

Groups may be 'open' or 'closed' in their membership. An example of an open group would be a monthly People First meeting, which is open to anybody with a learning disability in the area. The function of this type of group, which may have a large membership (25–40 people), is to emphasize taking action collectively, e.g. lobbying the local authority about services. In contrast, another group which is independent may have a close-knit membership of 10 or 12 individuals, who use part of their meeting to solve problems on behalf of members. Trust and confidentiality are important in this setting; obviously a large membership would negate some of the effectiveness of the group. It is a common practice in this type of group for existing members to consider the interest of a new person when a place does become available. The applicant may come to an initial meeting so that everyone can get an impression of how they will 'gel' with the group.

Some groups may be aimed at women only, so membership is obviously restricted. There are particular issues which women who have a learning disability wish to discuss in a safe, supportive setting.

Groups which are specifically for people from black and ethnic minorities also exist. The question of dual discrimination is considered under collective representation.

It is therefore essential to think about the type of group which is needed and envisaged in an area before embarking on the new venture of setting up a new group.

GETTING STARTED

You may be aware of service users who you believe would benefit from a self-advocacy group, but no such group is running in the area. In these circumstances you may wish, along with potential group members and supporters, to think about getting an initiative going.

You may well find that your employer, whether a statutory or independent sector provider, will support the development. Consumerism reigns supreme in the 1990s: an NHS Trust, social services department or independent sector provider which can demonstrate its flexibility and responsiveness to users' wishes is likely to have a future. The establishment of a users' forum locally will fit the objectives of a forward-looking organization. The process of considering a new group, discussions with potential members and the search for an appropriate venue are part of an interesting and rewarding (though time-consuming) process. Planning the group, negotiating with staff of venues can be an enriching learning experience for prospective group members and supporters. The foundations of a successful, active self-advocacy group are to be found in a small nucleus of people who are concerned about their rights and wish to achieve changes in their lives, including local services.

Potential members may know others, probably through the services they use in the area. They will have an interest in, and commitment to, meeting regularly for about 2 hours. Meetings might range from weekly to monthly. At this stage the emphasis is on spending time together and enjoying one another's company. From social beginnings, and the discussion of common interests and concerns, the group begins to form.

Major points to consider at this stage include finding a suitable venue; identifying members and advisers; investigating the possibility of obtaining funding; organizing transport if needed.

Developing valued roles

A central tenet of self-advocacy is that the agenda is set by the service users. Another is that they occupy the official roles in the group and have the opportunity to practise and develop the meeting skills, e.g. chairing a meeting. Typically, a self-advocacy group would have elected officers in the roles of chair, deputy chair, secretary and treasurer. Advisers to groups are in a position to support service users in these roles. A new chairperson might need help in asserting order in a meeting; a recently elected secretary may need assistance in taking minutes (tape recording a summary of discussions and decisions is a very useful strategy).

Gains include:

- Growth and confidence
- Trust
- Self-valuing
- Identity
- Determination
- Responsibility
- Ability and knowledge
- Sensitivity to others
- Finding a voice (Williams & Shoultz 1982).

ADVISING A GROUP

An effective adviser concentrates on helping group members to acquire the skills which are needed to run meetings properly. Helping members to generate agenda items and supporting the discussion of issues and possible courses of action is crucial.

In our groups we have support. That helps us make decisions (User's view, Dawson 1995).

The adviser should be responsible to the group. The person may have been interviewed by service users for this position, and should be at the group's disposal. Group members might ask the adviser to leave the meeting at times.

I have found that group members value the support of an adviser greatly. However, if there is more than one adviser in a group, one must be wary of interaction between or by advisers dominating the meeting. I would recommend that a self-advocacy group of eight or nine members should have only one adviser present, unless an individual requires one-to-one support in order to participate in a meeting. Advisers should have knowledge of local services and of learning disability issues.

Often advisers are interested workers from local services. Commitment is crucial: the adviser should *want* to be at the meeting, not *have* to be there (Dowson & Whittaker 1993). Although there is an argument which suggests that advisers should be completely independent of services (because of the potential for conflict between the role of adviser and their service role) suitable people are not necessarily available. Also, I think that this somewhat misses the point: the characteristics and skills of the adviser are much more important than whether he or she is independent. In some situations the link with services can be an advantage. People do value the support of advisers who know about their lives, providing that this contact is not too close. There could be tension if, for example, a member of a group who lives in a staffed home has a member of his house staff acting as adviser. This may inhibit his freedom to talk in the group. He may wish to comment to members of staff on the service he receives, but this belongs in a different type of group, i.e. a users' committee.

People in the group will need help in finding out who to contact and what to do in order to answer their queries. An adviser who is part of a network will be in a strong position to enable group members to become more independent. The practical aspect of this is that service users may not have access to a telephone during office hours, possibly on account of their own timetable at work experience, day centre or college. A key skill for the adviser is the capacity to demonstrate how to do things – not to actually do them for the group, but there may be times when it is the only practical solution because of time or resource constraints.

Listening is very important, as has been discussed already. In the group context, including less assertive members is important. There are strategies for achieving this, for example doing a 'round' of the group.

Complex issues and impenetrable jargon-laden documents need to be 'translated' into an accessible form which retains the essence of the original meaning – quite a skill!

Raising awareness of possible options in a situation, including the strengths and weaknesses of each, is a process which the adviser can facilitate, but ultimately, the group is responsible for its own decisions, including mistakes. The adviser will have helped to explore consequences, particularly on major issues (see Box 14.1).

COLLECTIVE REPRESENTATION

Involving service users

In recent years there has been increasing acknowledgement that users have valid views about their lives, including the type and quality of services they receive and how these should be provided. Realization is growing that service users have a valuable role to play in the planning, monitoring and evaluation of those services. In the service culture of the 1990s the consumer is king. Although there may be debate about who exactly the consumer is (some would assert that the purchasing authority is the true customer), there is no doubt in my opinion that the involvement of users in learning disability services can significantly enhance those services.

People with a learning disability have always been a rich source of information about their own lives and aspirations (Atkinson 1988). The growth of the self-advocacy movement has brought new opportunities for people to express themselves and to listen to the concerns of others. Opportunities for people to participate in conferences, meetings and small group discussions have increased (Whittaker 1990).

Commissioners and providers of services, including NHS Trusts, social services departments and independent organizations, have much to gain by involving users in an appropriate way. It is clear that service users have a very positive contribution to make. They must, however, be supported through the process and have access to information that is presented in a comprehensible way, and have enough time to understand and form a view on it.

A potential trap here is for planners to think that user involvement is a 'good idea', and to carry this out in a tokenistic way. Think of the following example of how not to involve the user in a fair or constructive way. This would be to invite the individual, perhaps a self-advocate, with a learning disability to a locality planning meeting at short notice with a large group of professionals and others who are well versed in the process and politics of such meetings. The user sits, bewildered, in the committee room, struggling to make sense of a wordy document which others have received in advance and had time to assimilate. In this case, the invitation for a user to speak, e.g. 'What do you think of our strategy document, John?' is unlikely to be more meaningful than a rubber-stamping exercise.

It is vital to be aware of the pitfalls of such potentially token involvement. People should not be exposed to the type of scenario described above. There are major questions about putting

---

> **Box 14.1 Supporting a self-advocacy group: features of support**
>
> Enhancing mastery and control for self-advocates
> Learning to be on their side (e.g. people with a learning disability) in seeing problems
> Commitment
> Belief in people
> Knowing, and enjoying the company of, group members
> Emphasizing positive qualities
> Sharing skills and information
> Monitoring own communication
> Learning to assist without control or power
> (Brechin & Swain 1987)

Activity 14.3

Self-advocacy and user groups
Are there clients whom you support who would like to participate in a self-advocacy group?
    How do you think they might benefit?
    Do self-advocacy groups exist in the local area? Are these based at social service department day centres, or within NHS Trusts? Are there any independent groups or People First groups in the area?
    If groups do not function locally, would you or a colleague be prepared to help set up a new initiative with users?

one person in the position of speaking as a representative for all users in an area.

This is not to suggest that it is not appropriate for users to attend such meetings: however, there should be at least two people involved (for peer support) and they must have proper preparation before and support during the meeting.

A stronger approach would be for service planners to elicit users' views by meeting them in an advocacy group context. In this way, a wider range of views would be gathered and service users would be less daunted by being in a familiar setting. There are significant differences between consumer participation and advocacy. Although common concerns undoubtedly do exist, e.g. housing, support, work and transport, we must not lose sight of the individuality and diversity of the needs and wishes of people with learning disabilities.

Coventry Social Services Department has a cohesive strategy for the representation of users' views. A number of local self-advocacy groups, including a women's group and a black group, provide members who attend a representatives' group. Service users in Coventry have had opportunities to put their questions directly to a panel of 'top people' (chair of social services committee, director and assistant directors) from the social services department at a conference. Concerns were expressed about cuts in services and low levels of pay at day centres and workshops (1994).

Northeast Warwickshire has developed the 'New Ideas' learning disability equal access project, which seeks users' views by consulting them on key issues such as independent living – including support required – and work, educational and leisure opportunities. A project worker and other professionals with an interest in advocacy facilitate the process, working with groups in the local communities of Bedworth, Nuneaton and Rugby.

In Oxfordshire, workers from the NHS Learning Disability Trust support a group of service users who come from advocacy groups across the county. The group holds monthly open meetings at a community centre. Members express their views about, for example, service quality, to the managers of the Trust.

Things that will help us to get involved (Service User Groups in the West Midlands, 1995):

- Being clear about what we can do
- Involving us from the start
- Go at our pace
- Make us an important part of the organization
- Keep our involvement going
- Give us choice about how we are involved
- Use places we know and which are easy to get to
- Make sure that we feel relaxed
- We are the best judges of our wants and needs.

RESEARCH AND SERVICE EVALUATION

There has been considerable growth in user-oriented research in the learning disability field since the early 1980s. Increasingly, researchers have recognized that the views expressed by people with a learning disability about their own lives and experiences represent a valid perspective (e.g. Malin 1983, Flynn 1989). Open-ended questions are favoured (Sigelman et al 1980); yes/no questions are considered to have serious limitations because of acquiescence and overreporting; in either/or questions a tendency to select the second option is a potential pitfall (Sigelman & Budd 1986).

People may find it difficult to answer direct questions. Work involving people living in group homes has concluded that less structured interviews may produce richer information from respondents because they are able to talk more freely (Malin 1983). Semistructured and unstructured interview techniques have emerged as being valuable. A major study by Flynn (1989) of 88 people in the northwest effectively utilized unstructured tape-recorded interviews as the key method of data collection, supplemented by other approaches including information from social workers, case records and a 'house environs and living facilities measure'.

Service users have much to contribute to the process of service evaluation, given their perspective as consumers. It has been reported that certain conditions need to be in place for successful user-led service evaluation (Whittaker et al 1991). As well as appropriate support and training for people with a learning disability who are involved in the process as consultants, commitment from service managers and frontline staff is important. A key principle is that service users should be involved at every stage. A great deal of time and thought will need to be invested in the planning and execution of the service evaluation.

Preparation is crucial because consultants will be involved in the process of devising interview schedules, for example, along with a supporter, and developing their skills in interviewing and recording information. Potential consultants might possess some of the required skills already, but will need to be ready to work as part of a team.

SERVICE USERS AS TUTORS

Service users have a considerable amount to contribute as staff trainers and authorities on learning disability issues (e.g. Drage & McNally 1995). They are experts on their own lives and aspirations, possessing a potential which has not been used properly to date. Clearly, it is appropriate for people with learning disabilities to talk about self-advocacy rather than for professionals to describe developments on their behalf (Sutcliffe 1990). There are significant gains for students in caring professions in learning about services from the user's perspective. I have seen that people with a learning disability can gain a great deal in terms of increased self-esteem from these encounters.

CONFERENCES

In a discussion of collective representation, questions of information sharing and networking need to be considered. Members of this client group tend to have relatively few opportunities to meet service users from other parts of the country in order to share their ideas about services and how these are developing. A lack of suitable events, finance and difficulties with support and transport are some of the reasons for this. Supporting service users in conference settings tends to be stimulating and rewarding; these events are beneficial (learning about advocacy, developing networks) for both clients and supporters. There are, however, some user-oriented conferences: do go to a workshop or conference in partnership with a service user if you have the opportunity.

The annual Self-Advocacy Skills Workshop which takes place at the Hayes Centre, Swanwick, Derbyshire, is a notable example. It is organized by the Self-Advocacy in Action: Working Together and Helping Others to Speak Out group. The event has grown in size and importance since it began in 1990, and provides a valuable networking opportunity. Service users select a topic from a choice of workshops and work together with peers for 3 days (McNally 1996).

People First holds a national conference annually. The British Institute of Learning Disabilities has some user-centred sessions at its annual conference.

COUNTERING DUAL DISCRIMINATION

A discussion of representation must address the needs of people with a learning disability from ethnic and cultural minorities. These people are vulnerable to dual discrimination (Baxter et al 1990): it is widely acknowledged that people from black and ethnic minorities may suffer discrimination, and people with disabilities are also vulnerable to discrimination. The fact that antidiscriminatory legislation exists bears witness to this.

The phenomenon of dual discrimination – i.e. the doubling effect of being a member of a disadvantaged minority twice over – has attracted some attention in recent years. The evidence indicates that ethnicity and culture have significant implications for the provision of services to people with a learning disability. Concern exists regarding the under-use of services by families from black and ethnic minority communities. Gunaratnam (1993) reports that the most significant stereotype applied to Asian carers is that all Asians live in extended families, where clearly defined roles and responsibilities exist and 'caring for ill or disabled family members is a natural function' (p.115).

In setting out to provide flexible, individualized services for *all* clients with learning disabilities, it is important that service planners have an accurate profile of the local community (the 1991 census should provide a basis for this). By establishing a demographic profile of the community and monitoring the use of services, it is possible to estimate the level of unmet need (Baxter et al 1990). Consultation with black professionals and other members of the Afro-Caribbean community, for example, would be invaluable for this purpose.

Existing services must develop to meet the needs of ethnic minority clients. These services must be accessible both physically and in terms of communication.

The key questions here for the service user might be:

- Is the resource (e.g. day centre) within a reasonable distance of my home?
- Is there a worker whom I can see at home or at the centre who speaks my first language?
- Do the staff understand the cultural implications for my needs? There are several dimensions here: physical care, e.g. personal hygiene, hair care, food and drink; social and emotional care; access to users of one's first language; presentation of self; and spiritual care.

Services have tended to be based on the needs of clients from the white British population. Also, the label of learning disability has tended to mask issues such as ethnicity and culture, as though everyone with a learning disability had the same set of needs.

Action is necessary to ensure that the needs of people from black and ethnic minorities who have a learning disability are met.

Black People First groups can be influential in this. There are some successful local developments, but the national approach needs to be more unitary, properly funded by the

Activity 14.4

User involvement in services
Does your organization have a forum in which users can express their views?

Do people with a learning disability have the opportunity to contribute to the locality Strategy for People with a Learning Disability or Community Care Plan?

How would you ensure that users' views could be represented, e.g. in the local strategy for meeting the needs of people with a learning disability?

What links exist for clients whom you support, e.g. with People First or BILD?

Government and mediated via agencies which embrace antiracist policies and procedures.

CONCLUSION

What is the future for representation? Professionals and carers have an influential role to play in supporting empowerment through self-advocacy for people with learning disabilities. Support comprises encouraging choice making and expression of views. It may involve assistance in forming a partnership with an independent citizen advocate, or in becoming a member of a self-advocacy group.

Citizen advocacy is a valuable approach which can do much to promote the identity and dignity of the individual. Unfortunately, it seems that there are far fewer citizen advocates than people who carers feel could benefit from their input.

Because citizen advocacy is a voluntary, unpaid activity for which an advocate could expect only to receive expenses, it requires a level of financial security and a commitment of time and energy which many would find too demanding.

The indications seem to be that the self-advocacy movement is growing rapidly. This can be seen not only in the increasing numbers of self-advocacy groups in the country (Crawley 1988), but in the development of independent groups, as well as those which are based within services (Whittaker, 1991). It is to be hoped that the potential of service users to participate in the development and delivery of the local services and policies which affect their lives so profoundly will be recognized and utilized. This will happen through the consultation process involved in formulating community care plans, for example. The future should also see a greater utilization of users' skills and experiences in conducting service evaluations and acting as trainers, and being paid for operating in these roles.

KEY POINTS

- Representation is part of citizenship: it is important for all people, including those with a learning disability.
- Representation is linked with concepts of autonomy and empowerment.
- Self-advocacy and citizen advocacy are approaches which assist representation.
- Nurses and other professionals and carers can support empowerment of clients through advocacy.
- Nurses can identify, initiate and support self-advocacy groups in partnership with service users.
- Nurses can help clients to develop partnerships with citizen advocates.
- Collective advocacy can be valuable, both locally and nationally.
- Professionals must be aware of the dual discrimination which confronts service users from ethnic and cultural minorities, ensuring that such clients have access to services which meet their needs.
- Users have a valuable part to play in research, including service evaluation.
- Users can contribute positively to programmes of training and education: their experiences and thoughts are potent teaching tools.

REFERENCES

Atkinson D 1988 Research interviews with people with mental handicaps. Mental Handicap Research. BIMH 1(1): 75–90

Barton Empowerment Group 1994 The empowerment group guide-lines part 1: listening. Oxfordshire Learning Disability NHS Trust, Oxford

Baxter C, Poonia K, Nadirshaw Z 1990 Double discrimination. King's Fund, London

Bogdan R, Taylor S 1989 Relationships with severely disabled people: the social construction of humanness. Social Problems 36(2): 135–148

Brechin A, Swain J 1987 Changing relationships: shared action planning with people with a mental handicap. Harper and Row, London

Campaign for People with Mental Handicaps 1987 Values into action. Talking Points 5.

Chamberlain P 1985 The STEP Staff Training Package. British Association for Behavioural Psychotherapy, Rossendale

Clare M 1990 Developing self advocacy skills. Further Education Unit, London

Conroy J, Bradley U 1985 A five-year longitudinal study of the court-ordered deinstitutionalization of Penhurst. Temple University, Philadelphia

Crawley B 1988 The growing voice: a survey of self-advocacy groups in adult training centres and hospitals. CMH, London

Davies B, Challis D 1986. Matching resources to needs in community care. Gower, Aldershot

Dawson P 1995 Report on visit to self-advocacy groups for Department of Health. EMFEC, Nottingham

Dawson P, Palmer W and East Midlands Further Education Council 1991 Self-advocacy at work – training materials. EMFEC, Nottingham

Department of Health 1989 Caring for People. HMSO, London

Department of Health 1995 Continuing the commitment. Report of the Learning Disability Nursing Project. HMSO, London

Dowson S, Whittaker A 1993 On one side – the role of the adviser in supporting people with learning difficulties in self-advocacy groups. Values into action/King's Fund Centre, London

Drage H, McNally S 1995 The experience of advocacy. Part 2: A group member's perspective. British Journal of Nursing 4 (8): 451–452

Edgerton R 1967 The cloak of competence: stigma in the lives of the mentally retarded. University of California Press, Berkeley

Flynn M 1989 Independent living for adults with mental handicap. Cassell, London

Gadow S 1979 Advocacy, nursing and new meanings of aging. Nursing Clinics of North America 14(1): 81–91

Gadow S 1980 Existential advocacy: philosophical foundation of nursing. In: Murphy C, Hunter H (eds) Ethical problems in the nurse–patient relationship. Allyn and Bacon, Boston

Gates R 1995 Advocacy: a nurse's guide. RCN/Scutari, London

Gathercole 1986 cited in Butler K, Carr S, Sullivan F 1988 Citizen advocacy: a powerful partnership. National Citizen Advocacy, London

Gathercole C 1988 Involving people with learning disabilities. In: Towell D (ed) An ordinary life in practice. King's Fund Centre, London

George M 1996 Too little too late. Community Care 5–10 January: 19

Gibson C 1991 A concept analysis of empowerment. Journal of Advanced Nursing 16: 354–361

Goode D 1984 Socially produced identities, intimacy and the problem of competence among the retarded. In: Tomlinson G, Barton L (eds) Special education and social interests. Croom Helm, London

Gould C C 1988 Rethinking democracy: freedom and social cooperation in politics, economy and society. Cambridge University Press, Cambridge

Gunaratnam Y 1993 Breaking the silence: Asian carers in Britain. In: Bornat J, Pereira C, Pilgrim D, Williams F (eds) Community care: a reader. Macmillan/Open University, London

Jowell T 1991 Community care: a prospectus for the task. Joseph Rowntree Foundation, York

Kinsella P 1994 Who's in control. Mencap News April: 6–7

Malin N 1983 Group homes for mentally handicapped people. HMSO, London

Marshall T H 1950 Citizenship and social class. In: Turner B (ed) Citizenship and social class and other essays 1991. Pluto Press, London

McNally S 1995a The experience of advocacy. British Journal of Nursing 4 (2): 27–29

McNally S 1995b Is the new disability bill radical enough? British Journal of Nursing 4 (22): 1299–1300

McNally S 1996 Self advocacy skills workshop: a report. British Journal of Nursing 5 (2): 99–103

Monach J, Spriggs L 1994 The consumer role In: Malin N (ed) Implementing community care. Open University Press Buckingham

Moxley D 1989 cited by Challis D Care management. In: Malin N 1994 Implementing community care. Buckingham Open University Press

O'Brien J 1981 Learning from citizen advocacy programs. Georgia Advocacy Office, Georgia, USA

O'Brien J 1987 A guide to personal futures planning. In: Bellamy G, Wilcox B (eds) A comprehensive guide to the activities catalog: an alternative curriculum for youths and adults with severe disabilities. Paul JH Brookes, Baltimore, USA

Parsloe P, Stevenson O 1992 Community care and empowerment. Joseph Rowntree Foundation, York

Phoenix NHS Trust 1993a A guide to using symbols. Connect, Bristol

Phoenix NHS Trust 1993b Are you happy with the help you get? Connect, Bristol

Rappaport J 1984 Studies in empowerment. Prevention in Human Services 3: 1–7

Rogers C 1967 The interpersonal relationship in the facilitation of learning. In: Kirschenbaum H, Henderson V (eds) The Carl Rogers reader. Constable, London

Royal College of Nursing 1995 Advocacy and the nurse. RCN, London

Sang B 1984 Citizen advocacy in the United Kingdom – a first attempt. In: Sang B, O'Brien J (eds) Advocacy: the UK and American experiences. King's Fund (Project Paper 51), London

Self Advocacy in Action Group – Working Together and Helping Others to Speak Out 1994 Speak up for yourself: some ideas about self advocacy groups. Fairdeal, Leicester

Service User Groups in the West Midlands 1995 Together we can get what we want. BILD, Kidderminster

Shevin M, Klein N 1984 The importance of choice-making skills for students with severe disabilities. Association for Persons with Severe Handicaps 9(3): 159–166

Sigelman C, Budd E 1986 Pictures as an aid to questioning mentally retarded persons. Rehabilitation Counselling Bulletin 29: 173–181

Sigelman C, Schoenrock C J, Spanhel C, Hromas S, Winer J, Budd E, Martin P (1980) Surveying mentally retarded persons: responsiveness and reponse validity in three samples. American Journal of Mental Deficiency 84 pp. 479–484

Simons K 1992 Sticking up for yourself – self advocacy and people with learning difficulties. Joseph Rowntree Foundation, York

Simons K 1995 Empowerment and advocacy. In: Malin N (ed) Services for people with learning disabilities. Routledge, London

Sutcliffe J 1990 Education for choice and empowerment. NIACE, Leicester

Tyne A 1991 A report on an evaluation of Sheffield citizen advocacy. Sheffield Citizen Advocacy National Development Team, Manchester

West Midlands Learning Disability Forum 1994 Planning for change. BILD, Kidderminster

Whittaker A 1990 Involving people with learning difficulties in meetings. In: Winn L (ed) Power to the people. King's Fund Centre, London

Whittaker A 1991 How are self-advocacy groups developing? King's Fund Centre, London

Whittaker A, Gardner S, Kershaw J 1991 Service evaluation by people with learning difficulties. King's Fund Centre, London

Williams P, Shoultz B 1982 We can speak for ourselves. Souvenir Press, London

Wilson E 1992 Contemporary issues in choice making for people with a learning disability. Part 1: Underlying issues in choice making. Mental Handicap 20 (1): 31–33

Wintersgill C 1991 Separate identities. Social Work Today 17 October: 22

Wolfensberger W 1972 The principle of normalization in human services. National Institute of Mental Retardation, Toronto

Wolfensberger W 1983 Social role valorization: a proposed new term for the principle of normalization. Mental Retardation 21: 234–239

Sexual and personal relationships

P. Oakes

INTRODUCTION

The kind of support we give to people who are learning disabled depends on the answer to one simple question: is the person with a learning disability a full and complete person? If not, we should probably be kind and make a reasonable effort to meet their basic physical needs, but we do not really have to do much more than that. If a person with a disability is fully a person, there are massive implications for the care and support which we provide. Much of this book is about answering 'yes' to this question. All of the guiding philosophies of care begin with the answer 'yes' to this question, and one of the most significant implications of a positive reply is in the area of sexual and personal relationships.

This chapter has been written to help those who are involved in the care and support of people with learning disabilities explore some issues which can be challenging and controversial, and yet which can have the most significant impact on the quality of life of such people. There will be opportunities to explore the experience of people who receive services and to relate it to that of people who do not receive support with their sexual and personal relationships. The main body of the chapter will be devoted to looking at the ways in which basic philosophies such as normalization can be related to the needs, hopes and wishes of people. This will then be put in the context of the history of approaches, before moving to the main dilemmas and opportunities that face modern services. The final section will consider the role of direct carers and other professionals as providers of those services.

WHAT'S THE BIG DEAL?

Why should sexual and personal relationships be enjoying such attention? Are they really very important to the people for whom we provide? To answer this it is important to consider two of the great themes of our lives, and then to reflect on our own experiences.

Increasing independence is a theme of growing up. It begins with a child's first words and the ability to move without being carried. It strengthens at school, with a programme of learning outside the home which is mirrored by increasing independence in most aspects of personal care. It moves on with trips to the shop, going on buses and developing a taste in music, humour, hobbies and so on. Independence is often a hard-won prize, for there are many struggles along the way. These are made all the more difficult because those who resist our independence do so out of love and care, with a deep concern for our safety and wellbeing. The relationships which have underpinned the security of early years can thus become a source of conflict.

It is these relationships which form another great theme of our lives. We begin completely dependent yet well equipped to elicit the love and care of other people. In the essential early days of childhood key relationships develop from the giving and receiving of care, and our experience of these sets a pattern for much of our lives. During early childhood toddlers seem simply to bounce off one another, yet the seeds of close relationships are being sown. School years bring best friends – and hating the very idea of kissing anyone. As the teenage years arrive huge amounts of energy are spent on trying to look our best and understanding the tiniest signals from other people. Then come the rituals of meeting people, dancing, talking and experimenting all the time. This leads to ever closer contact as we set our own boundaries and explore the boundaries of others. Enormous energy and personal commitment is put into the making, keeping and breaking of relationships.

It is here that we see how the great themes of independence and relationships are intertwined. Children and young people experience a growing wish to build close relationships with other people. This is best achieved when people come together having already established their own independence and power.

Issues of relationships and independence are not confined to childhood and young adulthood: they simply have their roots there. Studies throughout adult life, from the early years of parenthood to older age, describe the importance of close personal relationships and the sense of control which leads from independence (see Activity 15.1).

Having thought through your own experiences, consider the person with learning disabilities. The two great themes of relationships and independence are now explained in turn. First, the question of relationships. There is no reason in argument or evidence to suggest that relationships are any less important for people with disabilities. There are many ways of understanding learning disabilities, yet they are basically a matter of intellectual functioning and its impact on coping with the challenges of everyday life. The idea that relationships assume greater importance for people who are more able or intelligent is patently absurd. Equally, the range and type of relationships to be engaged in are a function of

Activity 15.1

Memory lane
Having read thus far you have been reminded of some times in your own life. Take some time now to think some more about this. Remember the great themes of independence and relationships. Take some key times, say ages 7, 12 and 17, and now as an adult. Remember and note down the people, events, music, TV programmes and activities that were important to you at those times. Think about the importance of relationships – people you looked up to, people you learned from and people who were special to you. Think about the struggle for independence and recapture the emotions ranging from excitement and determination through to frustration and blind panic. Pause to go through this exercise now.

personality, experience and opportunity, not intellectual ability. Every person has a unique range of relationships, from the most distant to the most intimate. People with learning disabilities are not limited in the range and types of relationship that they can engage in.

In the second great theme, that of independence, the differences are striking. A child of 7 with learning disabilities may have only recently learned to walk, and may still need help with toileting. Perhaps the child can say just a few single words. Needing support in each of these areas is certain to make the struggle for independence even more difficult. At every stage during the formative period of development, this struggle will have a completely different character and will be limited by practical realities. This reduces neither the need nor the desire for independence: it simply limits their expression.

It was noted earlier that the opportunities to make relationships are a factor in determining the kind of relationships people become involved in. This is a key point at which the themes of independence and relationships meet. People with learning disabilities are likely to have attended a special school and may have had few opportunities to meet and experiment in the ways other children do. It is also possible that the opportunity to learn the ways of making relationships from friends and peers may be limited in a special educational setting. Firth and Rapley (1990) reviewed a range of literature about the opportunities and experiences of people with learning disabilities. They found that the early experience of segregation marked the beginning of a process which led to isolation in adulthood, where a substantial minority of adults are reported to have no close friendships or very poor social networks.

Returning to the question of the importance of relationships and the reason why the issues are receiving such attention: it is clear that people with learning disabilities have no reason to value the whole range of possible relationships any more or less than anyone else. This is a great theme of life for all people. However, it is intertwined with another great theme: that of independence and control. An individual's difficulty

in learning is likely to disrupt the struggle to become independent. There are a host of reasons why people with learning disabilities may need support to reduce the impact of dependence on the development of all kinds of relationships. Having established the importance of providing such support, it is necessary to understand a philosophical framework within which it can thrive.

PHILOSOPHIES OF CARE

Over the past 30 years services for people with learning disabilities have been changed and guided by a small number of philosophies of care. These are principles that set out the way in which a person is to be understood and supported in all aspects of the services he or she receives. Perhaps the best known and most important of these philosophies is what is known as normalization (Brown & Smith 1992). A central tenet of normalization is that people who receive services have the same human value as anyone else. It follows from this that service providers should work with people who are learning disabled, to achieve the ordinary things in life that are valued by us all (e.g. somewhere nice to live). It is also important that support is provided in a way that would be appreciated by anyone (e.g. with a certain amount of respect).

There is also a new set of ideas that can be summed up under the heading 'empowerment' (Orford 1992). This incorporates some of the ideas of normalization but takes them forward. It stresses the value of the differences between people, seeing them as positive. It further encourages people to learn to speak up for themselves, both individually and in groups. The last major element of empowerment is an emphasis on the importance of 'community'. This means understanding people in the context of the community to which they belong, and enabling the community to learn to help itself and to support those who are vulnerable. Care and support throughout this model are local and informal. Formal and central services are rejected (Cocks & Cochram 1995).

It important to understand the relevance of these philosophies to the issue of sexual and personal relationships. Services may receive their structure and direction from these philosophies, which have also been influential in the forming of Government policy and the requirements of service purchasers. Work in the area of sexual and personal relationships must be consistent with, and indeed spring from, the philosophies if it is to acquire the support it needs from managers and purchasers.

There are four main areas of the main philosophies of care which will guide work in this area.

- **People are fully human.** This is the starting point of all current philosophies of care. It may seem self-evident, yet the section about the history of services tells us that this basic truth has not always been accepted, and may be under threat. Services are still underpinned by some key declarations of the human rights of people with learning disability. The most influential is that proposed by the United Nations (1983), which states clearly that people with learning disabilities have the same human rights as anyone else.

- **Relationships are important.** Teaching from normalization tells us to concentrate on the aspects of life which are valued by people in everyday life (O'Brien 1987). The first part of this chapter has demonstrated that sexual and personal relationships are highly valued as a great theme of life. Community is also about people relating to each other. A strong community is more likely where there are effective and fulfilling relationships.

- **Growing through life.** The early Scandinavian proponents of normalization talked about the normal patterns and cycles of life being of great importance (Nirje 1980). This means that services are to encourage full involvement in these cycles and engaging in the opportunities and challenges of each of the stages of life (e.g. childhood, adolescence, adulthood). It also involves learning, changing and doing things you have never done before.

- **Power.** Applying these philosophies of care has meant giving people choice and control over the things which are important to them. This began with rather low-key issues such as food, drink and bedtimes. However, services are now

Activity 15.2

What matters most?
Make a note of the 10 things you most admire in people. What is important to you when thinking about the people you like to spend time with? Now consider how many of those attributes are related to intelligence and the ability to cope with the challenges of everyday life.

recognizing the need to extend this work to the fundamentals of life, including relationships with other people. Central to the issue of power is the abuse of power. Recent years have seen the long-overdue recognition that the abuse of power in respect of people with a learning disability has not been confined to restriction of opportunity and overprotection: it has also included active sexual abuse. This issue will be considered in more detail later (see Activity 15.2).

The vast majority of things which set us apart as human beings and which we value in each other are unrelated to learning or intelligence. This notion brings life to the bare facts of a philosophy such as normalization. Humour, gentleness, loyalty, honesty, openness and sensitivity are deeply attractive human qualities which are fully available to a person with a learning disability. Qualities such as these are also at their best when enjoyed between people at the heart of close and personal relationships.

It can be seen from the discussion so far that there is an important link between helping people with their relationships and applying recent philosophies of care to direct work with people. Any service seeking to develop along lines set by the philosophies of normalization and empowerment is bound to consider the issues of sexual and personal relationships. It is also necessary to make sense of work in the area of close personal relationships by referring to the guiding philosophies that can be seen in services for people with learning disabilities.

A BRIEF HISTORY

Before moving to the current professional issues

in the area of sexual and personal relationships, it is important to set these in the context of history. This is particularly the case as the century – indeed the millennium – draws to a close. It was around 100 years ago that services for people with learning disabilities were set for a positive move to supportive residential and day services. These would quite possibly have created opportunities to develop close and meaningful relationships, but sadly, this was not to be the case and a dramatic change of direction was made. However, the story starts a little before these great events and should be told in its proper order.

There is a detailed account of the history of our response to people with learning disabilities in Chapter 1. This section focuses instead on the main changes that have been related to helping people with a learning disability to build close personal relationships.

This account begins in the middle of the last century. Literature prior to that time has little or nothing to say about relationships. Rather, it is concerned with people's disposal under law (Gostin 1986), the conditions and regimens of residential services and the process of political change (Skultans 1979). It seems that the mid-19th century brought references to masturbation and the idea that it violated natural law. Indeed, it was seen as both a cause and a result of learning disabilities, with accounts of various attempts to stop the practice in institutions (Rhodes 1993). However, there developed at this time a sense of benevolence and professional paternalism, which began to influence services. This seemed to arise from the work of a key French pioneer, Sequin. He introduced the idea that a person with learning disabilities can be helped to learn and to develop. Small schools were established and these ideas took hold across Europe and the United States. Issues of sexual and personal relationships were ignored, but the conditions were favourable for the introduction of teaching and support in these areas of life.

At the same time, however, Darwin was setting out his theories of evolution, and his cousin Francis Galton was developing the idea of eugenics (from the Greek for 'well born'). Rhodes (1993) tells us that these ideas began to drive a new movement that was particularly important in the United States. Other parts of the emerging scientific approach to people and their behaviour were also put to use by the leaders of this movement. Again, in France, Binet had developed the earliest assessments of intelligence. These tests were applied to a series of research projects (Kempton & Kahn 1991) which embarked on major descriptions of extended families. The most notorious of these were the Jukes family and the Kallikaks. Researchers attempted to trace the extent of criminal behaviour in these families and used the new tests to help them in their task. They were attempting to prove a three-point argument: that criminal behaviour was inherited; that learning disability was inherited; and that criminal behaviour was linked to learning disability. Apparently startling results were obtained. The Kallikak family comprised 480 descendants, 143 of whom reportedly had learning disabilities and 75% were said to be 'degenerate'. A remarkable change can be seen in the reporting of data gathered about the Jukes family. In 1877, a study concluded that poor environmental conditions were largely responsible for high levels of criminal behaviour. The study was published again in 1915, this time claiming instead that 50% of the family had a learning disability and that all those who committed crimes came from this half of the family (Rhodes 1993).

These projects had a clear political agenda: they were used to give credibility to a set of ideas called Social Darwinsim. It was claimed that the human race depended on a healthy pool of genes, which could be contaminated by learning disabilities and any form of deviant behaviour. These threats were reportedly inherited and were all the more threatening because the people involved were said to be engaging in a good deal of sexual activity. The picture was a frightening one: a group of people were procreating faster than anyone else, and by so doing were spreading the contamination of the human gene pool.

Social Darwinism became the dominant idea in the first 20–30 years of this century, and effectively contaminated the excellent work that had begun in a range of settings for adults and children with learning disabilities. Services now had a new objective: to halt this frightening decline. The measures taken were fairly predictable, given the understanding of the problem which was to be solved. Men and women with disabilities were taken away to large, separate and usually isolated institutions. The populations of the various institutions increased massively and programmes of enforced sterilization were begun. It must be said that these programmes were controversial and that they were always secondary to the use of institutions.

The options for people with learning disabilities at this time were extremely limited. Most were to live a life which was celibate and separate. The ultimate expression for these ideas was found in Nazi Germany. Jewish people were not the only group of whom the Nazi Party sought to rid the world: people with learning disabilities also suffered terribly at the hands of those who conducted programmes of experiment and extermination.

The end of the tunnel?

With the defeat and rejection of fascism came the end of Social Darwinism. Programmes of sterilization were abandoned and some people were released from institutions; although the overall populations remained at a peak until the mid 1960s. It is in the mid to late 1960s that the seeds of change in respect of working to help people with sexual and personal relationships can be found. Learning disabilities were becoming increasingly better understood in terms of adaptive behaviour and community skills, in addition to intellectual ability. The philosophy of normalization was also introduced, and a small number of workers began to propose help and education for people in these parts of their lives. The 1970s and 1980s saw a proliferation of teaching and support materials available to direct staff, along with a full acceptance of the importance of close personal relationships.

In the 1990s, services have become aware of the implications of attempting to respond to close personal relationships. The acknowledg-ment of the issue and the development of teaching resources have been significant steps forward. The early ideas and materials have been reasonably straightforward. However, the complexity of the task has begun to challenge service providers in new ways. A range of issues have to be confronted. These include:

- Marriage
- Parenthood
- Consent
- Risk
- Abuse.

What have we learnt?

Before moving on it is important to see what can be learnt from this account. In many ways this involves returning to the link between dependence and close personal relationships. Throughout history, if a person has had learning disabilities other people have taken decisions about many aspects of that person's life. These include everything from when they might have a bath, through to where and with whom they might live. It is this freedom to take decisions that is guarded so jealously by people who do not rely on services. The area of sexual and personal relationships is one of the most treasured parts of a person's life, and it is here that some of the most heavy-handed control has been exercised, either by failing to acknowledge this part of a person's life or by curtailing the opportunities available to such people. In modern services there remains a reluctance to enable people to take their own decisions and act upon them in respect of sexual and personal relationships. This represents a long history of control and must be understood as such.

The second major point which can be drawn from a study of history is the extent to which services are influenced by the wider political scene: people with learning disabilities have always been the object of social policy. This again represents the dependence of individuals who need others for support to cope with the challenges of everyday life. Thus if social policy is concerned with the purity of the gene pool or the economic viability of services, there will be serious consequences for people who are disabled. This remains the case so long as people with learning disabilities are not helped to work together to influence the policies that affect their lives.

Change has come about through the actions of researchers, sociologists, politicians and journalists. This increases the vulnerability of new developments to changes in social and political policy. It may be that those who support people with learning disabilities could usefully spend more time assisting them to exert greater influence on the policies that govern the most personal and intimate parts of their lives.

The final lesson that can be learned from the history of services is the ever-present threat to the very existence of people who are learning disabled. David Potter and others have drawn attention to the increasing drive to 'prevent' learning disabilities (Potter 1993). The notion of positive eugenics has significant implications for the sexual and personal freedoms of people with learning disabilities. Women with severe disabilities have undergone sterilization where consent for such an operation cannot be obtained (Campion 1995). The law now distinguishes between the unborn child with learning disabilities and the unborn child who has no identified disability. There is a time limit after which a child who is not thought to have learning disabilities cannot be aborted. This time limit simply does not apply to the unborn child with a 'serious disability', who can be aborted until the pregnancy is at full term.

These moves to restrict the population of learning-disabled people strike at the heart of any philosophy that seeks to value such people as being fully human. Without that basic foundation, work to empower people in their close personal relationships is unlikely to succeed. This is so, not least because much of our ability to develop relationships depends on our own sense of security or self-worth. If a person lives in a community which believes that he or she should not exist, or at least should have been prevented from existing, such self-worth will remain a distant hope.

CURRENT ISSUES
Long-term partnerships

In considering close, personal and sexual relationships, people are faced with two positive options. A person may choose to enter into a long-term partnership with another individual. That partnership is characterized by a number of features, three of which are identified here:

- Sharing the opportunities, challenges, tasks and decisions of life
- Agreeing that the relationship is special and that each person is committed and faithful to it
- Expressing the closeness of the relationship by intimate sexual contact.

Alternatively, a person may choose to remain single where 'single' is understood as not being involved in a long-term partnership. This does not exclude casual or short-term relationships, nor does it exclude long-term friendships.

Although for many people this decision is made just once, others will take this decision on a number of occasions in their lifetime. It is very important to be clear that either option can be seen as a positive choice and a valued lifestyle.

In discussing marriage, Pitceathly and Chapman (1985) note that this choice has not been available for people with learning disabilities, initially because of the traditional link between long-term relationships and the bringing up of children. Given the ideas presented earlier in the history of services, this was clearly not an option for people with disabilities. However, changing attitudes and the development of contraception means that this positive choice is available to such people. There is certainly no reason why the elements of sharing commitment and intimacy cannot be engaged in by people who are learning disabled.

Interestingly, discussions of this subject just 10 years ago focused on the extent to which a long-term partnership might be successful, in terms of the likelihood of breaking up and so on (Pitceathly & Chapman 1985). This is an example of a way of thinking which is often seen in the field of learning disability: somehow, it is felt that a person with a learning disability should not make the same mistakes as other people do. Decisions are examined in the minutest detail and the person seems to have to attain far higher standards than those required of other people when making those decisions.

This discussion of long-term partnerships begs many questions. Some will be addressed in later sections (e.g. the role of direct staff, issues of consent, parenthood and risk). However, it is important to draw attention to two specific points.

- Good care practice dictates that an individual should be helped to take an overall look at the support he or she receives on a regular basis. This may be called life planning, individual planning or care review. Does this or any other process in direct care support people as they seek to make a positive choice about a long-term partnership?
- To what extent are residential services designed to enable people to follow the positive decision they may have made?

Study Box 15.1 and reflect on the likelihood of such a scenario.

Parenthood

It has already been established how the eugenics movement and the setting up of long-stay institutions have effectively outlawed the making of close personal relationships and stable partnerships for people with learning disabilities. Reducing the possibility of people with learning disabilities becoming parents has been both a cause and an effect of these ideas and practices. However, recent years have seen a significant increase in the number of people with learning disabilities who have become parents. This is a natural consequence of work to enable such people to live and make choices, like others in the community. Modern practice has given people new opportunities, and they have taken them in increasing numbers.

Clearly the growing numbers of parents who have learning disabilities represent a challenge to services, not least because of the prejudice that they encounter when they interact with chil-

---

Box 15.1

The year is 2007 and Britain is governed by a new and extreme political party. The fabric of society has been breaking down for a number of years, with record levels of broken families, youth crime and unemployment. The new Government has been voted in on a wave of despair and uncertainty about the future.

The touchstone of the Government's manifesto has been to take control of people's close personal relationships. It is argued that stable long-term relationships are the foundation of society, and that their breakdown has caused society to begin to crumble. Few disagreed with that. The next step of the argument was more controversial. Because of this cycle of breakdown, it was argued, people had lost the ability to make and maintain long-term relationships. Somehow our cultural instinct to commit ourselves to other people had been lost. The only solution was to impose such a commitment and to teach people how to restore their lost instincts.

A massive programme of training is introduced to set up a group of personal relationship overseers (PROs). Every citizen is to be assigned to a PRO, who will take control of all close personal relationships. Everyone will attend individual and group sessions to learn and develop skills and attitudes in this area. The PRO will arrange meetings and opportunities to mix with people who are similar to each other. Each person will have a 6-monthly review of relationship needs, hopes and wishes, at which progress will be monitored and plans will be made. Clearly, the citizen will only attend part of the meeting and the PRO and his or her senior PRO will continue the discussions in confidence.

On hearing the news of this policy in detail, many are disturbed and a few minor splinter groups attempt to point out the dangers of such a radical approach. However, a desperate situation calls for desperate measures. The Government obtains backing from the media and the programme begins. Existing relationships are assessed, and those with the potential to remain stable are allowed to do so. Partners still have to undergo training and all aspects of the relationship are monitored closely. For others, the slow process of learning begins. New relationships are not allowed until all parties are considered to be ready. This can take a number of years. Once a new relationship begins, it has to be closely monitored. Emotional, social and physical assessments are made at every stage. The closest scrutiny is reserved for intimate contact of any kind.

---

dren's services. Although research to help understand and meet this challenge has been scarce, a small number of workers have produced work of the highest quality. These include Booth and Booth (1994a,b) and McGraw (1994) in Britain; Feldman (1994) in Canada; and Tymchuk (1992) in the United States.

Activity 15.3

Future perfect?
Read Box 15.1 and then attempt to undertake this activity. Imagine you live in 2007 and that you are about to be assigned to your PRO. Note down your thoughts about the following issues:

- What fears, hopes and concerns might you have?
- You may have many objections to such a regime, but try to think about one or two absolutely basic problems.
- If you were about to meet your PRO, what kind of person would you want her/him to be and what kind of person would you not want him/her to be?
- In what ways does this picture of life in 2007 mirror the experience of people with learning disabilities today?

The first and most consistent finding of research in this area is reported by Booth and Booth (1994b): it is absolutely clear that there is no link between intelligence and the ability to be a parent. There is no point on a scale of intelligence below which a person becomes a bad parent. There is equally no point on a scale of intelligence above which a person becomes a good parent. It follows that treating people with learning disabilities as a homogeneous group is as inappropriate here as it is in every other area of life.

Research does however, seem to suggest that people with learning disabilities may have difficulties in bringing up children, and may be at greater risk of becoming involved in child protection issues (Feldman 1994). The difficulties reported include being sensitive to the child's development and providing a stimulating environment in which to learn and play. Also noted are problems in expressing love and affection and maintaining good discipline, along with physical safety (Feldman 1994, Booth & Booth 1994b).

However, this work has many weaknesses. The first and most important is an assumption that these difficulties arise from the learning disability. However, the evidence does not warrant the claim of a causal link, because there are so many other possible reasons why someone can run into difficulties with bringing up a child.

Studies seem to be based on small groups of parents, with little attempt to control for key factors such as social and economic circumstances (Campion 1995).

Booth and Booth (1994b) note a number of other reasons why research is weak. These include a tendency to study parents who are already in some trouble and known to services. There is also an enormous conceptual difficulty in defining good, bad or adequate parenthood.

Despite the problems with much of this research, it does seem clear that people with learning disabilities require support of various kinds if they are to have a rewarding and successful experience of parenthood. This support is beyond that which is available to parents who are not learning disabled, even though the reasons why such support is required may not actually involve the learning disability itself. Four main areas of support can be identified.

- **Making sense of it all** The first kind of support is in the area of practical help and teaching. McGraw (1994) has produced a series of booklets to help people with a learning disability to learn about the tasks of parenthood. The areas covered are as follows:

- What's it like to be a parent?
- Healthy food
- To be clean, healthy and warm
- To be safe
- To be loved
- To learn right from wrong.

Fundamental to this and other support is that it is given in a form which can be understood by people with learning disabilities. It will be important to use the special methods of helping communication, such as Makaton signs and symbols. It is also essential to match the level of information to the ability of the person for whom it is intended.

Another element of communication is the support a person may require to understand the workings of official bodies such as the Departments of Social Services and Social Security. It is possible that parents will fall foul of these bodies, simply because they do not understand what is being asked of them. For example, a social worker may become concerned because a parent does not attend a crucial meeting at school. The reason may be that the parent has been sent a letter about the meeting which he or she could not read.

● **The answer's no: now, what's the question?** The second area of support required by parents who have a learning disability lies in the attitudes of professionals and the services they represent. An important movement in general services has fought to ensure that a person with a disability is seen as a person first, with a consideration of their strengths and abilities next. Only after that should the disability and the support required be looked into. The same is true in the area of parenthood. People with disabilities who have children should be given their full and proper status as parents first (Booth & Booth 1994b). Areas of strength and ability should then be recorded. This can be followed by an assessment of the support needed to maintain the parental relationship, which should not be based on assumptions about people with learning disabilities. It will be unique to the family.

● **Stand up and be counted** The third area of help involves the need of all parents to stand up for themselves and make supportive relationships with friends in the local area. Research suggests that this need is particularly relevant to parents who have a learning disability (Campion 1995, Booth & Booth 1994b). At times of stress it is important that parents do not become dependent on services and professionals; rather, workers should be helping people to get together with others in the same situation. Booth and Booth (1994b) make particular mention of the help which can be gained from a 'benefactor' (relative or friend) who does not have a learning disability.

● **First things first** The final area of support which may be needed by parents is environmental. Parents with learning disabilities are susceptible to the same stresses and pressures of modern life as everyone else. It seems that they are also more likely to experience the social conditions of poverty, poor housing and so on. The load is often made heavier by the effects of prejudice and victimization, which people may experience as a result of their learning disability. Although professionals may be able to do little to lighten these particular loads, it is essential that they understand their impact on a struggling family.

To read the books and articles about parents who have learning disabilities is an encouraging task, and it would seem that the long night of prejudice has passed and the new dawn has begun. Sadly, however, the experiences of many people with a learning disability who have children suggest that this is a false dawn. Campion (1995) notes that more and more people require the approval of others to bring up a child, and people who have a learning disability are increasingly under the scrutiny of those who give such approval. Much more work needs to be done to ensure a just outcome for those people and their children.

Making decisions

People make hundreds of decisions every day of their lives, ranging from the smallest detail, such as whether to have a cup of tea or a cup of coffee, through to decisions of enormous importance such as a change of job or a move to a new place. Thinking about decisions is not just a matter of the importance of a particular course of action: there are other dimensions. Some decisions affect only the person making them; others may affect lots of people; still others will affect a small number of people in a very significant way. Then there is the quality of a decision that is to be taken: some are practical, others are emotional, others are moral or spiritual.

A particular decision is likely to involve a number of these dimensions, and the person has to weigh up the different consequences of each option. Important decisions tend to have a whole series of pros and cons. The last confusing piece to this jigsaw is the fact that everybody makes decisions in a different way according to different criteria.

Perhaps the most complex area in which

everyone makes decisions is that of close personal relationships. For many people such decisions are the most significant in their lives. People with learning disabilities may need support to reach a decision and to take the resulting action. This raises a series of issues for the people who provide that support.

Service providers are bound by law, and by the demands of good practice, to consider the extent to which a person with a learning disability can make decisions. There are two aspects to this. The first involves deciding to engage in a close relationship and the business of placing boundaries around it. This means that a person must decide whether to become involved with another person and how intimate and/or physical that involvement should be. The second is about the treatment or clinical intervention a person might be receiving. There are a number of options for a person with a learning disability in this area of life. These include teaching and assistance with personal and intimate matters. Also there may be various forms of contraception available (e.g. vasectomy or sterilization), or the use of medication to reduce sexual drive or potency, either deliberately or as a possible side effect.

In considering the ways in which people make these important decisions a number of legal concepts have to be understood. These can then be set alongside the professional issues which are relevant to the making of decisions. Extensive discussions of the legal aspects of these issues can be found elsewhere (Carson 1987, 1991, Gunn 1994). However, some important principles can be set out here.

The main legal issues that surround decision making are known as capacity and consent. Children become able to make decisions in law at different ages for different actions. At 16, a young person can consent to heterosexual sex and to entry into a mental health hospital. Other forms of treatment can also be consented to at 16, although this can be earlier depending on the individual. At 18, a person can decide to vote and to enter into a contract (there are some exceptions to this). At 18 a person can decide to have homosexual sex.

The law is formally concerned with biological age. Once a person has reached these ages it is assumed in law that she or he is capable of making the decisions. However, if a person has some form of mental 'disorder', and it can be demonstrated that he or she is not capable, then different rules apply. Here a person must be able to understand the nature of the action and its consequences to be able to take a legal decision. It is important that the assessment is to be of the person's understanding, not their wisdom (Law Commission 1991).

Allied to the notion of a person's capacity to make a decision is the notion of consent. Issues to consider here are the differences between approval and non-objection, the way a person communicates, and the time at which a person has the opportunity to give consent. It is important to note that consent can be undermined by fear, force or fraud. Consent can also be undermined when a position of authority is used to ensure submission or acquiescence.

Given the complexity of decision making and the fact that people with learning disabilities are likely to require support in this area, what are the issues for clinical practice?

- **Legal** It is clear that all practice must be within the law. This is to be achieved by a responsible group of professional people working alongside the person and her or his advocate. These people will require the support of the various organizations involved in the support of that person.

- **Choice** It is essential that work is carried out to understand how a person makes and communicates choices. Following from this, the ways in which a person understands the nature and consequences of a course of action must also be understood. This is certain to involve a consideration of the verbal and non-verbal means of communication the person uses.

- **Personal context** Support in this area is to be given in the context of an understanding of the person as a whole. This is to include issues of development, background and personality.

- **Service context** The philosophies of normalization and empowerment are widely accepted as a means of helping individuals make decisions when communication and understanding are difficult.

- **Assertiveness** A decision usually boils down to saying yes or no to a particular course of action. However, to do this a person must have experience of making decisions, and these decisions must have been respected by others. To say yes or no, a person needs to believe that he or she is of some value, and that it matters if he or she says yes or no. A person with a learning disability may lack both the experience and the belief. It will be the prime task of carers to help people develop this vital sense of personal value.

Risk

There is an element of danger whenever people come close to each other. The words 'getting hurt' may have become overused and overdramatized, but as people make close relationships with each other they can come to real harm, which can be emotional, psychological or physical. It is possible, though not proven, that people with learning disabilities may be more vulnerable to the dangers involved in close personal relationships. There are two reasons why this assumption may be true. First, a person with a learning disability may have experience of coming to harm in relationships. Such experience can form a pattern in a person's life. Secondly an individual may have found it difficult to learn the cues which help us to determine whether another person is sincere and is engaging in an equal relationship. These factors are likely to result from the kind of environments in which people live. These may be settings where key relationships are with members of staff, who are paid to be there and who can move on at any time. There may also be few opportunities to make and learn from relationships.

The next section will deal with the abuse of people. Prior to this, it is important to consider the ways in which people with learning disabilities can be positive about situations which might be harmful. There has been an increasing amount of attention given to the concept of risk in recent years. In the field of learning disabilities, this work has been led by David Carson (Carson

1990). A risk can be defined as any activity that can have more than one outcome, and where at least one of those outcomes is harmful to the person. This is different from a dilemma, where there are no options which are free of harm and where delay is also harmful.

Carson (1990) has produced an excellent method of dealing with risk, which can be applied to all risk situations, including those involved in sexual and personal relationships. The risk is assessed in terms of the exact nature of the proposed activity and the benefits that are available to the person taking the action. This is followed by an assessment of the possible harm that may result from the action. These benefits and harms are given values to help weigh them up. If the group of people agree that the benefits outweigh the harms, the risk is taken, along with any other possible actions which might reduce the likelihood of harm. This last process is known as risk management.

It is important that risk assessment and management do not occur in isolation. The organizations involved in a person's support will need to have considered the wider aspects of risk. This will lead to a policy to guide and support those involved in risk work, and an overall strategy to take an overview of risk (Carson 1990).

Abuse

Perhaps the most significant harm that can be survived by a person is to be abused. Whereas the subject of physical and sexual abuse of children has been taken seriously for some time now, the abuse of people with learning disabilities has been a relatively recent addition to mainstream thinking. Indeed, the early papers tackled the subject as a great taboo, with titles such as 'Thinking the unthinkable' (Brown & Craft 1989) representing one of the earliest treatments of the issue in the United Kingdom. Even in 1994 a paper about working with members of staff to help confront issues of sexual abuse needed to be called 'Alarming but very necessary' (Brown et al 1994). However, the issue is now on the agenda and has been extensively reviewed and discussed (Turk & Brown 1993, Brown et al 1995). It has also been encouraging to note that the National Association for the Protection from Sexual Abuse of Children and Adults With Learning Disabilities (NAPSAC) has been formed to assist with this work.

Definition

Brown and Turk (1992) adapted some earlier work in defining sexual abuse. They relied heavily on the ideas of consent that were discussed earlier in this chapter, including the factors that can undermine the person's capacity to give consent. Following this, two main categories of abuse were suggested (see Box 15.2).

Brown et al (1995) made some minor amendments to this work in a follow-up study. They included the idea that people can be victims to a number of different perpetrators, either in the same incident or over time. Equally, one perpetrator can have more than one victim.

Characteristics

The pattern of abuse seems to have been fairly consistent across studies. A detailed study was carried out by Brown et al (1995). Over a 4-year period 228 reports of sexual abuse were analysed, 169 of which were shown to be proven or highly suspected to be proven. Although it is difficult to work out the national incidence from a regional sample, the study suggests that some 1400 cases of sexual abuse can be expected in the United Kingdom each year.

Men and women are at risk of abuse to an almost equal degree, but the vast majority of perpetrators (96%) were men. It seems that the majority of victims have moderate to severe

learning disabilities and have additional difficulties. The perpetrators are generally known to the victim, and other people who receive the service made up the largest group. This was followed by members of staff, other known adults and members of the family.

Response

The first thing to say here is that the action taken in response to abuse was inconsistent, with few prosecutions and disciplinary actions. The implications of this work for practice in services across the country have yet to be recognized and acted upon. This can be seen from the survey results (Brown et al 1995). However, there is a reasonably simple set of measures that could be put together to improve matters significantly.

Turk and Brown (1993) stress the importance of ensuring that sexual abuse is recognized, recorded, responded to, reported and remembered by services. This will increase the likelihood of abuse being taken seriously, and assist in changing the culture of services to one which impedes rather than promotes abuse.

This issue of service culture was taken up by Furey (1989) in a paper about general abuse. It is clear that much can be done to reduce the likelihood of people being abused. Members of staff need support to reduce stress at work and to avoid situations which might lead to abuse (e.g. late-night sessions of one-to-one work). All staff need to be taught to be particularly vigilant, so that perpetrators may expect to be caught. Procedures need to be clear so that perpetrators can expect the most serious outcome following abuse. These issues should fall within a policy which will cover all those who are abused or who are vulnerable to abuse (Fruin 1994).

Individuals who receive services will continue to need support to say yes and no, as mentioned earlier. This will be combined with work to help people who have suffered abuse. Individual and group work with survivors of abuse will be an essential part of the therapeutic work of the future. There are the beginnings of a literature about this (Synason 1994). However, it will be necessary to extend the skills of working in this

---

Box 15.2 Types of abuse

Non-contact abuse	Contact abuse
Pornography	Touch
Indecent exposure	Masturbation
Harassment	Penetration/attempted penetration

way to those who have direct contact with people. It will also be necessary to enable people to get together as survivors of abuse. Current research and writing seem very well intentioned, but there is still a sense of the person who is abused as 'subject'. So far the 'subject' has been studied and surveyed. Sometimes the 'subject' is given therapy. Maybe the 'subject' could be helped to throw off the role of subject, for that has too many parallels with the role of victim. It may be time for survivors to get together, take control of the services, the writers and the researchers and tell them what should be done about sexual abuse.

ROLE OF DIRECT STAFF

Having considered a range of issues, it remains to pull together the role of direct staff in addressing this area of a person's life. This can begin with the overall requirements of good practice and move to discuss a model of direct work in respect of close personal relationships.

The basics

It is essential that people work within a full legal and policy framework, which means that members of staff will be guided by and accountable to a clear policy. This policy will address specific issues such as sexual intercourse, masturbation, consent and so on. It will ensure that everyone knows exactly how decisions are to be taken within the policy. Nobody will be uncomfortable with actions that they are expected to take. This will all be contained within a legal and philosophical framework. Policies on sexual and personal relationships will include or be related to policies on abuse, risk taking and health and safety.

The second overall requirement concerns the need to maintain general standards of good practice. Members of staff require regular and effective supervision. People who receive the service will be active participants in a care planning process that addresses their needs, hopes and wishes. Procedures need to be in place which ensure that the service has an effective

---

Box 15.3

At the beginning of every year it is hard to imagine the big news of the year to come. Yet each year seems to bring its share of great events which shape the world and the way we think about it. It may be an outbreak of war, a declaration of peace, a massive earthquake, a cure for common yet lethal disease, or yet another technological breakthrough. Each year also brings its human stories of triumph or tragedy, which touch us all and then disappear to make way for the next one. None of these events is predictable and few of us are directly affected.

One such event in the next few years may lead to reports like the following. The gradual deterioration of the earth's atmosphere has led to the wheat and barley in our fields producing tiny quantities of a previously unknown chemical. This chemical, known as LD3, has no effect on 99% of the population. However, the remaining 1% are affected by the gradual onset of a general intellectual disability. A person's ability reduces over a 6-month period and then remains stable, with the possibility of gradual improvement over the rest of the person's life. This leaves the person unable to talk fluently and needing help to care for personal health and support in community life. During the early stages sufferers have been moved to special hospitals for observation and study. Widespread public fear and ignorance has meant that most people are rejected by friends and society as a whole. Families, on the other hand, have stayed loyal and concerned, but feel very guilty about the role they may have played in the person falling victim to LD3. There is some evidence that susceptibility to LD3 is passed on to the children of sufferers.

Activity 15.4

The kind of help I need
Read Box 15.3 and then attempt to undertake this activity.

Imagine that you have fallen victim to the chemical LD3. You have just a few weeks to describe the kind of support you would wish to receive as the disability takes hold. Consider particularly the kind of support you would need to begin to make close personal relationships again, and work through these questions:

● What kind of people should support you and what should they do?
● What would you expect to really help and what would definitely not help?
● What are the most important things that our future service will need to know about you to help you to get this part of your life right?

means of getting to know the people who receive it; this may include diary work and reliable recording.

All services will have given thought to the ways of maintaining the health and safety of people who receive them. This will be balanced with the danger of overprotection, but will include specific help to ensure that people engaged in sexual relationships remain safe through the use of condoms etc.

Direct care staff are those who care for people with learning disabilities on a day-to-day basis. This involves actual social or physical contact. The role of direct staff can be divided into four main areas of activity, each of which can be related to working alongside people to develop close personal relationships. A discussion of some of these issues can be found in Craft and Brown (1994).

• **Doing** In a number of situations a member of direct staff is required to do something for the person with learning disabilities. Examples of this should be kept to a minimum. However, if a person is unable to move their arms and legs someone will need to dress them and place food in their mouth. In view of the imbalance of power in the relationship between staff who are paid by a third party and people receiving the service, and the enormous vulnerability of both groups to exploitation, members of staff cannot become involved in this intimate part of a person's life.

• **Teaching** There are many resources to assist with individual and group teaching. These are of great benefit to people, although it is important that they have the opportunity to learn about relationships at all times (Craft & Brown 1994). This will involve members of staff setting appropriate examples and intervening if inappropriate activities are being pursued. Learning is always

improved if it takes place in a natural setting. Social settings and gatherings can provide many opportunities for such learning.

• **Facilitating** This is about making sure that people who receive the service have the opportunities to meet people, spend time with them and develop close relationships, both inside and outside the home setting. A key issue here will be the need to be alone and not interrupted.

• **Advocating** It will often be necessary to speak up on behalf of learning-disabled people. It may be that there are objections and resistance to the idea of such a person becoming close to another. A service may lack the policy framework or the facilities to enable them to develop close personal relationships. It is also possible that the community at large objects to such people making relationships. Here the member of staff may need to speak up and encourage change. It is important to remember, however, that it is essential to help people to speak up for themselves and to take control of these issues.

CONCLUSION

Life without being close to other people is hard to imagine, yet easy to impose on others. This chapter has described the reasons why such an imposition is so devastating for learning disabled people, and has charted its history in services for such people. It is now possible to discuss, with reference to all sorts of books and resources, the ways in which this imposition can be lifted. However, the day-to-day experience of a very large number of people with learning disabilities is certainly not one of closeness and intimacy. The ideas, the words and the good intentions need to be turned to action in settings right across the country if they are to prove to be of any real value.

REFERENCES

Booth T, Booth W 1994a Parenting under pressure: mothers and fathers with learning difficulties. Open University Press, Buckingham
Booth T, Booth W 1994b Working with parents with

mental retardation: lessons from research. Journal of Developmental and Physical Disabilities 6: 23–41
Brown H, Craft A (eds) 1989 Thinking the unthinkable:

papers on the sexual abuse of people with learning difficulties. Family Planning Association, London

Brown H, Smith H 1992 Normalisation: a reader for the nineties. Routledge, London

Brown H, Turk V 1992 Defining sexual abuse as it affects adults with learning disabilities. Mental Handicap 20: 44–55

Brown H, Hunt N, Stein 1994 Alarming but necessary: working with staff groups around the sexual abuse of adults with learning disabilities. Journal of Intellectual Disability Research 38:393–412

Brown H, Stein J, Turk V 1995 The sexual abuse of adults with learning disabilities: report of a second two year incidence survey. Mental Handicap Research 8:3–24

Campion M J 1995 Who's fit to be a parent? Routledge, London

Carson D 1987 (ed) The law and the sexuality of people with a mental handicap. Southampton University Law Faculty, Southampton

Carson D 1990 (ed) Risk taking in mental disorder: analyses, policies and practical strategies. SLE Publications, Chichester

Carson D 1991 Clarifying the law on mental responsibility. Health Service Journal 16 May: 14–15

Cocks E, Cochram J 1995 The participatory research paradigm and intellectual disability. Mental Handicap Research 8: 25–37

Craft A, Brown H 1994 Personal relationships and sexuality: the staff role. In: Craft A (ed) Practice issues in sexuality and learning disabilities. Routledge, London

Feldman M A 1994 Parenting education for parents with intellectual disabilities: a review of outcome studies. Research in Developmental Disabilities 15: 299–332

Firth H, Rapley M 1990 From acquaintance to friendship. Issues for people with learning disabilities. BIMH Publications, Kidderminster

Fruin D 1994 Almost equal opportunities … developing personal relationships: guidelines for social department staff working with people with learning disabilities. In: Craft A (ed) Practice issues in sexuality and learning disabilities. Routledge, London

Furey E M 1989 Abuse of persons with mental retardation: a literature review. Behavioural Residential Treatment 4: 143–154

Gostin L 1986 Mental health services – law and practice. Shaw and Sons, London

Gunn M 1994 Competency and consent. In: Craft A (ed) Practice issues in sexuality and learning disabilities. Routledge, London

Kempton W, Kahn E 1991 Sexuality and people with intellectual disabilities: a historical perspective. Sexuality and Disability 9: 93–111

Law Commission 1991 Mentally incapacitated adults and decision making: an overview. HMSO, London

McGraw S 1994 How to be a good parent. BILD, Kidderminster

Nirje B 1980 The normalisation principle. In: Flyn R J, Nitsch K E (eds) Normalisation, social integration and community services. University Park Press, Baltimore

O'Brien J 1987 A guide to lifestyle planning. In: Wilcox B, Bellamy G T (eds), Comprehensive guide to the activities catalog. Paul H. Brookes, Baltimore

Orford J 1992 Community psychology: theory and practice. Wiley, Chichester

Pitccathly A S, Chapman J W 1985 Sexuality, marriage and parenthood of mentally retarded people. International Journal of Advanced Counselling 8: 173–181

Potter D C 1993 Mental handicap: is anything wrong? Kingsway, London

Rhodes R 1993 Mental retardation and sexual expression: an historical perspective. Journal of Social Work and Human Sexuality 8: 1–27

Skultans V 1979 English madness: ideas on insanity 1580–1890. Routledge and Kegan Paul, London

Synason V 1994 Working with sexually abused individuals who have a learning disability. In: Craft A (ed) Practice issues in sexuality and learning disabilities. Routledge, London

Turk V, Brown H 1993 The sexual abuse of adults with learning disabilities: results of a two year incidence survey. Mental Handicap Research 6(3):193–21

Tymchuk A 1992 Predicting adequacy of parenting by people with mental retardation. Child Abuse and Neglect 16:165–178

United Nations 1983 Human rights: a compilation of international instruments. United Nations, New York

FURTHER READING

Booth T, Booth W 1994 Parenting under pressure: mothers and fathers with learning difficulties. Open University Press, Buckingham

Craft A (ed) 1994 Practice issues in sexuality and learning disabilities. Routledge, London

Craft A, Members of the Nottinghamshire SLD Sex Education Project 1991 Living your life: a sex education and personal education programme for students with severe learning difficulties. LDA, Cambridge

3

Supporting the family in learning disability

16

Interventions in a family context

O. Barr

INTRODUCTION

The majority of people with learning disabilities live at home with their families. Consequently, family members often make a major contribution to their care. Parents, brothers and sisters and, at times, members of the extended family provide accommodation, as well as aspects of day care, nursing care, social care, education and social support. Current community care policies rely heavily on the input of family members.

The need to involve family members in care is not a new idea: Manthorpe (1995) notes that attention to the needs of families was incorporated into the 1913 Mental Deficiency Act, and it has been clearly stated in most reviews of legislation and policy documents between 1971 and 1995 (Welsh Office 1971, DHSS 1995). The rationale for this can be viewed from both practical and social policy perspectives. The statementing process within the Education Act (1993) and the Education and Libraries Order (NI) (1986) indicates clearly how parents should contribute to the assessment of the child's abilities and needs. The parents have the right to challenge the final assessment report and the proposal for education if they disagree with it (see Chapter 7).

The Carers (Recognition and Services) Act (1995) which was implemented on 1 April 1996, for the first time provided carers with the legal right to have a comprehensive assessment of their own needs in relation to the care they provide. The NHS and Community Care Act (1990) introduced comprehensive assessment and care management as one system of care coordination.

The consideration of the abilities, needs and views of the carers is a key requirement in this approach. The Code of Professional Conduct for Nurses, Midwives and Health Visitors requires each registered nurse, midwife and health visitor to 'work in an open and collaborative manner with patients, clients and their families...' (UKCC 1992). On a practical level, Hornby (1995) points out that parents both have needs and can contribute to the care process. All parents have communication needs, most have liaison needs, many require education about their child, and some require the services of counselling and support groups. Parents can also make valuable contributions to services. All parents can provide information, most are interested and capable of collaboration, and are a resource in the provision of care. Further to this, some may be willing to contribute to the formulation of policies on a local and national level through their involvement in joint planning ventures and support groups.

Dale (1996) provides a comprehensive rationale for parental involvement in relation to children with special needs which can be expanded to include adults with learning disabilities and other family members (Box 16.1). Much of the literature to date focusing on family involvement in care relates to the role of parents (often more specifically the mother), but it requires more than this and must consider the role of both parents and siblings and the effect of the impact on the extended family.

Involvement should mean more than the professionals unilaterally collecting data from family members and then deciding priorities, which are then explained to the family. Active involvement sees the family as valued contributors and not merely as passive recipients of services.

The recent changes in legislation, professional guidelines, policy statements and practical considerations mean that the involvement of family members must be an integral part of the assessment, planning, implementation and evaluation of services offered to them. Active family involvement does not require the person with learning disabilities to be living at home (although it is often thought of in this way). Even

---

Box 16.1 The case for parental involvement in the care process (adapted from Dale 1996)

- The professional needs family cooperation to do their own job effectively.
- Family members are a potential resource for helping the person with special needs.
- Parents and other family members need support and guidance to help them carry out their parenting and care of the person with learning disabilities.
- Unless professionals work alongside family members supportively, their actions can have a disabling effect on the person with learning disabilities and the family unit.
- The family has a key role in the life of the person with learning disabilities.
- People with learning disabilities are individuals with their own needs, wishes and feelings.
- Families provide continuity for children throughout their childhood, and for many adults with learning disabilities.
- The abilities and needs of the person with learning disabilities cannot be separated from the family process and functioning.
- Carers want to be more involved in activities and decisions on services provided to the family members with learning disabilities.

---

when they live in a residential facility family members can still play an active part in their life.

In order for active family involvement in care to become a reality of service provision professionals must recognize that there are many different types of family, and how the diagnosis of learning disability in a member will influence this complex structure.

WHAT IS A FAMILY?

As individuals we have a variety of family backgrounds. During conversations with friends and colleagues, similarities and differences in our family circumstances are often commented on. These include areas such as the size of the family, the number and gender of children, and our ordinal position within the family. Discussions between friends and colleagues about our relationships with our parents and siblings, their abilities and needs and how our parents related to each other will have provided insight into the differences between many families. Often these differences have their origins in cultural, religious and ethnic beliefs. Consideration will probably have been given to whether our family is very close to each other, and whether it is an extended family with grandparents and aunts, uncles and cousins in regular contact, or a much smaller unit consisting only of parents and their children. It is possible that the rules and roles within our family were a topic of discussion and at times much debate, both inside and outside the family setting. During conversations about our families there is an assumption as to what a family is. Despite variations in definitions it is generally accepted that a family involves the following broad areas:

- A defined membership
- Agreed group values
- Relationships between members
- Roles
- Structure
- Functions
- Stability over time.

The emphasis given to each area will be greatly influenced by the values, beliefs and cultural background of the family.

Current state of the family

The structure, function and role of the family in society has long been a topic of discussion and is widely covered in sociology texts (Giddens 1992, Haralambos & Holburn 1995). Gittins (1993) outlines two opposing views when she states that 'some argue that the family is the foundation of society...others maintain it is the source of most of our problems and unhappiness' (p. 1). The idea of a stable family containing two healthy parents who are supportive, loving and involved with the interests of their children remains the image largely portrayed by the media, but is this really the case? Some insights into the family in the UK can be gleaned by reviewing the number of marriages, divorces, births and who children live with.

Evidence as to the 'health' of the family in society at present is conflicting (Table 16.1). These figures reflect the changing nature of families requiring services. Marriage remains popular and the majority of children live with both natural parents, who are married. During 1992, in 37.6% of marriages one or both partners had previously been married. This results in an increased number of step-parents and step-siblings, although the reported number is small at present.

Table 16.1 Current state of the family in the UK (adapted from Social Trends 25, CSO 1995)

Marriages
In 1992 there were 350 000 marriages; of these
62.4% were first-time marriages for both partners (85.6% in 1961)
21.0% were first marriages for one partner
16.6% were subsequent marriages for both partners

These figures reflect a 24% drop in marriages since 1971.
There was a 100% increase in divorces recorded over the same period.

Live births
68% inside marriage
32% outside marriage

The number of live births outside marriage has increased by 300% since 1971

Children under 16 living with natural parents
With two parents
Both natural parents
75.5% (within marriage)
2.7% (cohabiting)
2.1% (also with stepchildren)
One natural parent
3.9% (within marriage)
1.9% (cohabiting)
With single parent
14.8% (with mother – 36.8% never married, 31.6% divorced)
26.3% (separated, 5.3% widowed)
1.8% (with father)

Activity 16.1

- Define in your own words what the term family means to you.
- Compare and contrast your definition with that of colleagues, and consider why you have defined a family as you did.
- Following discussion with colleagues, prepare a list of the components of a family as identified in the discussion.

In 1992, lone parents with dependent children made up 21% of families with dependent children in the UK. Despite the image of lone parents as single mothers who have never been married, the figures available show that 62% of lone parents in 1992 had previously been married.

In extended family networks grandparents, aunts, uncles and cousins may be very much part of the family and involved in the care of the person with learning disabilities. The impact of support from grandparents and other relatives must be recognized. When they offer practical and psychological support this can increase the coping abilities of the parents and siblings. Grandparents are affected by the birth of a child with learning disabilities: they often feel the pain of their son or daughter, and may find it difficult to cope with their own emotions, thereby reducing the provision of active support. They may have limited understanding about the care of a child with learning disabilities, or very different views on learning disabilities from those of their son or daughter.

Information about people with learning disabilities should be available to grandparents and, if necessary, other relatives. This should help them talk with the child's parents and reduce the possibility that they will try to cope by not talking about the child's difficulties, by blaming either parent, or holding unrealistic expectations of the person with learning disabilities or their son or daughter.

Variations of the extended family concept referred to earlier include a three-generation family, in which grandparents live along with the family in the one home. Another possibility is an extended family in which brothers and sisters and their respective families live together, either out of necessity or as part of a cultural tradition.

With the need to travel for employment – indeed, some families move to gain access to what they believe to be better services – a situation can arise where family members are a considerable geographical distance apart. Even so, they can remain actively involved in the decisions and life of the family. Equally, just because family members live nearby, it must not be assumed that support will be forthcoming.

Some families may move regularly from one location to another for various reasons, such as employment, career prospects, housing, personal interest or as part of a way of life within a specific culture, as in the itinerant population. This can mean that they slip through the services net. They are also not established in a neighbourhood, and therefore do not benefit from the informal community support available because they are not known in an area.

An increasing number of people with learning disabilities are being cared for either by foster parents or by adoptive parents. The challenges faced by these families may at times be different from those faced by natural parents, but they remain considerable. It is an unwarranted assumption to believe that adoptive or foster parents will cope better than natural parents because they knew the child had learning disabilities prior to caring for him. In the case of adoptive parents this is often not the case, as they generally take the child from a very young age, but even with advance notice, the same practical difficulties of care arise.

Families are complex and fluid structures which change regularly. This raises the question of whether it is possible to identify a clear definition to cover all families. New family structures will continue to emerge, requiring services to adapt. Family units with partners of the same gender are starting to be acknowledged, and as more people with learning disabilities have children, yet another type of family structure will develop.

Family membership is defined by other family members and can vary greatly according to place and time. People with learning disabilities in residential care often view the people they live with as their 'family'. Unfortunately, this has not always been appreciated in plans for developing new accommodation. Crude measures, including original address, ability level, contracted places and the desires and self-interests of some managers of new services have on occasions been applied, resulting in the destruction of such 'families'.

It is no longer desirable to have a static definition of the 'family', as it runs the risk of perpetuating the stereotype of what a family should be, the difficulty being that, when a family fails to match our preconceived idea of what it should be, judgements are placed on its worth. Such judgements could have serious implications for the availability, delivery and evaluation of services for people with learning disabilities and their families, and therefore must be carefully guarded against.

In conclusion, it would be more practical to obtain up-to-date information on the key components that provide an understanding of the individual nature of each family and reflect its current functioning. Regular revision of the initial information collected must be undertaken to ensure that the changing nature of the family is accommodated in any interventions.

PERSPECTIVES ON FAMILY FUNCTIONING

'Family functioning' refers to how the family is structured, its aims, objectives, priorities and purpose, and the strategies used to achieve these. If services are to be effective and family members actively involved, it is important that the intervention strategies used by nurses, social workers and other professionals are compatible with the functioning of the family. Varying perspectives exist on how a family operates, each emphasizing different aspects of the process. All frameworks have implications for the involvement of the family in care. The developmental, ecological and family systems frameworks outlined below offer differing yet complementary perspectives on family functioning.

Activity 16.2

- List the factors inside and outside the family which you believe influence its function.
- From the list you prepared, describe the effect of four factors (two inside and two outside the family) and what implications this may have for nurses of people with learning disabilities.

Developmental approach

This perspective presents a set of stages to be passed through, in sequential order, and each stage is considered to be qualitatively different from the others. Thus a framework is provided in which to understand the goals of the family at any given time during the family lifecycle. Gelles (1995) highlights the fact that the number of stages in a developmental framework varies depending on the author of the work (Rodgers 1962: 10 stages, Duvall 1967: 8 stages, Rubins 1976: 4 stages). Despite these variations, each framework follows a remarkably similar path. The age of the eldest child is taken to be an indicator of the developmental stage of the family. However, it is necessary to consider that families may be attempting to achieve a number of goals simultaneously from various stages, depending on the age range of their children.

Viewing the family and its members within a developmental model can provide the nurse with some insights into the impact of a person with learning disabilities on family development (Table 16.2). This will differ according to the stage of family development. However, irrespective of this, families have to grapple with 'changed expectations for the child, altered perceptions for the future and an acknowledgement of being a different family' (Manthorpe 1995).

There are limitations to using this framework to coordinate services, as all stages are not directly applicable to families of people with learning disabilities. The framework is based on the belief that adult sons and daughters leave home, but this may not be the case for many people with learning disabilities. It has been demonstrated that adults with learning disabilities often remain at home with their parents until the parents can no longer manage (Conliffe 1993). This scenario is likely to become more common with the implementation of current Government policies aimed at maintaining people at home for as long as possible. Therefore the final three stages need to be reconsidered for such families.

Developmental goals have been shown to differ for families which are not 'traditional' in their structure (i.e. two healthy heterosexual

Table 16.2 Family developmental tasks and additional considerations

Stage	Developmental task to be achieved	Considerations when a family member has learning disabilities
1. Setting up home	Establish relationships (marriage/cohabiting) Integrate with partners relatives and friends Priorities identified (children, career, home) Roles evolve in relationship	
2. First child arrives	Learn about and adjust to new roles Care of the child Keeping time for self and each other Maintaining work plans Readjusting priorities	Increased stress due to care needs. Fears over future children. May be unable to return to work. Blaming partner or oneself if genetic cause is found. Financial pressures. Regular appointments to be kept with increasing number of professionals. Social isolation may develop owing to difficulties with child minding or reluctance to go out socially.
3. Out to school	Encourage integration with peers Support child's learning Liaison with teachers sharing child's care Seek employment (if desired)	Assessment process undertaken. School confirms degree of disability (possibly for first time). Difficulty in nursery and school place. Additional programmes of work and appointments. Child development overtaken by siblings, cousins or other children born at same time.
4. Living with an adolescent	Readjust boundaries of responsibility Adapt to new peer group Reducing supervision Maintaining educational and vocational progress Facilitating choices and risk taking	Puberty may be delayed. Difficulties in explaining physical & psychological changes. Concerns over sexual expression and risk of exploitation. Unsure of further opportunities. Adult size, possibly with additional physical care needs for parents. Pressure on time owing to additional supervision needs of person with learning disabilities. Conflict as son/daughter realizes that some opportunities of adolescence are not open to them.
5. A new freedom	Children leave home Parents readjust to free time and increased living space Provide financial support in higher education Pursue new goals and hobbies Maintain open communication with son/daughter Possible new role as grandparent Reappraisal of life Revise plans for career, possibly consider early retirement Reinvest time in marital relationship	Person with learning disabilities may leave home for independent living or because of increased care needs or possibly limited day-care facilities. Remains at home, imposing new restrictions on parents' time. May be only son/daughter remaining at home. Concerns over further care increasing. Limited time for new interests. May have to explain to other children about risk of learning disabilities in their children. Additional burden of care may fall on siblings (especially eldest sisters).
6. Together to the end	Leave work, enter retirement, adjust to changes in physical and mental ability. Require support from family members	Alternative care required, separated from son/daughter with learning disabilities. Feeling of failure if residential care is required may be strong for some parents. Expectation that siblings will take over care of person with learning disabilities.

parents with children). Additional developmental tasks have been reported for adoptive, separated, single-parent, remarried and stepfamilies (Johnson 1992). Revised developmental frameworks have also been reported for divorced, reconstituted, dual-earner and low-income families, and families of people with alcohol dependence (Carter & McGoldrick 1989). Care must be taken in transferring these new 'norms', developed in the USA, to families within the UK, as the structure, function and development of families has been shown to differ across cultures (Giddens 1992).

Despite the limitations of the developmental model it does provide an outline of what might be happening in the family at any given time. In using it, the nurse must also consider the influence of external factors (legislation, politics, economics, conflict) that alter the position and role of the family within society, at both the micro and the macro level.

Ecological model

The ecological model, as reported by Hornby (1994, 1995), overcomes some of the difficulties highlighted in respect of the developmental approach. Family functioning is placed at the centre of the social context. Four levels of influence are noted (microsystem, mesosystem, exosystem and macrosystem) which affect family functioning and therefore require attention at all stages of the care process (Table 16.3).

The nuclear family is at the centre of this model (microsystem). All the personal characteristics of the family members have a direct impact on the family. This makes it necessary to ascertain from the family members what they consider their personal characteristics to be, and what impact these have on the functioning of the family. The abilities and needs of a person with learning disabilities and his or her carers will be a major part of this assessment.

Discussions with family members invariably point out other influences on the family, such as the extended family, friends, workmates and the professionals involved (mesosystem). Such people can be a critical component in the coping abilities of a family with a person with learning disabilities, and their impact should never be underestimated. Practical, emotional and possibly financial support from relations, friends and workmates will reduce the isolation of the family and assist in maintaining their energy and moti-

Table 16.3 The ecological model of family functioning (adapted from Hornby 1994, 1995)

Microsystem	Parent factors (e.g. age, status, health education, socioeconomic status) Child factors (e.g. age, abilities, needs, cause of disability, prognosis) Sibling factors (e.g. number, birth order, gender, abilities, needs)
Mesosystem	Impact of extended family, friends, neighbours, colleagues, other parents, nurses, social workers, teachers, psychologists, other therapists. Involves impact as individuals and in relation to professional services, the degree of coordination, cohesion and conflict
Exosystem	Images portrayed by local and national television, radio, newspapers. Voluntary/support groups – availability, resources and response to people as individuals.
Macrosystem	Influence of larger social forces and how these affect family unit and individual family members. Involves the influence of community, culture, ethnicity, religion, economics, politics and the legal system

vation. On the other hand, the diagnosis of learning disabilities in a family member can also result in the fragmentation of previous relationships, leading to lack of support, increased isolation and further demands. The pain of long-standing friends and colleagues failing to talk about or to the child with learning disabilities will be remembered by parents and siblings for a long time.

As the move to inclusive services gathers momentum, resources in the wider community (the exosystem) will exert an increasing influence over the abilities of families to care for the person with learning disabilities. Although services in most areas are reasonably comprehensive for children, adults continue to encounter major problems. Access to open employment, choice of accommodation on leaving home (or hospital), integrated recreational facilities continue to be patchy and inadequate.

On the last level (macrosystem) the impact of political decisions and the resourcing of services needs to be considered. At a local level nurses should involve family members and people with learning disabilities in project groups to develop new services or policies. At a national level, voluntary organizations can provide valuable insights into policy decisions and should be used.

The ecological model also provides a relevant framework to guide intervention, and has the advantage of orientating services to the wider issues affecting the lives of families. In doing so it challenges staff to respond on all levels, not only within the microsystem. Although external factors are important, care must be taken to ensure that the family remains central to the whole intervention process, and does not get lost within the response to wider long-term issues.

Family systems theory

Family systems theory differs from the two preceding theories in that its focus is on the interaction within, as opposed to outside, the family. Although it acknowledges both the environment outside the family and the stage of family development, the essential component is considered to be the relationships between family members.

A series of interactions between two or more family members is considered not only to bring about a change in the members involved, but also in the overall functioning of the family. Equally, a change in the abilities and needs of a family member, such as the development of learning disabilities, illness, leaving home and starting or leaving school or employment, will have an impact on all the other members and the functioning of the family. The family system conceptual framework has four interrelated components, namely family characteristics, family interaction, family functions and the family lifecycle (Turnbull & Turnbull 1990) (Table 16.4). Any changes in the family life are recognized as potentially having a major impact on family functioning.

Consequently, within this framework any intervention, to be effective, must concentrate on the nature of interactions within the family, instead of focusing on one particular member. The aim of intervention is to bring about changes

Table 16.4 Components within family systems model of family functioning (adapted from Turnbull & Turnbull 1990)

Family characteristics (inputs)	Physical, psychological and social characteristics of each individual member. Physical, psychological and social characteristics of family as a unit. Special challenges faced by the family and the resources available to meet these
Family interaction	Degree of cohesion and adaptability in interrelationships within the family between parents, siblings, marital relationship and involvement and relationship of the above groups with the extended family
Family lifecycle (change process)	Developmental stages and transitions. (Remember possible impact of having family member with learning disabilities) Change in family characteristics (new members, people leaving, alterations in health, socioeconomic status)
Family functions (outputs)	Priorities among functions of economic, daily care, affection, leisure, socialization, education, reproduction

in the overall family system and not in any one particular person. Family systems theory is relevant to the care of people with learning disabilities as such a diagnosis in a family member will lead to alterations in family characteristics (abilities and needs of child and parents, time, money, energy, motivation required to maintain previous functioning). Family interaction between the parents as a couple, parents and siblings, siblings with each other or friends and the impact of the extended family may alter. The increased physical and emotional demands on the family resources (the need to keep appointments, run new programmes of care, changes in working practices) may lead to a change in priorities among family functions.

The issues encountered during the lifecycle and strategies for responding will be influenced by the changes noted above. Teaching new skills for physical care or the response to 'challenging behaviour' occurs within a family context. Therefore, the best results will be achieved when any intervention acknowledges family functioning. A focus on the person with learning disabilities in isolation may at best result in inconsistent progress. At worst, the failure to consider the family context will increase rather than reduce the challenges faced by the family. When intervention fails to achieve its stated aim, professionals must carefully examine how family centred the care process was. It is not sufficient to attribute the failure to a lack of interest or commitment among family members. Limited resources, lack of explanation, confusion, little or no encouragement and fatigue are only some of the reasons for unsuccessful care programmes.

Summary

The models of family functioning make it clear that it is not possible to provide care to the person with learning disabilities in isolation from the family context. The context of family life is dynamic, and has many influences that need to be taken into account. Models of family functioning provide some starting points and frameworks to guide intervention. The key task is to select the model that fits best with the family at the time of the intervention(s). It must always be remembered that these are guides to assist practice, and not absolute commands written in tablets of stone.

Although accepting the individuality of families, research into how families respond to the diagnosis and care of people with learning disabilities provides further insights which are helpful in applying the models of family functioning.

Activity 16.3

- Review the models of family functioning and identify which one is predominant in the delivery (not the promotional literature) of the service in which you work.
- Evaluate how effective you feel the current approach to be, providing examples to illustrate your points.
- Consider whether another approach might have contributed to the intervention.

THE IMPACT OF LEARNING DISABILITIES ON THE FAMILY

Diagnosis

Only a minority of parents have definite advance warning that their child is going to have learning disabilities, possibly from ultrasound scan results, amniocentesis (performed in high-risk mothers) or other tests undertaken because of a previous genetic history. Unless a definite physical abnormality or characteristic signs (as in children with Down syndrome) are present at birth, or a traumatic delivery has taken place, learning disabilities are often not suspected or diagnosed at birth. Even if clear signs are present it can take several days to confirm test results. It should be remembered, however, that these tests cannot predict the degree of learning disability with accuracy, and for this reason, conclusive statements relating to the possible degree of disability should not be made. A major determinant in the eventual level of functioning of the person is dependent on their environment after birth. Some mothers report having a feeling during pregnancy that things were 'not right', but had no hard evidence as to what was wrong. However, the vast majority of parents have no inkling that their child will be learning disabled before it is born.

Learning disability is most often diagnosed in early childhood, when the child fails to reach developmental milestones. During the developmental period parents may have concerns over their child's progress and suspect that a problem exists. It is foolish and unprofessional of those (e.g. GP, health visitor, paediatrician or other nurses) in contact with the parents at this time to dismiss these concerns and label the parents 'overanxious' or 'overprotective'. Value judgements such as these have no place in nursing. If it is thought that a parent is unnecessarily anxious the staff involved should record exactly what makes them believe this. In doing so, nurses often realize that parents' concerns make sense. Many parents who have a child with learning disabilities report feeling that they have been 'fobbed off' by professionals (Leonard 1994). Nurses should accept that parents spend a lot of time with their children in daily activities, and therefore see how the child is progressing and become aware of minor fluctuations in progress. Therefore, nurses must start from the position that parents' concerns usually have some substance.

It is essential that such concerns are taken seriously, are clearly noted, factual information gathered and that parents are assured that they have been listened to. A regular check should be kept on the child's progress (more often than the usual screening checks) and clear records kept. It is a relief to both parents and professionals to be able, after a period of observation, to show that the child is achieving normal milestones.

Parents do not expect professionals to have all the answers, and are heartened by an honest answer that admits limitations in knowledge and an agreement to provide the information when available. Parents are deeply hurt and the prospects for partnership damaged by the illusion of expertise. The memory of how the diagnosis was given to the parents remains fresh in their minds for many years: some parents state that it will never leave them. The prospects of active family involvement will be damaged in the short term, and possibly for several years, when a diagnosis of learning disabilities is confirmed after repeated concerns have been dismissed or received little attention.

The bereavement process

The diagnosis of a child with learning disabilities has been compared to bereavement, in which parents, siblings and grandparents mourn the loss of their 'dream child' (Allan 1993, Maxwell 1993). Models have been presented to explain the process that follows a diagnosis of learning disabilities. These models focus on a series of stages that parents are considered to pass through as they progress from the initial shock and confusion to a state of adaptation to their new situation (Table 16.5). Progression is not always forwards and family members may find themselves oscillating between different stages at times of difficulty.

There are poignant accounts by parents which graphically illustrate the challenges that families encounter in adjusting to living with a child with learning disabilities (see Further Reading at the end of this chapter). Such accounts provide valuable insights for nurses into the complexities of family life, with clear evidence of the difficulties and the joys encountered.

Positive and negative effects

Some effects will span all family members, others will be specific to one or two members. Although parents may have common abilities and needs, 'as individuals' mothers and fathers can have very different concerns and coping strategies. Siblings may have concerns similar to their parents about the health, abilities, needs, future achievements and care of their brother or sister. Further to this, there may be specific concerns for either parent or the siblings as individuals. It is necessary to take time to gain a clear understanding of how all family members perceive their situation, and the coping strategies employed by individuals and the family as a functional unit. In doing so a more accurate picture of family interactions and priorities is gained (Powell & Gallagher 1993).

As noted, the presence of a person with learning disabilities in a family affects the interrelationships within the family. This impact is often envisaged as being negative, but positive consequences have also been reported. These are:

- Increased knowledge and care skills
- Increased contacts and confidence
- Fewer persistent family problems
- Increased family cohesion
- Effective response to challenging situations
- Increased life satisfaction
- Promotes personal growth and wellbeing of parents and siblings (increased warmth, empathy, compassion, increased tolerance of differences)
- Strengthens religious beliefs
- Career choice in caring professions (adapted from Barr 1996).

It has been shown that the family as a unit may gain from living with a person with learning disabilities. However, family members who have

Table 16.5 Models of adaptation to diagnosis of disability

Hornby (1994) Stage	Associated emotion	Miller et al (1994) Stage	Associated emotion/behaviour
Shock	Confusion Numbness	Surviving	Shock, fatigue, physical symptoms, feelings of weakness, fragility and vulnerability. Feelings of grief, helplessness, aloneness, sadness, depression, confusion and chaos, uncertainty and ambiguity, preoccupation with child, worrying, asking questions that
Denial	Disbelief Protest		appear to have no answers. Guilt, self-absorption, self-pity, self-doubt, shame and embarrassment, resentment and envy, blaming, feelings of betrayal, chosen and unconscious denial (seems to last for ever).
Anger	Blame Guilt	Searching	Begins while you are still surviving. Outer searching: quest for diagnosis, search for a label, contact with other families, new awareness, gaining competence and control
Sadness	Despair Grief		Inner searching: forced self-development, redefining life goals and priorities, asking questions of self, being realistic about child's abilities without giving up hope. Acknowledging that you are not
Detachment	Emptiness Meaninglessness		the same person as you would have been if your child did not have special needs, and deciding whether this is a disappointment, a challenge or a blessing.
Reorganization	Realism Hope	Settling In	Realization that there are no quick cures or easy answers, realize that some of your questions do not have answers, you become aware of regular progress in your child's development, sense of urgency, establish new priorities in your life and child's life, you get on with the rest of your life, balancing changes, developing new knowledge and skills, find out what works for you, develop a
Adaptation	Reconciliation Coming to terms		network of people, increased flexibility and adaptability in responses
		Separating	Giving some control over to child and others, admitting you cannot make the disability go away, pride in seeing your child achieve goals, getting 'tough' making decisions and sticking to them.

limited interactions with the person with learning disabilities may well not develop the attributes noted above. The person with learning disabilities can bring an added dimension and depth to family cohesion which for other people can be difficult to understand.

Nurses and other team members should recognize and reinforce the qualities and abilities that can result from having a family member with learning disabilities. This is the first step towards developing the mutual respect, understanding and trust of family members, which is a prerequisite to an effective partnership.

There are also negative consequences, and these must be recognized and responded to. They include:

- Chronic sorrow and levels of depression, particularly in the mother
- Emotional turmoil and confusion for siblings (mixed feelings of guilt, anger, frustration, jealousy, embarrassment)
- Challenging behaviour in siblings, requiring professional intervention
- Perceived external locus of control
- Increased social isolation
- Perceived lower social acceptance of family, parents and siblings
- Perceived lower life satisfaction
- Parents' fears of the future (continuing care, finances, care after they die)
- Siblings' fears of the future (inheritance risks, care of sibling)
- Raised expectations by parents of siblings in all areas of life (as a compensation for having a child with learning disabilities) (adapted from Barr 1996).

Mothers and eldest sisters appear at most risk of physical and mental health problems because of the responsibility of caring for the person with learning disabilities (Damrosch & Perry 1989, Andersson 1993). The level of disruption to the life of siblings, together with information about their brother or sister's condition, are critical factors in their adaptation process (Powell & Gallagher 1993).

The presence of difficulties is not inevitable, and care must be taken to distinguish difficulties which are part and parcel of normal family life from those which are a result of having a family member with learning disabilities. The nurse's awareness of potential negative consequences will help her to recognize these quickly and respond appropriately to reduce the impact.

The reality in most families is that a combination of consequences exists. No matter how well parents or individual family members are coping, the nurse will do well to remember that 'it never gets easy' (McCormack 1992). The impact on the family spans physical, psychological and social domains, and therefore to be effective intervention must do the same.

Activity 16.4

- Think of a person with learning disabilities with whom you are currently involved, and write down the names and approximate ages of the members of their family.
- List the attributes of the family and its members which you feel are as a result of living with a person who has learning disabilities.
- Select three of the attributes you listed above and outline why you feel they are a result of there being a person with learning disabilities in the family.
- Share your results with colleagues (and family members if possible) and assess the strength of your observations and explanations.

Variables influencing the impact of living with a person with learning disabilities

Key variables that can affect the balance of positive and negative consequences can be grouped under four headings: the characteristics of the child, of the parents, of the family and the local environment (Table 16.6). There is debate as to the impact of a child with learning disabilities on the strength of a marriage, and whether her or his presence increases the likelihood of divorce or separation. When a marriage or a cohabiting relationship breaks up and there is a child with learning disabilities, it is often seen by onlookers as the critical factor in the breakdown. The risk of scapegoating the child is great. The strength of the relationship prior to the birth is considered the most accurate predictor of whether a relationship will survive the birth of a child with learning disabilities.

Many other factors can influence the eventual outcome of a marriage or cohabiting relationship, and the total picture must be examined and not simply focus on the child with learning dis-

Table 16.6	Variables which may affect the ability of a family to care for a member with learning disabilities
Parents	Appraisal of the situation
	Perceived locus of control
	Perceived life satisfaction
	Reported previous coping strategies, individually as parents and together as a couple
	Perceived abilities and needs
	Response to other children
	Strength of relationship
Person with learning disabilities	Communication abilities
	Degree of continence
	Mobility
	Presence of challenging behaviour
	Physical health
Family	Family health/vulnerability
	Level of disruption to previous family functioning
	Level of training and competence of family members in care tasks
	Financial stability
	Number of children
	Reaction of grandparents and other relatives
Environment	Level of social support activity available and used
	Values, beliefs, culture
	Acceptance of the family
	Acceptance of the person with learning disability
	Availability and quality of services
	Professional response (optimistic/pessimistic)

abilities as a causative factor (Mathias 1992). Parents who see their circumstances as a challenge, and believe that they have control over their future (internal locus) will manage stress more effectively than those who perceive a threat and little or no control (external locus). An internal locus of control can be encouraged by asking parents to work in partnership with professionals and by valuing their abilities. The reaction of professionals in the early days can be critical in determining how the family views their situation. Pessimistic professionals will make a difficult situation worse. Although at times progress may be painfully slow, there is always something which can be a realistic objective. If they are clear, realistic and achievable within a few months, objectives can provide motivation for family members, professionals and the person with learning disabilities. The characteristics of the child have been associated with the level of stress experienced. In particular, the reduced ability to communicate, incontinence, physical illness or the presence of challenging behaviour has been noted to increase stress levels. Therefore, equipping parents and siblings with the knowledge and skills to manage these situations is a priority.

Wider issues within the family and extended family will have a bearing on the balance between positive and negative consequences. The disruption to lifestyle, together with the perceived fairness of parents in managing siblings, is crucial. Brothers and sisters must continue to have their own interests and hobbies; their birthdays, clothes, possessions and activities should as much as possible remain individual to them. If the siblings consider that they always take second place to their brother or sister with learning disabilities, the cohesion of the family will be reduced. Siblings may assist in practical tasks but resent this 'duty' and withdraw from it at the first opportunity.

A local community that takes an interest in the person with learning disabilities, and welcomes him or her into its homes and shops, will help families achieve integration. Conversely, when the family feels isolated and unsupported, stress will be increased. This can be a particular difficulty for families who are new to, or poorly integrated into, an area.

Practical considerations, including accessibility to GPs, nursing, social work, nursery and education provision, are important. Access to public transport or a car will be important if the child has regular appointments to attend. It is not unheard of for families to move house to improve their access to services, although being in a new community can compound their isolation. The provision of flexible respite care services and introducing families to support groups in the local area can be keys to reducing their social isolation.

COLLABORATION WITH FAMILY MEMBERS
Moving towards collaboration

Active family involvement in care requires collaboration between several groups of people. Family members must assist each other and there must be strong partnerships between family members and staff within both statutory and independent (private and voluntary) organizations. Staff within statutory and independent organizations must be committed to working effectively with each other. Active family involvement does not necessarily require the person with learning disabilities to live at home. People in hospitals, community residences or living independently may desire family involvement (Blacher & Baker 1992). When a person with learning disabilities leaves home it should not mean that their family no longer has any significance in their life.

Collaboration does not come about simply by putting people together, or because a family 'needs' nursing services. Hennemann et al (1995) identified the antecedents for collaboration as individual readiness, understanding, acceptance, recognition of the boundaries and confidence in one's own role. These qualities must exist within a culture of trust and respect, and among people who value participation and interdependence. These authors outline 10 defining variables by which collaboration in action can be recognized:

- Joint venture
- Cooperative endeavour
- Willingness and participation
- Shared planning and decision making
- Team approach
- Contribution of expertise
- Shared responsibility
- Non-hierarchical relationships
- Power sharing based on knowledge and expertise versus role or title
  (adapted from Henneman et al 1995).

The degree to which family members wish to be involved in aspects of care can vary greatly. The level of interest will be influenced by the abilities and needs of family members (including the person with a learning disability), the time available, urgency of action and the professionals involved. No assumption should be made that family members will rush to be totally involved, and no obligation should be placed on them to take on tasks they do not feel prepared for. Pressure to become involved and exploitation of family members' willingness to assist is just as undesirable as deliberate exclusion. Active involvement is a gradual process, starting with small manageable decisions and proceeding to larger, more complex decisions that may involve challenge and conflict.

Obstacles to active family involvement

When real difficulties have been identified they need to be overcome if partnership with family members is to become an integral part of the service. These barriers can be categorized as follows:, professional and family interactions, policy considerations and family characteristics.

Parents and professionals may view the same situation very differently. In identifying family needs professionals have been shown to give too much emphasis to the need for counselling and clinical services, while underestimating the need for parent education and access to services. Lack of appropriate information for parents is a consistent finding (Sloper & Turner 1991, Heyman & Huckle 1995). The individuality of each family

may bring with it challenges to be overcome to make family involvement a reality.

Family members may require assistance, advice and at times guidance, but they always require respect. An interaction with any member of the multidisciplinary team which does not show respect for the opinion of family members can have a detrimental effect, which may last for years. Lack of respect does not necessarily involve the nurse being abrupt or unpleasant: failure to listen attentively; dismissing parents' concerns; always offering advice or instructions; treating parents as 'just another parent'; not keeping appointments or not apologizing for delays; showing little interest in the person with learning disabilities; and many more apparently minor instances will signal lack of respect (Maxwell 1993). Family members are not easily fooled and can quickly recognize when non-verbal behaviour does not match apparent understanding and empathy of the words being used.

The use of professional language can exclude family members from decision making. Dale (1996) illustrates how words used regularly in reports (e.g. peer group, self-image, cognitive, fine motor, auditory), which many nurses would not consider jargon, are open to misunderstanding by parents. Negative attitudes towards family members (often based on information from others and not direct contact) held by professionals will prevent any effective partnership developing. Wolfensberger and Thomas (1994) argue that professionals are at times 'unrealistically prideful of their own capacities, their supposedly specialist knowledge, education and training ... and deeply distrustful of ordinary citizens, sceptical and pessimistic as to what such citizens can and will do'. Further to this, seven negative attitudes (by definition based on assumption, speculation and value judgements) towards parents have been noted by Hornby (1995). These involve viewing parents as problems, adversaries, vulnerable, less able, needing treatment, the cause of the difficulties experienced, and the need to keep a professional distance.

Leonard (1994) states that a consequence of inappropriate attitudes is that parents report that their concerns are not taken seriously, that they are 'fobbed off' and 'labelled'. Also, the information given them often does not match their needs at the time. It may be too little too late, or, conversely, too much too soon. A careful assessment of the individual parents' and family members' current level of understanding and identification of the areas in which they feel they require more information is essential. This will increase the probability that information provided is seen as significant. Some parents report suspecting collusion, deceit and the closing of ranks among professionals. Whether proven or not, beliefs such as these among family members will seriously limit their active partnership in care.

Further to the above, rigid inflexible criteria for assessment, priorities in care, complex forms to be completed, restricted access to information and no involvement of family members in the evaluation of care impede any attempt to develop partnership. Meetings should be negotiated with practical considerations in mind such as location, timing and how they fit in with the other commitments. A disregard for practical considerations can reduce the time taken for discussions and lead to a reduction or absence of active family involvement.

Lack of knowledge may be a consequence of lack of information and will reduce involvement in decision making. Many family members need to be taught new skills which can be used when providing care. These can be as diverse as behavioural management strategies and the passing of a nasogastric feeding tube. Without skills specific to their situation, family members will be unnecessarily reliant on services. Great caution must be exercised in the teaching of new skills, as when nurses teach new skills to family members they are accountable for the quality of their instruction. If family members are poorly instructed or misinformed, and their competence is not assessed, the 'teacher' can be held accountable. This makes it necessary for clear records to show how the nurse followed a structured educational programme and was satisfied that family members were competent in the skills. If, after instruction, family members make an error though lack of attention or taking short cuts in safety procedures, the accountability

rests with them. Therefore, instruction is best provided within a structured yet individualized approach.

The attitudes of family members may not be welcoming to professionals (with or without good reason). This is not a reason to respond by keeping them out of decision making, but makes it imperative to change these attitudes by demonstrating the merits of partnership for all involved.

Models of collaboration

The nature of the collaboration entered into with family members can be clarified by considering a continuum of models relating to family involvement in care. Because of variations in family composition, nurses may be working with both parents or single parents, and partnership may develop with some or all family members. The principal foci and priorities of the models are transferable to situations where the nurse is working with one or both parents, or with siblings, or with any combination of these people. The models may be compared on seven characteristics:

- Role of family member
- Role of professional
- Nature of interactions
- Location of control in decision making
- Identification of the problem
- View of conflict
- Criteria for a successful outcome (Table 16.7).

 Activity 16.5

- Think of the family members of two people with learning disabilities with whom you have recently worked in which active family involvement in care was limited (despite the wishes of the family).
- List the obstacles, and their origins, to active family involvement in care.
- Describe the nature of the impact of these obstacles on their involvement in care and relationships with staff.
- What was the solution (actual or potential) to these obstacles?

Table 16.7 Comparison of some key characteristics of models for working with parents and family members

Model	Identification of problem	Role of parent	Role of staff	Nature of interactions	Control in decisions	View of conflict	Desired outcome
Expert	Selected by staff based on their expertise	Obeys instructions Passive & accepting of decisions	Make decisions Inform parent Give instructions	View of parents not valued Mainly one-way communication from staff to parent Compliance of parents	Totally with staff	Undesirable Suppressed Expert knows best	Compliance with prescribed care
Transplant	Selected mainly by staff, parents may have some limited involvement	Participates in care, actively learns new skills	Facilitates parent learning, resource person. Retains expert role to a lesser extent	Two-way flow of information. Opinions, knowledge & skills of parents respected, valued to some degree	Staff and parents consult but final decision by staff	May arise in discussion not valued	Family learn new skills & parents become a resource
Consumer (Cunningham & Davis 1985)	Parents and staff	Active in discussions. Full control over decisions	Combination of roles. Consultant, instructor, facilitator	Two way dialogue. Abilities of parents acknowledged.	Parents and staff contribute, but final decision is made by parents	Challenge to staff expected & viewed as part of negotiation process	Partners in care Increased control of resources & decision by parents
Empowerment (Appleton & Minchom 1991)	Selected by parent and professional	Active in decisions, degree of involvement selected by parent	Facilitates parent control. May act as expert, instructor, resource person to help empower parent	Two-way dialogue which includes social network of parents. Aims for partnership	Shared between staff and parents Parents' control promoted but possible need for staff to make decisions to assist parents	Viewed as part empowerment Valued as creative Acknowledged & channelled into action	Partners in care Parents have more control Social network recognized
Negotiating (Dale 1996)	Problem of mutual concern agreed by parents and staff	Consumer role recognized. Active participation encouraged. Recognizes differing levels of involvement desired by parents	Variety of possible roles (expert, instructor, consultant, facilitator) Selected roles agreed with parents. Major listening role	Both parties can learn from each other. Family, community & ethnic differences catered for	Joint control neither party has total control Both parties may undertake expert, instructor or facilitator roles depending on the decision	Conflict a possibility – part of the process Dissent & failure to agree common purpose may result in suspension of partnership	Jointly agreed decision on issues of mutual concern

Expert

The expert does not provide active partnership for family members. In this model their role is passive and obedient to the instructions of professionals. Such an approach provides a short-term intervention in emergency situations, or at the earliest stages of family involvement. Beyond this it is limited and does not desire active family involvement in decision making. This model can feel safe for professionals and is visible in services long after initial interventions. This can be damaging to longer-term plans for partnership.

Transplant

The central focus of the transplant model is teaching family members new skills (which are transplanted from the professionals) to enable them to care for the person with learning disabilities. As noted earlier, many family members desire new knowledge and skills, and therefore this model has a place in interventions. However, a major limitation is that it is often the professionals and not family members who decide the skills to be taught. This can result in the specific needs of family members not being addressed, particularly in light of the dichotomy between what professionals view as important to parents and what parents view as important to themselves. It is also essential that the risk of family members acquiring new skills and then being left unsupported by services is acknowledged and guarded against.

Consumer

The consumer model provides a degree of partnership, recognizes the abilities of family members and the changing role of professionals, and in theory the final decision is left with the parents. Two issues need to be considered; first, if this results in unilateral decisions by parents it resembles the expert model, with the parent as the expert, and has similar limitations; secondly, if the decisions are left to family members it must be clear that the interests of the person with learning disabilities are seen as paramount, and

are not secondary to the desires of other family members. This model does not justify professionals abdicating their responsibility by stating that family members made the decision and not them. Partnership will only result if family members are enabled to implement or see the implementation of the decisions they have made.

Empowerment

The empowerment model seeks to move closer to active partnership. Both family and professionals are recognized as having expert ability and needs, and both are involved in decision making. The implementation of this model requires relevant information to be accessible to family members, and can result in a longer time being necessary for decisions to be reached that will have implications for service resources. It also requires professionals to be open to having their advice questioned, disregarded and not always accepted. Gibson (1991) highlighted the need for self-determination, a sense of control as well as motivation, to exist within the client for empowerment to evolve. Some of the visible indicators of empowerment in nurse – client interaction are trust, empathy, mutual goal setting, participation in decision making and overcoming organizational barriers. Braye and Preston-Shoot (1995) emphasize that empowerment must move beyond tokenism. This may require a review of service values, models, policies and procedures, and an investment in staff education and monitoring.

Building on her earlier work, Gibson (1995) proposed a model for the development of empowerment within mothers of chronically ill children. In this she noted the preconditions of commitment, a bond with the child, love and the influencing factors of beliefs, values, determination, social support and experience. The presence of frustration with the situation was considered to be the driving force in achieving empowerment. Empowerment was recognized as having both positive and negative outcomes. An increased purpose and meaning in life, self-development, satisfaction and mastery over the challenges were viewed as positive. In contrast, rejection by professionals, becoming overloaded with responsibility, and having reduced support because of managing so well, were negative consequences. In light of this nurses must continue to provide opportunities for empowered family members to ask for help without feeling that they are failing. Dale (1996) built on the empowerment model (in which she viewed professionals still having the final decision) to develop the negotiation model. There are crucial differences between the two. The starting point of the empowerment model is the identification of a problem of mutual concern, not a professionally selected problem. The possibility of conflict and temporary suspension, or indeed the breakdown of partnership, is recognized, as are the interchanging roles of both professionals and family members. Working in partnership with family members and facilitating their involvement in decision making is the stated policy aim of most services. However, it is important to recognize the range of possible levels of collaboration and their usefulness. The model of involvement must match the abilities and needs of the family members and professionals at any particular time, and may vary with time and the challenges faced. This flexibility is incorporated into the negotiation model, which accepts the need for expert roles at times but requires them to be agreed by all involved, and not unilaterally by either professionals or family members. Forcing an empowerment model on a family who is not yet able to respond as required by this model, can be just as damaging as adhering to an expert model in a situation where empowerment or negotiation models could be implemented.

GUIDELINES FOR PROVIDING SERVICES IN A FAMILY CONTEXT

The practical considerations for assessing, planning, implementing and evaluating care remain important when working with family members. In addition, specific considerations are necessary (see Box 16.2). Each model of family participation provides a broad framework for collaboration. Although there are differences in the degree of active involvement of family members across the various models, some guidelines for practice

Activity 16.6

- Obtain two information leaflets on services for people with learning disabilities and their families within your locality. (These must be obtained from a public place and should not need to be obtained from offices or people to which family members do not have free access.)
- Evaluate the leaflets in relation to the accuracy of the information they contain (e.g. names, phone numbers, roles, services available).
- Evaluate the leaflets in relation to the usefulness of the information they provide that would assist family members in making informed decisions. What percentage of leaflets does this make up?
- If possible, have family members evaluate the leaflets on the above criteria and compare their findings with yours. Explain any differences that exist between the evaluation by family members and your evaluation.
- Make recommendations (if required) for improvements to the leaflets in the light of this exercise.

span all models. It must be clear to all family members that the nurse is interested in and capable of helping the person with learning disabilities and other family members in the challenges facing them. Without this discussions about nursing and proposed interventions may be viewed as just another thing to do, and, depending on priorities, may or may not be done. Interest is demonstrated through small details of practice, rather than policy statements and glossy pamphlets. Talking and listening attentively, touching, holding (if appropriate), joining in activities and being prepared to learn from the person with learning disabilities and family members acknowledges their value, whereas an aloof and distant approach will do little to set the scene for understanding the complex dynamics of each family and its members.

Support for family members must be practical and relevant to their situation. Central to effective intervention is an understanding of the nature of the structure, functioning and priorities of the family. Providing services based on fixed ideas of what a family needs is unwarranted, ineffective and potentially damaging for the person with learning disabilities, family members, the family as a unit, and ultimately for services.

Box 16.2   Practical considerations for active family involvement in care.

C Collaboration requires two-way communication
A Assessment of abilities/needs of all family members and the family unit
R Recognition of +/– aspects of caring
E Empathy with person with learning disabilities and family members
R Respect for opinions, concerns and cultural diversity in families
S Support: physical, psychological, social

I Individualized approach to interventions and the provision of information
N No abuse of commitment/negotiation of roles undertaken by professionals and family members
V Values and priorities of intervention agreed
O Organizational policies and procedures may need to be reviewed
L Link person/liaison known and accessible to family members and professionals
V Voluntary and private organizations (local and national) known about
E Existing networks utilized but not exploited
M Mothers often primary carers. Careful not to overburden
E Evaluation of structure, process and outcomes involving family members
N Nurses' accountability for actions and omissions
T Teamwork necessary for coordinated services

Information gathering over the first few weeks will provide a baseline understanding from which to proceed. People as individuals and families as units are dynamic, and for this reason information must be kept up to date if intervention is to be effective.

The relationship with family members must be based on respect for their right to have views. Central to this is honesty, which means an acceptance that you do not know all the answers. Any pretence or deceit will eventually be uncovered and exposed as a disrespect for family members as well as the role of professionals. Confidentiality is a critical component to the development of trust and respect in partnerships. Family members must be aware of who will have access to the information they provide. It is important that only people who require information should receive it. Casual talk in offices, meetings or public places must not disclose confidential information.

Nurses and other team members must be prepared to acknowledge limitations and mistakes, as well as being willing to learn. As the relationship develops information will be more forthcoming and a deeper understanding will be gained. An authoritarian approach, on the other hand, often leads to family members telling professionals what they think they want to hear, and concealing their real views, abilities and needs. Assessment must lead to visible action, with the information obtained guiding intervention.

Trust, interest and motivation generated by team members will quickly wane if the long discussions, and sometimes the detailed self-disclosure by family members, do not result in tangible progress.

Family members will vary in their interest and willingness to be involved in care planning and delivery. Although interventions should respect and utilize existing family resources, pressure should not be placed on family members to participate in activities in which they do not feel confident or competent. Procedures which appear straightforward to nurses (because of their education and experience) can appear dangerous, unpleasant or disrespectful to family members. The willingness of family members to be involved in the care process should never be assumed or exploited for any reason (especially to reduce costs, or to overcome service deficiencies), but should be agreed in relation to specific aspects of care. Everyone involved must be aware of the expectations, requirements, the support available, the advantages and possible limitations of undertaking the roles agreed. This agreement should be reviewed regularly to provide opportunities to alter the level of commitment without the person feeling (or being made to feel) that they have let someone down. Irrespective of the model of involvement being applied, care should be coordinated. It should always be possible for family members and the professionals involved to identify and easily contact the person responsible for the coordination of the care package. This may be a nurse, care manager, social worker, doctor or another person acting in a key worker role. Loose partnership structures that result in vague accountability, uncertain management and poor channels of communication are confusing, wasteful and unnecessary. Practical support must be available, the nature of which will vary, but family members will assess whether it is practical or not. For this reason they should be involved in decisions about the priorities of care and the interventions. It is no longer acceptable to determine the needs of people with learning disabilities and their families based only on what is currently available. A 'needs-led approach', as envisaged within the NHS and Community Care Act (1990), emphasizes the need for services to be clear about families' abilities and needs and to design individualized packages of care (Nolan & Caldock 1996). Support will mean different things to different family members. For some it will be advice and someone to talk to; for others it may mean practical assistance with care tasks, respite care or financial assistance. The involvement of family members in project groups to develop new policies, and in evaluation activities in respect of services they receive, can provide valuable information and suggestions for developing better services, and increasing the needs-led approach.

Specific attention should be given to building up relationships with all family members. Specific appointments can be offered to family members who are not usually at home when home visits are made, or for those hard to meet during usual contact. By doing so, a balanced perspective of the family is obtained and the differing abilities and needs of individual members, be they parents or siblings, noted.

Family members often gain tremendous support from contact with other families of people with learning disabilities. Nurses and other multidisciplinary team members should have up-to-date knowledge of voluntary and private organizations available locally and nationally, which may be of assistance to the person with learning disabilities and their family members (see Chapter 17). Care must be taken to present an objective opinion of the service available, if asked.

CONCLUSION

Family involvement in care is the stated aim of many services and their policy documents. Although some progress towards this important goal has been achieved, much remains to be done. At times family members wish for greater involvement than seems practical: on other occasions they may want limited or no involvement. Family members may also appear to have expectations that the professional services cannot meet, and the interaction between the parties becomes strained.

Attitudes to professionals can vary from sincere appreciation to distrust, and should be seen as a product of how family members perceive their situation and not as a deliberate unchangeable position. For either party to make value judgements and label each other as overprotective, disinterested, unmotivated, hostile, pushy or uncaring can be the greatest barrier to active family involvement. By noting the facts and discussing individuals' perspectives on situations it is often possible to come closer to understanding their actions and omissions. The life of the person with learning disabilities is of paramount importance in all interventions. There may be differences of opinion between professionals, family members and the person with learning disability about the preferred course of action, but negotiation can normally lead to an agreement about how best to proceed. However, negotiation requires time, openness, honesty, respect, confidence and a willingness to achieve an understanding of all perspectives.

There is no getting away from the fact that people with learning disabilities are members of families. Therefore, the role of family members in their lives must be acknowledged, respected and become an integral part of service provision. The development of services which actively involve family members is not easy, but it is well worth the effort.

Acknowledgements

I would like to sincerely thank D. Linton (parent), V. Maxwell (parent) and P. McLaughlin (CNMH) for their comments on an earlier draft of this chapter, and for their support and encouragement over several years.

REFERENCES

Allan I 1993 View of the family. In: Shanley E, Starrs T (eds) Learning disabilities. A handbook of care, 2nd edn. Churchill Livingstone, Edinburgh

Andersson E 1993 Depression and anxiety in families with a mentally handicapped child. International Journal of Rehabilitation Research 16: 165–169

Appleton P, Minchom P 1991 Models of parent partnership in child development centres. Child Care, Health and Development 17(1): 27–38

Barr O 1996 Developing services for people with learning disabilities which actively involve family members. A review of recent literature. Health and Social Care in the Community 4(2): 103–112

Braye S, Preston-Shoot M 1995 Empowering practice in social care. Open University Press, Buckingham

Blacher J, Baker B L 1992 Toward meaningful family involvement in out of home placement settings. Mental Retardation 30 (1): 35–43

Carter B, McGoldrick M 1989 The changing family life cycle, 2nd edn. Allyn and Bacon, Boston

Central Statistics Office 1995 Social Trends 25. HMSO, London

Conliffe C 1993 The burden of care. Institute of Counselling and Personal Development, Belfast

Cunningham C C, Davis H 1995 Working with parents. Frameworks for collaboration. Open University Press, Milton Keynes

Dale N 1996 Working with families of children with special needs. Partnership and practice. Routledge, London

Damrosch S P, Perry L 1989 Self reported adjustment, chronic sorrow, and coping of parents of children with Down syndrome. Nursing Research 38(1): 25–30

Department of Health and Social Services 1995 Review of policy for people with a learning disability. DHSS, Belfast

Duvall E 1967 Family development 3rd edn, J B Lippincott, Philadelphia. Cited in Gelles R J 1995 Contemporary families: a sociological view. Sage, Thousand Oaks, California

Gelles R J 1995 Contemporary families. A sociological view. Sage, London

Gibson C 1991 A concept analysis of empowerment. Journal of Advanced Nursing 16(3): 354–361

Gibson C 1995 The process of empowerment in mothers of chronically ill children. Journal of Advanced Nursing 21(6): 1201–1210

Giddens A 1992 Sociology, 2nd edn. Polity, Cambridge

Gittins D 1993 The family in question, 2nd edn. Macmillan, London

Haralambos M, Holburn M 1995 Sociology. Themes and perspectives, 4th edn. Collins Educational, London

Hennemann E A, Lee J L, Cohen J L 1995 Collaboration: a concept analysis. Journal of Advanced Nursing 21(1): 103–109

Heyman B, Huckle S 1995 How adults with learning difficulties and their carers see 'the community'. In: Heyman B (ed) Researching user perspectives on community health care. Chapman Hall, London

Hornby G 1994 Counselling in child disability. Skills for working with parents. Chapman & Hall, London

Hornby G 1995 Working with parents of children with special needs. Cassell, London

Johnson R 1992 Family development. In: Stanhope M, Lancaster M (eds) Community health nursing, 3rd edn. Mosby Year Book, St Louis

Leonard A 1994 Right from the start. Looking at disclosure and diagnosis. Scope, London

Manthorpe J 1995 Services to families. In: Malin N (ed) Services for people with learning disabilities. Routledge, London

Mathias P 1992 Family vulnerability, support networks and counselling. In: Thompson T, Mathias P (eds) Standards and mental handicap. Keys to competence. Baillière Tindall, London

Maxwell V 1993 Look through the parents' eyes. Helping parents of children with a disability. Professional Nurse 9(3): 200–203

McCormack M 1992 Special children, special needs. Families talk about living with mental handicap. Thorsons, London

Miller N B, Burmester S, Callahan D G, Dieterle J, Niedermeyer S 1994 Nobody's perfect. Paul H. Brookes, Baltimore

Nolan M, Caldock K 1996 Assessment: identifying the barriers to good practice. Health and Social Care in the Community 4(2): 77–85

Powell T H, Gallagher P A 1993 Brothers and sisters – a special part of exceptional families, 2nd edn. Paul H. Brookes, Baltimore

Rodgers R 1962 Improvements in the construction and analysis of family life style categories. Western Michigan University Press, Kalamazoo. Cited in Gelles R J 1995 Contemporary families: a sociological view. Sage, Thousand Oaks, California

Rubins L B 1976 Worlds of pain: life in the working class family. Basic Books, New York. Cited in Gelles R J 1995 Contemporary families: a sociological view. Sage, Thousand Oaks, California

Sloper P, Turner S 1991 Parental and professional views of the needs of families with a child with severe physical disability. Counselling Psychology Quarterly 4(4): 323–330

Turnbull A P, Turnbull H R 1990 Families, professionals and exceptionality: a special partnership, 2nd edn. Merrill Publishing Company, New York

Welsh Office 1971 Better services for the mentally handicapped. HMSO, London

Wolfensberger W, Thomas S 1994 Obstacles in professional human services culture to the implementation of social role valorization and community integration of clients. Care in Place 1(1): 53–56

UKCC 1992 Code of professional conduct, 3rd edn. UKCC, London

FURTHER READING

This is a selection of books/chapters written by parents of people with learning disabilities. Tremendous insights into the practicalities of family life with people with learning disabilities can be gained by reading and thinking about the messages in these texts.

Allan I 1993 View of the family. In: Shanley E, Starrs T (eds) Learning disabilities. A handbook of care, 2nd edn. Churchill Livingstone, Edinburgh
Boston S 1994 Too deep for tears. Pandora, London

Fitton P 1994 Listen to me. Jessica Kingsley, London
Hannam C 1988 Parents and mentally handicapped children, 3rd edn. Classical Press, Bristol
Miller N B, Burmester S, Callahan D G, Dieterle J, Niedermeyer S 1994 Nobody's perfect. Paul H. Brookes, Baltimore
Vagg J 1992 A lifetime of caring. In: Thompson T, Mathias P (eds) Standards and mental handicap. Keys to competence. Baillière Tindall, London

17

Helping agencies for the family

K. Baillie   J. Clutterbrook   M. Dearing
A. Kent   I. Tweddell

INTRODUCTION

History suggests that people with learning disabilities have always been alluded to in a negative manner. The Mental Deficiency Acts of 1913–1927 used derogatory terms such as 'idiot', 'imbecile', 'feeble minded' and 'moral defective'. Even the Mental Health Act (1959) failed to recognize the degrading nature of labelling, referring to the 'severely subnormal', for example (see Chapter 1).

Many people with learning disabilities were seen as misfits and problems, and were often put away in institutions or care colonies. These moves were often justified by people saying that they needed the care and protection offered by such havens. However, many of these people could have been cared for in their own homes, with the right amount of support. Over the last two decades many reports and Government White Papers have supported this view. With the closure of long-stay institutions, the need to provide comprehensive community resources is imperative.

In his report entitled *Community Care – an Agenda for Action*, Sir Roy Griffiths (1988) supported this view. He recommended that services should be tailored to meet individual needs, rather than attempting to fit the person within the available resources.

In 1994 the Government implemented legislation via the NHS and Community Care Act (1990), which stated that 'wherever possible people should be cared for within their own homes'. To enable this to happen, certain legal requirements were introduced, one of these being the right of people to have a community care assessment. Many voluntary organizations provide additional services not normally provided by the statutory agencies, and many health authorities/NHS Trusts provide community services for people with learning disabilities that sometimes include the following features:

- Community teams provide practical advice and support to children and adults with learning disabilities and their carers. The services provided vary from area to area and may comprise:
  - a multidisciplinary team of registered nurses for people with a learning disability, occupational therapists, physiotherapists, psychologists, speech and language therapists and often social workers
  - a purely nursing service
  - a specialist service providing, for example, advice and support to people with a learning disability who also have challenging behaviour
- assessment and treatment facilities for people with a learning disability who may also have mental health needs or challenging behaviour
- specialist respite services
- some specialist residential provision.

This chapter will endeavour to identify these voluntary agencies, giving examples of how and why they may be accessed and used by carers. It seeks to provide a practical overview of a range of services that learning disability nurses may wish to recommend to clients and/or carers. The case studies in this chapter present authentic life experiences that community learning disability nurses have encountered. Each of the case studies is accompanied by a reader activity and a suggested outcome of referral as to how the community learning disability nurse might best respond.

WORKING WITH FAMILIES AND CHILDREN

Outcome of referral for Case study 17.1

When the community nurse looked at Marie's identified needs the following interventions were used.

Case study 17.1

Working with families and children
Marie Blake is 4 years old; she lives with her mother, who is a single carer, her brother Jack is 6 years old and attends the local primary school, and her younger sister Katy is 18 months old.

Approximately a year ago Marie's mother attended her local health centre because of her concern about the difficulties she was experiencing with Marie. Ms Blake explained that, although Marie walked when she was 11 months old and had begun to talk when she was 14 months, in recent months her developmental progress had plateaued and she now appeared to be losing some of the skills that she had attained. In fact, the playgroup that Marie attends was finding it so difficult to cope with her boisterous behaviour that she now only attends for three mornings a week instead of five.

After Ms Blake had spoken with her GP and health visitor Marie was referred to a consultant paediatrician, who felt it necessary to refer Marie and her family to a geneticist. Investigations have now revealed that Marie has a rare mucopolysaccharide disorder (see Chapter 2). As a result of these recent investigations and diagnosis, Marie has been referred to the community team for learning disabilities.

Activity 17.1

Now that you have had the opportunity to read and digest information on Marie's profile consider the following. You should undertake this activity in the assumed role of a community learning disabilities nurse. The purpose of the activity is to facilitate your understanding of community agencies and their roles.

- Identify the helping agencies that will play a core function in Marie's care.
- Formulate a care plan that will take into account the following:
  - Marie's health needs.
  - The social support that Marie and her family may require.
  - The practical support that the family may need to assist them in caring for Marie.
  - The financial help that may be available, not only helping the family to care, but also to enhance Marie's quality of life.

Health needs

Working with children who have learning disabilities and their families, the community nurse would have to undertake a careful and detailed assessment of Marie's health needs. This should also give details of Marie's present level of development. As Marie's condition is progressive, this could be used in the future as a baseline measure to ascertain the skills that Marie is able to maintain, and also act as an indicator for areas in which she has started to deteriorate.

Marie may need assistance in the future in managing her continence. She may also require help in coping with frustration, as she could have problems making herself understood verbally, and may therefore require an augmented method of communication.

Her boisterous behaviour could mean that she is more prone to accidents through stumbles and falls, and therefore may need to be provided with a safe environment. Marie's family may need advice on how to cope with her behaviour.

Her mobility may deteriorate and she may experience difficulties with her coordination and balance. Marie may also find it difficult to feed herself, and experience problems with chewing and swallowing.

It is important that the community nurse refers Marie to other health professionals, such as an occupational therapist, a speech and language therapist, a psychologist and a physiotherapist to enable Marie's needs to be met holistically.

Social support

Discovering that your child has a special need or disability is probably one of the most devastating experiences that a parent can live through. The feeling of physical and emotional isolation can be acute. The pressures of having a child with a mental and/or physical handicap in the family are widely documented in the literature (Olshansky 1962, Erickson 1989, Mathias 1992, Gates & Wray 1995). The effects of caring can be stressful upon the family, and therefore the special networks that a family is able to establish are important. There are a number of agencies that recognize and develop support for carers: for example, the Carers National Association encourages carers to recognize their own needs, provides appropriate support for carers, and also

provides information and advice for carers. Contact a Family is a national charity that aims to encourage mutual support between families whose children have specific disabling conditions and link them together on a one-to-one basis. Caring for a child with a learning disability is time consuming, and parents often feel they do not have enough time to spend with other children in the family. This issue can be helped by Barnardos, a national charity which offers support not only to parents, but to siblings. They arrange playgroups and outings during the school holidays, where the children get the chance to be the centre of attention and forget the pressures at home for a while. In some areas Barnardos have a caravan or holiday chalet that they are able to let to families for a small fee, enabling them to have a break from the routine of caring.

Financial support

Marie's mother is not in full-time employment, and therefore is entitled to benefits for herself and her children from the Department of Social Security. To ensure that she receives all the benefits she is entitled to, she should be helped to access the Disability Rights Service. This association is recognized as the leading independent authority on social security benefits for disabled people, and is able to provide advice and information to people with disabilities and their families.

Ms Blake could also access the Family Fund on behalf of her daughter. This was originally established by Joseph Rowntree and its aim is to provide financial assistance.

If special equipment is required to enhance Marie's quality of life, there are a number of trusts and charities that may be of assistance. These can be accessed through a book published by the Family Welfare Association entitled *Charities Digest*, which is available in most public libraries in the reference section.

Practical support

Nurses must remember that some families may feel that without practical support they would not be able to continue to care, whereas others may find someone coming into their home intrusive. It is important for professional carers to ascertain whether a family requires help, and if so the level of support they desire.

Recent legislation has now been enacted whereby a carer can apply to their local care management team for an assessment of their own individual needs. From this assessment social services may be able to provide practical support within the home. This may be a home help to assist with housework, thereby giving the carer more time to care. They may also be able to provide practical help in assisting carers with more intimate care needs, for example bathing.

Barnardos are also able to offer practical help with transport for hospital visits, for example. They can also provide a sitter service, where a sitter visits a family and looks after their disabled child for a few hours a week, giving parents time to do necessary chores like shopping.

Leisure

Leisure is not only important to a child who has a learning disability, but also to their parents, brothers and sisters. A number of voluntary groups have established leisure activities for children with learning disabilities, for example Gateway (see Chapter 13).

Some universities have volunteer groups that organize leisure activities for disabled children and their siblings. Charities such as Barnardos run outdoor centres where children with disabilities can develop their confidence going rock climbing, abseiling, canoeing and horse riding. In some cities Barnardos have organized playgroups for preschool children with disabilities, and after-school clubs in the evenings and weekends.

The types of supporting agencies that can assist families like the Blakes are shown diagrammatically in Figure 17.1.

FAMILIES AND PROFOUND LEARNING DISABILITIES

Outcome of referral for Case study 17.2

Health needs

The first step for a community nurse for people with learning disabilities, following initial contact with the family, would be to undertake a detailed assessment of Lisa's health needs, also

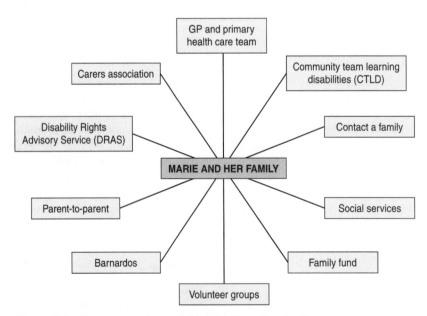

Figure 17.1 Support agencies available to Marie and her families.

Case study 17.2

Families and profound learning disabilities
Lisa is a 35-year-old woman with profound learning disabilities and physical disabilities that include cerebral palsy. Lisa also has epilepsy, and appears to be having a significant number of seizures on a daily basis.

Lisa lives at home with her parents, who are aged 64 and 69. They live in a three-bedroomed council house on a large estate. Both parents have health problems and are under increasing stress in caring for their daughter. The stress has now intensified with the news that Lisa's access to day services is under review and may be reduced in the very near future, owing to demand.

Lisa's disabilities affect her health and daily living skills in a number of ways. She is unable to walk and has very little movement of her upper body, and is therefore totally dependent upon her parents for all aspects of physical care, such as personal hygiene. Her parents are currently experiencing difficulty in lifting and handling Lisa at home. Pressure areas have developed and physical care has increased.

Concerns have been raised by Lisa's parents about the deterioration in her eating and drinking skills: she is unable to chew, and there has been significant deterioration in her ability to coordinate the movements required for swallowing. Her parents are having particular difficulties in ensuring that Lisa has an adequate intake of fluids.

Lisa is incontinent and suffers from constipation, which is further complicated by her poor diet and nutrition related to her eating and drinking difficulties.

Lisa also has communication difficulties: she is unable to speak, although her parents are able to interpret her needs, likes, dislikes and emotions through the different noises she makes, as well as her body language and facial expressions. However, staff at the day centre, or people who are unfamiliar with Lisa, sometimes have difficulties in communicating with her.

Lisa's general health and daily living have been further affected by an increase in her seizures. Lisa experiences both generalized seizures, mainly tonic – clonic, and absence seizures, although her parents had not recognized she was having absence seizures until another carer had pointed this out to them.

Lisa's parents want to continue caring for their daughter at home, but they realize the stress will increase without help and support.

Activity 17.2

You are a nurse working in a community learning disabilities team which provides a multidisciplinary service to adults with learning disabilities. Consider the following:

- Lisa's complex health needs and the specialist input that could be provided by yourself and the team
- The practical support that Lisa's parents may need for them to continue caring for her
- The social support networks/services that are available to Lisa and her parents
- The types of financial help available.

- Eating and drinking difficulties
- Nutrition
- Mobility
- Communication difficulties
- Incontinence
- Pressure area care.

It is important, perhaps in consultation with the parents, to identify or prioritize which need or needs they want to look at first.

- **Epilepsy** There is perhaps a need for education and information for parents in order to gain a more accurate picture of the number and types of seizures Lisa is experiencing, which will subsequently enable the GP or consultant to decide, with the parents, on the most appropriate antiepileptic chemotherapy.

There are tests such as CT and EEG (electroencephalogram) that can help in diagnosing epilepsy; however, the diagnosis and management of epilepsy is a clinical decision based on eyewitness detailed accounts of the seizures. Figure 17.2 is a proposed format for the recording of accurate details concerning her seizures.

The professionals involved in the care and treatment of Lisa's epilepsy could be the community nurse (RNMH), her GP, the practice nurse and a neurologist or specialist in epilepsy. The process outlined in this section is detailed in Figure 17.3. Information and resources are available from the professionals involved in Lisa's care, the National Society for Epilepsy and the British Epilepsy Association.

taking into account the needs of her parents, considering the amount of stress they are experiencing. The completion of detailed assessments can be time consuming but will identify, in Lisa's case, her complex health needs, as follows:

- Epilepsy

Date	Time	Description of what happened (i.e. movements seen, level of consciousness, unusual behaviours, etc)	How long did the seizure last?	Recovery following the seizure – how long and what happened

Figure 17.2 Accurate recording.

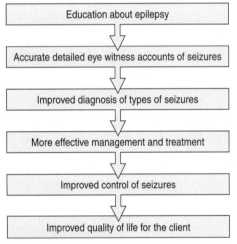

Figure 17.3 Managing epilepsy.

● **Mobility** Lisa's assessment may reveal a need for further assessment from other professionals. In the area of Lisa's mobility there may be a need for involvement from:

● **Physiotherapist:** for physiotherapy / exercises and training in lifting and handling for Lisa's parents

● **Occupational therapist:** assessment for aids and adaptations to make caring for Lisa easier for her parents when carrying out her activities of daily living, such as bathing, toileting, eating and drinking etc.

● **Community nurse:** advice regarding positioning, because of pressure areas which have developed.

Information and resources concerning mobility are available from the professionals involved, Disability Living Centres (demonstrations of equipment) and the Motability scheme. Vehicles can be bought or leased through the scheme using disability living allowance benefit.

● **Eating and drinking** There is clearly a need for involvement from the community nurse, occupational therapist, speech and language therapist and also the dietitian to identify Lisa's difficulties in chewing, swallowing and coordinating movements. An assessment to establish a baseline recording of fluid and foods eaten, so that her nutritional needs can be identified should be undertaken.

Advice can be sought from the speech and language therapist, along with an occupational therapist, regarding positioning and the type of seating required in order to aid the physical process of eating and drinking.

Further information can be obtained from PINNT (Patients on Intravenous and Naso-Gastric Nutrition Therapy). There are some people with learning disabilities who have chronic eating and drinking difficulties and are no longer able to take food or fluid orally; therefore, they are artificially fed. PINNT is a support group for people receiving parenteral or enteral nutrition. BAPEN (British Association of Parenteral or Enteral Nutrition) is an organization which can offer help and advice on nutrition therapy.

• **Communication** Here an assessment would be undertaken by the speech and language therapist in conjunction with both parents and the professionals involved in Lisa's care. The assessment should identify how Lisa communicates her needs, likes or dislikes, which may be achieved through the different noises or facial expressions she makes. The speech and language therapist would be able to help those involved in her care with how she communicates, and also suggest ways of improving this. Speech and language therapists can also provide assessment and information on communication aids (for example an Alphatalker) and the use of signs and/or symbols to facilitate communication.

• **Continence** This area would require an assessment to be carried out by a community nurse, but a continence adviser, dietitian and the GP may subsequently be involved. Baseline recordings are required to measure fluid input and output, how often Lisa's bowels are emptied, stool formation (whether she suffers from constipation), and information about her current diet. Advice could then be offered concerning the importance of an adequate volume of fluid, an increase of fibre in the diet, and help in recognizing when Lisa needs to urinate or empty her bowels. Some areas in the UK have a continence service that will provide various continence aids.

• **Practical support** Lisa's day care service is currently under review. Under the NHS and Community Care Act Lisa would be entitled to a community care assessment, which would be undertaken by social services (usually the local care management team), to identify the practical help and services required to meet her needs; Lisa's parents are also entitled to an assessment as carers. The community care assessment may request information from other professionals to be included.

Day and respite services may be offered. These are provided by the statutory agencies (social services and, in some areas, health services if a specialist service is required; also, the voluntary, not-for-profit and private sectors are increasingly becoming important providers of services in this area.

Other services available are Riding for the Disabled; local leisure facilities often provide activities specifically for people with disabilities; Gateway Clubs (contact Mencap); and respite (may be residential adult family placements of family-based respite, provided in the client's home).

Support in the home: the social services care management team could provide home help or a care officer to assist Lisa's parents in carrying out her activities of daily living, such as bathing. Specialist advice or practical support could be provided by the community learning disabilities team and other professionals working in the field of learning disability, such as occupational therapists, physiotherapists, speech and language therapists and psychologists. Some community teams provide a 24-hour service, and the social services usually operate an emergency duty scheme.

Social support: the National Carers Association could be approached regarding local carers' groups. Other agencies such as Mencap, Scope and Help the Aged promote carers' groups or schemes to support carers.

PEOPLE WITH MILD TO MODERATE LEARNING DISABILITIES

Outcome of referral for Case study 17.3

When the community nurse looks at Peter's identified needs it may be beneficial to use a holistic approach and divide the assistance required into four categories, i.e. help with health needs, practical help, help with financial needs and social needs.

• **Help with health needs** Peter was unable to come to terms with the death of his mother. This has prevented him from moving on and making positive plans for his future. Research has shown

Case study 17.3

People with mild to moderate learning disabilities
Peter is a 48-year-old man with mild/moderate learning disabilities. He lives in a local authority council house and until her death 8 months ago lived with his 76-year-old mother. Although Peter was very close to his mother, his brother and sister persuaded him not to attend the funeral as they felt he would only become upset and possibly disrupt the service. This appears to have had an adverse effect on his coming to terms with his mother's death.

Peter attended a school for pupils with moderate educational needs. His attendance was reported to have been very sporadic. He was easily led and appeared before the local juvenile court on three occasions for relatively trivial offences. Since he left school he has had no gainful employment and has been excluded from using day services, because of his poor attendance and disruptive behaviour.

Four years ago Peter was convicted of sexual offences against two girls under the age of 16. He was placed in a hospital for people with learning disabilities, under Section 37 of the Mental Health Act (1983). After 3 years, and following a multidisciplinary care conference, Peter was discharged under the Care Programme Approach. He was visited regularly by the community nurse who had been nominated as his key worker. Following the death of his mother the local housing department sought alternative accommodation for him, as the house he lived in was a four-bedroomed family house.

Clearly, to enable Peter to find suitable alternative living accommodation and for him to live as independently as possible, a whole range of statutory and voluntary helping agencies will be needed. Assessments carried out by both health and social services have indicated that Peter would be able to cope adequately with only medium support.

Activity 17.3

Now you have had the opportunity to read and digest the information in Peter's profile, carry out the following activities that will facilitate your understanding of community agencies and their roles.
- Identify the helping agencies that could play a key part in Peter's care.
- Formulate a care plan that meets Peter's needs in the following areas:
  - Practical help
  - Health needs
  - Social needs
  - Financial needs.
- After formulating a care plan, prioritize Peter's needs, identifying reasons for your decisions.

that people with learning disabilities need to go through the normal stages of grieving. Oswin (1991) has stated that people with learning disabilities 'have the right to grieve as individuals, the same right to consideration and to special help for particular difficulties'. However, Elliott (1995) has suggested that these individuals may not have had access to such interventions because of society's attitudes, parents' and carers' perceptions, and also the lack of appropriately trained bereavement counsellors.

Peter, who was very close to his mother, showed a number of signs that he was having difficulty in coming to terms with his loss. Examples of this were extreme anger, setting an extra place at the table, and generally being unable to cope with daily living events.

In Peter's case it was suggested that a community nurse would be ideally placed to support him following the loss of his mother. In the past, when addressing bereavement issues with a person with learning disabilities, medication was often used or, in some circumstances, a behavioural approach was taken, rather than addressing the bereavement issues directly.

After discussion, the community nurse, in conjunction with a trained bereavement counsellor from Cruse, took on the work using Worden's (1991) Task Model of Grief Counselling. This consists of the following:

- Accepting the reality of the loss
- Working through to the pain of grief
- Adapting to an environment in which the person is missing
- Emotionally to relocate the deceased and move on with life.

At the sessions the pace was dictated by Peter, and always ended with him saying he had 'had enough'. The sessions usually lasted about 40 minutes, and the next task was not moved on to until Peter and the counsellors felt success had been achieved. At the present time Peter appears to have come to terms with the death of his mother and is looking forward to life in the future.

- **Practical help** Although Peter and the professionals felt confident that, with the correct amount of support, he would be able to live independently, both his brother and sister had reservations. However, after in-depth work and encouraging the relatives to actively participate in constructing and implementing plans, using a wide variety of helping agencies, the community learning disabilities team enabled Peter's family to become the lead people in supporting him in his endeavours. Peter would need to have medium support to allow him to live as independently as possible. Following the decision of the local authority to look for alternative accommodation for Peter, the community nurse, in conjunction with Peter and his brother and sister, approached several housing associations in the local area. Peter was able to secure a two-bedroomed ground-floor flat, owned by a local church housing trust, that provided on-site warden support. The social services care coordinator arranged for a homemaker to visit twice weekly to help Peter prepare meals and keep the house clean and tidy.

• **Social needs** The need to provide positive and stimulating daytime activities was then looked at. Because of Peter's previous convictions, approaches were made to the National Association for the Care and Rehabilitation of Offenders (NACRO). This organization was able to offer a year's training, with a view to finding long-term employment. The training included working in an industrial laundry, a woodworking factory and a residential home for the elderly. Peter is assisting with domestic and cleaning duties, personal care and social activities with a number of residents.

In the evenings Peter has been able to access a number of voluntary services for social activities. He attends a social club on Tuesday evenings, organized by the Physically Handicapped and Able Bodied Society (PHAB), and on Fridays he attends a disco run by the local Mentally Handicapped Society (Mencap). Peter has also been able to participate in a befriender scheme run by local university students – Student Community Action (HUSSO). This enables him to go to the cinema, bowling and the pub, with his befriender June. All this has been beneficial in enabling Peter to become more assertive and decisive.

• **Financial needs** Peter had very limited knowledge of handling financial matters, as this had always been dealt with by his mother. Arrangements were made for his gas, electricity and rent bills to be paid on a weekly basis, and an appointment was made for Peter to see the local Disability Rights Advisory Service (DRAS), who were able to advise him on his statutory benefits

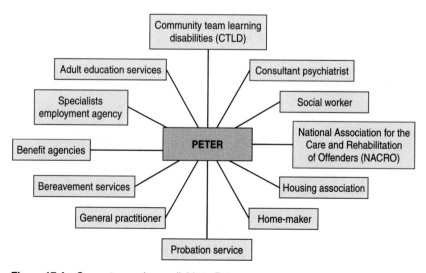

Figure 17.4 Support agencies available to Peter.

entitlement. After discussion with Peter, arrangements were made for him to enrol in the adult education classes looking at budget management, as well as reading and writing skills. Peter has also recently become part of a group looking at self-advocacy, which is run by a local advocacy forum.

• **Outcome of interventions** As demonstrated, Peter has been able to use a wide variety of helping and supporting agencies, both statutory and voluntary. Over a relatively short period, this has allowed Peter to take responsibility in planning and implementing all aspects of his life.

The range of helping agencies and support services are shown diagrammatically in Figure 17.4.

CONCLUSION

This chapter has endeavoured to provide the reader with a practical account of the various types of support that are needed, and which are available to people with learning disabilities and their carers. The agencies that have been identified are listed at the end of the chapter.

However, it must be remembered that these represent only a small proportion of those agencies in existence. It is recommended that the reader seeks out others from books and magazines, as well as using local information networks.

The use of agencies to help and support people living in the community will become even more important in years to come. With the closure of long-stay institutions, the safeguard of hospital admittance 'or a fallback position' is no longer available. This will mean that helping agencies will need to respond quickly and appropriately whenever a crisis or breakdown in care occurs. What is evident is that there is a fundamental obligation on the part of all helping agencies to assist and enable people with learning disabilities to lead positive, valued and fulfilling lives within their own communities.

Acknowledgement

The authors are grateful for the help and patience of Rita Bateson in preparing successive drafts of this chapter.

REFERENCES

Elliott D 1995 Helping people with learning disabilities to handle grief. Nursing Times 91(43): 27–29
Erickson M 1989 Chronic sorrow: a response to having a mentally defective child. Social Work 43: 190–193
Gates B, Wray J 1995 Support for carers of people with learning disabilities. Nursing Times 91(15): 36–37
Griffiths R 1988 Community care – an agenda for action. (The Griffiths Report) HMSO, London
Mathias P 1992 Family vulnerability, support networks and counselling. In: Thompson T, Mathias P (eds) Standards and mental handicap. Keys to competence. Baillière Tindall, London
Olshansky S 1962 Caretaking burden and social support: comparison of mothers of infants with and without disabilities. American Journal of Mental Retardation 94: 250–258
Oswin M 1991 Am I allowed to cry? Souvenir Press, London
Worden J W 1991 Grief counselling and grief therapy. Routledge, London

USEFUL ADDRESSES

BAPEN
For address contact PINNT

Barnardo's
Tanners Lane
Barkingside
Ilford
Essex IG6 1QG

Barnardo's work with 22 000 families, children and young people nationwide to tackle issues such as poverty, homelessness, disability, HIV/AIDS and sexual abuse.

Benefit Enquiry Line
0800 882200 (Freephone)

Free and confidential advice line for people with disabilities and their carers. The line is open Monday–Friday 8.30am–6.30pm and Saturday 9am–1pm.

British Epilepsy Association
Anstey House
40 Hanover Square
Leeds LS3 1BE

A national charity providing help and information for people with epilepsy, their families and those who care for them. Work includes advice, research and information.

Child Growth Foundation
2 Mayfield Avenue
Chiswick
London W4 1PN

A charity that is trying to ensure every child's growth is regularly assessed. Umbrella organization for growth hormone insufficiency, Turner syndrome, IUGR/Russell Silver, bone dysplasia, Sotos and PSM.

Contact a Family
170 Tottenham Court Road
London W1P OHA

Provides support for families who care for children with disabilities and special needs.

Croydon Epilepsy Society
Stanley Mews
71 Stanley Road
Croydon CRO 3QF

Disability Alliance
Universal House
88–94 Wentworth Street
London E1 7SA

The Disability Alliance provide useful publications on rights issues, benefits and policy publications

Disability Information Trust
Mary Marlborough Centre
Nuffield Orthopaedic Centre NHS Trust
Headington
Oxford OX3 7LD

Equipment for disabled people, price guides, manufacturers and bright ideas.

Disabled Living Centres
See telephone directory for local address.

Providing valuable information on aids and adaptations for people with disabilities and their carers/families to enable them to live as independently as possible.

Downs Syndrome Association
155 Mitcham Road
London SW17 9PG

The object of the association is to educate the public in all aspects of Down syndrome and enable people with Down syndrome to attain their full potential.

Epilepsy Association of Scotland
48 Govan Road
Glasgow G51 1JR
13 Guthrie Street
Edinburgh EH1 1JG

Family Fund
PO Box 50
York YO1 1UY

Provides financial assistance to families and individuals having difficulty in providing care for the person with disabilities. The finance is government money and not charitable donations.

Friedreich's Ataxia Group
Copse Edge
Thursley Road
Elstead
Godalming
Surrey GU8 6DJ

The group funds research into the causes of ataxia and associated conditions. It also publishes information and lists of local support contacts.

Independent Living Fund
PO Box 183
Nottingham
NG8 3RD

Irish Epilepsy Association
249 Crumlin Road
Dublin W12

Mersey Region Epilepsy Association
Glaxo Neurological Centre
Norton Street
Liverpool L3 8LR

Motability
Gate House
West Gate
Harlow
Essex CM20 1HR

National Autistic Society
276 Willesden Lane
London NW2 5RB

This society campaigns to offer advice and support for people with autism and their carers and families.

National Carers' Association
20/25 Glasshouse Yard
London EC1A 4JS

This is an association that provides information, networks and financial advice on benefits to carers of people with a disability.

National Society for Epilepsy
Chalfont St Peter
Gerrards Cross
Bucks SL9 ORJ

The society's objective is to advance the research, treatment, care, understanding and support of people with epilepsy nationwide.

PINNT
258 Wennington Road
Rainham
Essex RM13 9UU

Queen's Nursing Institute
3 Albemarle Way
Clerkenwell
London EC1V 4JB

Set up in 1887, its aim is to identify local health needs and encourage a multidisciplinary approach to healthcare.

Rathbone C.I.
1st Floor, Excalibur Building
77 Whitworth Street
Manchester M1 6EZ

An information resource to enable carers access to educational resources.

Remap
Hazeldene
Ightham
Sevenoaks
Kent TN15 9AD

Objective is to design and construct specialized equipment for disabled people that is not commercially available.

Resources for Learning Difficulties
Jack Tizard School
Finlay Street
London SW6 6HB

Provides educational teaching resources to be used in special schools, nurseries and children's own homes.

Riding for the Disabled Association
Avenue R, National Agricultural Centre
Kenilworth
Warwickshire CU8 2LY

The association works to provide the opportunity of riding to disabled people who might benefit in their general health and wellbeing.

Rompa
Goyt Side Road
Chesterfield
Derbyshire S40 2PH

Rompa provide specialist play, leisure, therapy and sports products for people with sensory impairments.

Sense
National Deaf/Blind & Rubella Association
11–13 Clifton Terrace
Finsburypark
London
N4 3SR

Sense is the national voluntary organization that works and campaigns for the needs of children and young adults who are deaf/blind, giving advice, support and information.

Scope
12 Park Crescent
London W1N 4EQ

Scope is the UK's largest charity working with people with disabilities. Formerly known as the Spastics Society, Scope works with people who have cerebral palsy and associated disabilities to keep them claim their rights and to lead fulfilling and rewarding lives and play a full part in society.

SPOD
The Association to Aid the Sexual and Personal Relationships of People with a Disability
286 Camden Road
London N7 OBJ

Works by providing a direct service to people with a disability and/or their partner who are experiencing sexual problems.

Wales Epilepsy Association
Ypant Teg
Brynteg
Dolgellau
Gwynedd LL40 1RP

Appendix

Legislation and social policy over the past 100 years   **311**

Legislation and social policy over the past 100 years

R. Gladden

This appendix, although not an exhaustive review of legislation and social policy, aims to highlight some of the sociopolitical influences that affect the lives of people with learning disabilities in the United Kingdom. The presentation is chronological, to allow the reader to track events and enabling consequential sociopolitical frameworks to be contextualized within the passage of time. It will be noted that terminology has changed throughout: this reflects the social beliefs and standards of specific eras. Although some of the legislation highlighted has been discussed elsewhere in this book, it is anticipated that this Appendix will provide students with a useful overview that could be used for revision and/or project work.

1900–1939

A Royal Commission that reported in 1908 suggested that the population of mental defectives had a considerable effect upon society. This Royal Commission accepted the eugenics argument that mental defectives were a threat to society because by their own reproduction they would pass on the undesirable traits of defectiveness. The Mental Deficiency Act of 1913 responded to this by creating a legislative framework that reinforced the segregation of people with learning disabilities from society. This Act placed mental defectives into one of four categories: idiots, imbeciles, feeble minded and moral defectives. It was believed that idiots and imbeciles required protection and were unable to attend to their own affairs. The feeble minded and moral defectives required care and supervision for their own and others' protection. It was popularly believed that moral defectives had tendencies towards vicious or criminal actions, upon which punishment had little or no effect. The Mental Deficiency Act of 1927 acknowledged that disease or illness could cause mental deficiency, enabling medical explanations to be taken into account.

This idea that people with learning disabilities posed a social threat continued to be believed into the late 1920s, when the Wood Committee (Board of Education and Board of Control 1929) approved the prevention of a radical disaster (the social fabric of society 'falling apart' without segregation of people with learning disabilities from the rest of society). Prior to the first world war the proposed solution to social problems and crime was segregation within institutions. The Wood Committee estimated that 300 000 mentally defective people resided in England and Wales, approximately 100 000 of these requiring segregation. In the mid-1920s the Board of Education reviewed its responsibilities towards defective children, agreeing with the Wood Committee's recommendations. This combination of legislation and reports in the early 1900s conspired against people with learning disabilities by promoting the idea that mental defectives created significant threats to their environments and to the future of the 'normal' population as a whole. Special school provision was established for some 'backward' children, although those excluded were classified as 'ineducable'.

The Local Government Act (1929) discarded the use of 'pauper', replacing it with 'rate-aided person of unsound mind'. Two new categories of people were acknowledged: the 'voluntary patient', who had the power to exercise a right, through written application, to treatment. Such individuals had the right to discharge themselves with 72 hours notice. The other new category was the 'temporary patient'. This category suffered from mental illness but was likely to benefit from treatment on a temporary basis, although at the time incapable of self-expression to indicate whether they wished to be treated.

The Mental Treatment Act (1930) made provision for people suffering from mental illness to be admitted into hospital on a voluntary basis. Officially patients had the opportunity to attend outpatient clinics at psychiatric hospitals, or to be admitted in to observation wards. The Act brought changes in terminology: the words 'asylum' and 'lunatic' were respectively altered to 'hospital' and 'person of unsound mind'.

1940–1950

The National Health Service White Paper (Ministry of Health and Department of Health of Scotland 1944), chaired by Sir John Hawton, highlighted two principles:

- The newly established National Health Service would provide comprehensive care and treatment for all.
- Provision of treatment would be free, with no implications related to individual income and the ability to pay. The Act had a considerable impact on the nation's health resources, although this legislation played an important role in the future care of people with learning disabilities.

The Universal Declaration of Human Rights (United Nations 1948) and the European Convention on Human Rights (Council of Europe 1950), provided principles underpinning human rights. The establishment and articulation of such rights has had profound implications for people with learning disabilities.

The Mental Health Act (1959) replaced previous legislation relating to mental health and the treatment of mental disorders, including the Mental Deficiency Acts of 1913 and 1939 and the Mental Treatment Act of 1930. It established new provisions relating to the treatment and care of people with mental disorders. A significant factor was the change of patient status from 'detained' to 'informal'. This Act made it an offence to ill treat or wilfully neglect patients' needs. The Act's new terminology, 'mental disorder', encompassed all of the disorders acknowledged within the Act. These disorders were subnormality, severe subnormality and psychopathic disorder.

1960s

The Seebohm Report (DHSS 1968), it is suggested, brought about effective family services within the community. In this report considerable emphasis was placed upon care by the community. There was recognition of the primary link between the statutory social services and informal carers. It was recognized that such innovative thinking would require considerable shifts in attitude to produce such a reality. The Seebohm Report recognized the need to define the 'community':

Community is usually understood to cover both physical location and the common activity of a group of people . . . the existence of a network of reciprocal social relationships which among other things ensures mutual aid and gives those who experience it a sense of well being.

Thus the report implicitly stated that equality lay within a community setting, although some may suggest that this completely eliminates people with learning disabilities from the community, when one considers society's attitudes towards this group of people.

During the 1960s a number of frightening reports emerged that depicted life within the long-stay hospitals. The Ely Hospital Inquiry, Cardiff (DHSS 1969), reported on complaints of ill treatment of patients, with inhumane and threatening behaviour employed by care staff.

Morris's (1969) report based on a national survey of mentally handicapped hospitals added considerable weight to the horrific reports from the Ely Enquiry. This helped establish that Ely was not unique, with poor conditions, low staff morale and organizational problems playing prominent roles in the reduction of care standards in mental handicap hospitals across the country.

1970s

The Education (Handicapped Children) Act (1970) made provision for all children to receive an education at school and eradicated powers stating that children with severe learning disabilities were not suited for an education at school. This legislation empowered all children to receive education, with official monitoring by local education authorities, regardless of their degree of disability.

The White Paper *Better Services for the Mentally Handicapped* (DoH 1971) enhanced opportunities for equality within the health services and community. A growing awareness of 'normalization' principles was beginning to develop. A greater involvement with the community was emphasized, with segregation occurring to a minimal extent. This paper called for more people with learning disabilities to live in community settings; the increased demands this made upon informal carers were appreciated, and the need for respite care services as well as community mental handicap teams acknowledged.

The Education Act (1971) provided a major turning point concerning education for people with learning disabilities. The responsibility for this was transferred from health authorities to education authorities, thereby providing enormous opportunities for people with learning disabilities to move away from a medical model of care. The Act also gave teachers a wider scope for implementing and enhancing educational methods and techniques.

The National Development Team was established by Barbara Castle, Secretary of State for Social Services in 1974. The National Development Team played an integral part in the development of national DHSS policies which highlighted the fact that many of the psychiatric hospitals had been neglected by the National Health Service. The National Development Team's role was to visit local authorities to inform, advise and monitor the implementation of DHSS policies, especially progress toward the provisions of the 1971 White Paper. The aims of the National Development Team were to ensure quality care that encompassed Government policies. As in the Court Report (Committee on Child Health Services 1976) (see later) the National Development Team emphasized that services for children with learning disabilities had diminished compared to their counterparts who did not have learning disabilities.

Although there was recognition of Government policies portraying the need for higher standards of living for people with learning disabilities, several disturbing reports were published. These contained horrific accounts of ill treatment and abuse in hospitals catering for such people, and it should be noted with some shame that such reports continued to surface throughout the 1970s. The report of the Committee of Enquiry into South Ockenden Hospital (DHSS 1974) highlighted understaffing, patient overcrowding and few physical resources.

The report of the Committee of Enquiry into Normansfield Hospital (DHSS 1979) provided detailed accounts of physical abuse, undesirable standards of living and ineffective leadership skills that set the precedents for the care for people with learning disabilities who resided there.

However, notable positive and far-reaching reports for improving the lives of people with learning disabilities also emerged in the 1970s: the Court Report (Committee on Child Health Services 1976) published recommendations recognizing that specialist expertise was required to accommodate the developmental needs of children with learning disabilities. It was recognized that such children, like others, had social, personal and emotional needs, but that these needs were frequently neglected. This issue was echoed by the recommendations of the Warnock Report (DoH 1978) (see later). The Court Report campaigned for a child and family-centred service which was readily available and accessible. Individuals with learning disabilities often required a multidisciplinary diagnosis, and so it was advocated that assessments of children should be related to any treatment and educational processes as an ongoing holistic approach. The Court Report also advocated that the new primary healthcare teams should be joined by personnel from child development centres who had specialist knowledge of children with learning disabilities.

The Warnock Report (DoH 1978) reviewed educational provision in England, Wales and Scotland for children and young adults with physical and learning disabilities. It also considered employment and the effective utilization of resources. The term 'children with special needs' was officially adopted, thus dispelling the concept of the educationally subnormal child. Skilled assessment and teaching programmes were recommended, with the integration and registration of children with learning disabilities into 'ordinary' schools.

The Jay Committee (DHSS 1979) considered the most appropriate model for the training of care staff for people with learning disabilities, who at the time were working within the National Health Service and local authority residential care settings. The Jay Committee initially considered the recommendations made by the Briggs Committee (DHSS 1972), which had suggested that the new caring profession should be introduced gradually. However, the Jay Committee stated that historically gradual alterations had not immediately produced valued lifestyles. The Committee's recommendations were to implement a radical financial change, involving staff, training and an overall reorganization of care provision. However, questions were raised concerning the role and aims of the existing registered nurse for the mentally subnormal along with other residential carers in respect of the developing Government policies. The principles of normalization were the guiding philosophy of the Committee, which identified three principles to which people with learning disabilities had a right:

- A normal lifestyle within the community
- Individuality
- Services to achieve individual potential.

Social aspects of care were considered the means of building upon an individual's proficiency, enabling people with learning disabilities to optimize their independence. A move towards the maintenance of community care was suggested, with greater emphasis on informal caring and care within the family home. Essentially, the Jay Committee found in favour of a social model of care, rather than the medical model that was prominent at this time.

1980s

In 1980 the King's Fund Centre published guidelines for services that provided residential care in the community. It was recommended that care establishments in the community should be ordinary houses supported by integrated care services.

In 1980 a report entitled *Mental Handicap: Progress, Problems and Priorities* was published by the DHSS that reviewed progress made on the 1971 White Paper *Better Services for the Mentally Handicapped*. The 1980 report examined the various roles of professional and voluntary services, and the extent to which they were providing coordinated care for the families of people with learning disabilities. Fostering schemes were recommended as an alternative to residential care, enabling more people with learning disabilities to take part in family life. Day care service provision, staffing issues and health service provision were all considered, and a number of suggestions were made for the improvement of future work. In-service training for staff was proposed, which would enable staff to ensure that the available resources were employed effectively.

At this time there were anecdotal claims that, following the publication of the 1971 White Paper, local authorities had improved their service provision in line with the initial recommendations. However, the 1980 review of progress described the development of community care as relatively inconsistent.

In 1980 the newly elected Conservative Government set up the Barclay Committee, which reported its findings in 1982. The main recommendation from this Committee was to build a 'community approach'; however, the Committee concluded that its findings provided little more than that which was highlighted by the Seebohm Report (DHSS 1968).

The Education Act (1981) created an official identification system that would encompass assessment as well as reviewing policies for all children considered to have special educational requirements. The official assessment, referred to as 'statementing', provided for extra or otherwise different facilities than were generally available in 'ordinary' schools. The assessment was to be multidisciplinary and involved coordination with parents and carers. Draft procedures were produced in order to provide an annual review assessment for each child that required special education. The Act gave parents of learning-disabled children greater involvement in all aspects of their child's education. Statementing related to a multidisciplinary assessment of children with severe learning disabilities within the first few years of life. During the early years of childhood it was the responsibility of district health authorities to refer children with special needs to the local education authority. Paradoxically, the multidisciplinary input may have had some negative effects, as professionals would advocate for specific educational needs that could not be met by the limited resources of the local education authorities. Nevertheless, the Act enabled children with learning disabilities to be taught in local mainstream schools, as long as the school could provide the education required to meet the child's needs, the child would not interfere with others' educational needs, and finally, the arrangements represented a sensible use of resources.

The DHSS report *Helping to get Mentally Handicapped Children out of Hospital* (DHSS 1981) endorsed the fact that large hospitals did not provide an appropriate environment for the health and development of children. Resettlement arrangements and the financial implications were initially considered by the DHSS in 1981 in a report that explored the movement of resources for care in England. The final arrangements for the shifting of resources were brought about through the DHSS report *Care in the Community and Joint Finance* (DHSS 1983). With the closure of long-stay hospitals for people with learning disabilities and the subsequent move towards care in the community, financial contributions needed this shift in order to make provision for care. Such payments were known as a 'dowry' and were paid to the local authority taking responsibility for the move from the hospital to the community.

The Mental Health Act (1983) redefined the legal categories of 'subnormal' and 'severely subnormal', replacing them with the categories of 'mental and severe mental impairment'. The new categories focused on the behavioural aspects, thus leading to a reduction in the use of such categories in learning disabilities. This new Act gave people with learning disabilities greater responsibility for their own lives, and for the most part effectively removed them from unnecessary legislation.

The Welsh Office All Wales Strategy for the Development of Services for Mentally Handicapped People (Welsh Office 1983) pursued the future development of integrated community-based multidisciplinary services. Health services, social services and the voluntary sector all aimed to combine their resources. The main philosophy for services providing residential care as 'homes' was that no more than four or five people with learning disabilities should reside in each home. The strategy considered small family units to allow individuals with learning disabilities to have a greater degree of empowerment and choice than if they lived in more heavily populated homes. One aim of the strategy was to provide a service to people with learning disabilities that was consumer-led, and this signalled a greater recognition of consumer- rather than provider-oriented values.

The Police and Criminal Evidence Act (1984) introduced the concept of an 'appropriate adult' as someone who could take responsibility if a person with learning disabilities or a mental disorder was taken into custody by the police. The appropriate adult's role is to observe, advise and to facilitate communication between the police and the person in custody during interviews. Although the Act and its codes of practice are not compulsory measures, it is the case that an appropriate adult must be present; if a confession is extracted without the presence of an appropriate adult then the statement must be considered with extreme caution.

In the mid-1980s the Social Services Select Committee published a report on service availability for people suffering from mental illness and learning disabilities, known as the Short Report (Social Services Committee 1985). This stated that prior to the discharge of an individual from hospital to a community setting, adequate care must be provided. The report also warned that community care was not to be considered as an economic windfall for service providers. Professional input was considered, and the role of the community mental handicap nurse was questioned. It was suggested that the community

mental handicap nurse should provide a long-term service with education and training, rather than just hands-on care. The DHSS responded through the Chief Nursing Officer in a report entitled *The Role of the Nurse in Caring for People with Mental Handicap* (DHSS 1985). This stated that the community mental handicap nurse embraced a role that was advisory and that would respond to a patient-led service.

The Cumberlege Report (DHSS 1986) stated that people with learning disabilities should use mainstream healthcare services.

In 1986, Sir Roy Griffiths was appointed to review the use of public finances in supporting community care policies, and in addition to recommend improvements in the use of finances, thereby creating more effective community care. The Griffiths Report (Community Care: an Agenda for Action 1988) commented upon the importance of flexibility in nursing and social work. It was suggested that by uniting expertise, networks could be formed that would open up support to people with learning disabilities and their families.

Griffiths recommended that:

- local authority social services should hold new powers, and he introduced the ideas of care management, purchasers and providers
- a new relationship should be developed that would involve interaction for service planning between social service authorities, health authorities and other service-providing agencies within the community
- local authorities should hold responsibility for the care of residents living in private, nursing or residential homes, thus enabling the best use of the available finances to produce the most appropriate care in respect of an individual's specific needs
- local authorities should work in conjunction with other caring professions, identifying opportunities to assess, arrange appropriate care and secure service delivery for people with learning disabilities.

The document *Community Care – Developing Services for People with Mental Handicap* (Audit Commission for Local Authorities in England

and Wales 1987) provided a basic outline for an audit of the services provided by local authorities for people with learning disabilities. The current challenges faced and future aims were detailed.

The 1988 Wagner Report (National Institute for Social Work 1988), although tackling issues concerning the elderly, was also concerned with the carers of people with learning disabilities. The report suggested that services within the community should attempt to contact all informal carers to discover whether support was required. If the situation did not appear to require regular support, then respite care was suggested as an essential element for the continuation of informal caring within the family home, thereby supporting an individual in the community. The stress and burden of caring for an individual around the clock was recognized, as was the problem of such situations creating potential health difficulties both for carers and those being cared for.

The White Paper *Caring for People: Community Care in the Next Decade and Beyond* (DoH 1989) aspired towards producing a framework for the present and the future to promote independence, and an opportunity for people with learning disabilities to obtain the services they required.

Six key objectives were developed to enhance service delivery:

- Promotion of the development of domiciliary, day and respite services. However, provision should be made for people to live at home whenever possible
- Support for carers to be the highest priority of the service providers
- Promotion of independent sectors alongside public sectors
- Define agencies' responsibilities, making them accountable for their actions
- Require proper assessments of people's needs and make provision for case management to ensure the highest quality of care
- Provide taxpayers with better value for money via the new funding system for social care.

Also during the 1980s the care of children by the NHS came under scrutiny and was highlighted in the Children Act (1989). For the first time, secure accommodation provided by the health service was regulated. A definition was produced as follows:

Any practice or measure preventing a child leaving a room or building of his own free will may be deemed by a court to constitute restriction of liberty.

This led nurses to explore their own practice and clarified that the only circumstances in law that would permit the restriction of a child's liberty were:

- a history of absconding, likelihood of abscondment if not detained, or is at significant risk if not detained
- the child is likely to self-harm or to injure others.

The Cullen Report *Caring for People: Community Care in the Next Decade and Beyond* (DoH 1989), attempted, at the request of the four Chief Nursing Officers of the United Kingdom, to review the demands made upon nursing staff caring for people with learning disabilities. The aim was to consider the development of a mixed structure of economic care. The phrase 'facility independence' was coined, acknowledging the fact that the role of the learning disabilities nurse transcended the structural environment in which he or she worked.

1990s

The NHS and Community Care Act (1990) provided a new legislative structure for the operation of the National Health Service, leading to:

- greater responsibility being delegated to local authorities, resulting in health and community services becoming more responsive towards individuals' needs and making community care more flexible for vulnerable people; providing relevant and responsive care related to local needs
- allowing hospitals greater freedom and flexibility to make decisions to benefit patients; self-governing status (National Health Trusts), financial and budgeting control; competitive roles encouraging services for wider populations

- new funding allowing financial assistance for patients within the community, incorporating primary healthcare teams, providing preventive health measures and assessment of patients' needs under their care
- stronger powers for the social services inspectorate of the Department of Health, and hospital-based staff had opportunities to transfer to the community-based services.

The Education Act (1993) stated that education authorities must identify children's requirements if they had difficulty before or after starting school. Parents appeared to be given greater powers concerning their rights of involvement. The Special Educational Needs Tribunal was also established by the Act. Parents were offered the opportunity to appeal against the local education authority's decisions concerning their child's special educational needs, thus giving parents greater control over the actions taken by the authorities.

The Mansell Report (DoH 1993) suggested that people with learning disabilities displaying challenging behaviour or mental health needs should have those needs met within their local area. Numerous recommendations were made for commissioners and the social services inspectorate, regional health authorities and the Department of Health. These covered the people involved, models of care, management commitment, agency responsibility, service development and value for money.

The Department of Health in 1994 published recommendations which stated that 'people suffering from a mental illness who were subject to the care programme approach should also be considered for inclusion on a supervision register'.

The supervision register aimed to:

- reduce levels of risk to the individuals themselves or others
- identify the numbers at risk
- aid future planning and development of the services.

This enabled people at high risk suffering from mental health problems to receive the highest priority in care, with active follow-up procedures, making sure correct care services were available, and enabling individuals to be traced if they moved between health authorities.

The criterion for inclusion in the supervision register is the significant risk of suicide, serious violence to others or serious self-neglect. Individuals placed on the register are reviewed at least every 6 months. Withdrawal from the register occurs when the person ceases to be considered at 'significant risk' of '… self neglect, violence or suicide'.

Following removal from the supervision register the documentation is transferred to the new community care provider.

The *Health of the Nation* strategy document (DoH 1995) for people with learning disabilities emphasized the move towards the use of generic services. This document developed five key areas that relate to the nation's targets for health:

- Coronary heart disease and stroke
- Cancer
- HIV/AIDS and sexual health
- Accidents
- Mental illness.

It suggested that these five areas were equally relevant to people with learning disabilities as they were to the general population, and recommended that health service providers should consider:

- health surveillance and health promotion programmes focused on the whole community, and therefore involving people with learning disabilities
- enabling people with learning disabilities to use health services available to all people in the community, but to have access to specialist services when required
- the encouragement of support services to enable people with learning disabilities to use health resources.

At the request of the Chief Nursing Officer a research project was set up and reported in 1995, entitled *Continuing the Commitment* (DoH 1995). This report aimed to examine the skills of nurses in the field of learning disabilities and to describe these, identifying initiatives used in practice. The report also gave advice to nurses on ways of producing coherent details informing purchasers, providers and other service users of the provision for people with learning disabilities. The report's recommendations were:

- Nurses' contributions should have greater links with health maintenance and enhancement of people with learning disabilities.
- Nurses' communication skills should be enhanced, to explain their roles to people with learning disabilities and their families.
- People with learning disabilities should be encouraged to advocate for themselves.
- Practices within residential homes should be reviewed and monitored via renewal of the Registration Homes Act.
- New ways to improve standards of care for

people with learning disabilities should continue to be developed.

CONCLUSION

Evidently there has been a gradual resettlement back into the community of people with learning disabilities. This century has witnessed a complete cycle of movement, from the community to institutions, and from the institutions back to the community. For nurses to move forward in promoting the care of people with learning disabilities will depend on the development of advanced nursing skills. In order to achieve such advanced skills, nurses will be required to apply research-based practice focused on the health needs of this group of people. However, it must be acknowledged that practice is mediated through and within a context: this Appendix has attempted to trace this context for the last 100 years.

REFERENCES

Audit Commission for Local Authorities in England and Wales 1987 Community care – developing services for people with mental handicap

Barclay Committee Report 1982 Social workers: their roles and tasks (Barclay Report). Bedford Square Press, London

Better Services for the Mentally Handicapped 1971. Cmnd 4683, HMSO, London

Board of Education and Board of Control 1929 Report of the Mental Deficiency Committee (Wood Report). HMSO, London

Children Act 1989. HMSO, London

Committee on Child Health Services 1976 Fit for the future (Court Report) Cmnd 6684, HMSO, London

Community care: an agenda for action 1988 (Griffiths Report). HMSO, London

Council of Europe 1950 Convention for the protection of human rights and fundamental freedoms. Council of Europe, Strasbourg

DHSS 1968 Report of the Committee on Local Authority and Allied Personal Social Services (Seebohm Report). Cmnd 3703, HMSO, London

DHSS 1969 Report of the Committee of Inquiry into Allegations of Ill-Treatment of Patients and other Irregularities at the Ely Hospital, Cardiff. Cmnd 3975, HMSO, London

DHSS 1971 Better services for the mentally handicapped. Cmnd 4683, HMSO, London

DHSS 1972 Report of the Committee on Nursing (Briggs Committee). Cmnd 5115, HMSO, London

DHSS 1974 Report of the Committee of Inquiry into South Ockenden Hospital. HMSO, London

DHSS 1979 Report of the Committee of Inquiry into Normansfield Hospital. Cmnd 7357, HMSO, London

DHSS 1979 Report of the Committee of Enquiry into Mental Handicap Nursing and Care (Jay Report). Cmnd 7468, HMSO, London

DHSS 1980 Mental handicap: progress, problems and priorities. HMSO, London

DHSS 1981 Helping to get mentally handicapped children out of hospital. HMSO, London

DHSS 1981 Care in the community: a consultative document on moving resources for care. HMSO, London

DHSS 1983 Care in the community and joint finance. HMSO, London

DHSS 1985 The role of the nurse in caring for people with mental handicap. Ref (No 855), HMSO, London

DHSS 1986 Neighbourhood nursing – a focus for care (Cumberlege Report). HMSO, London

DoH 1968 Health Services and Public Health Act. HMSO, London

DoH 1978 Report of the Committee of Enquiry into the Education of Handicapped Children and Young People. Special Educational Needs (Warnock Report). Cmnd 7212, HMSO, London

DoH 1989 Caring for people: community care in the next decade and beyond (Cullen Report). Cmnd 849, HMSO, London

DoH 1993 Services for people with learning disabilities and challenging behaviour or mental health needs: Report of a project group. (Mansell Report). HMSO, London

DoH 1995 Continuing the commitment. The report of the Learning Disability Project. HMSO, London

DoH 1995 Health of the nation: a strategy for people with learning disabilities. HMSO, London

Education Act 1971. HMSO, London

Education Act 1981 Special education needs. HMSO, London

Education Act 1993. HMSO, London

Education (Handicapped Children) Act 1970. HMSO, London

Health Advisory Service 1987 Bridge over troubled waters: a report on services for disturbed adolescents. HMSO, London

King's Fund 1980 An ordinary life. Project Paper No. 24, King's Fund, London

Local Government Act 1929. HMSO, London

Mental Deficiency Act 1913. HMSO, London

Mental Deficiency Act 1927. HMSO, London

Mental Deficiency Act 1939. HMSO, London

Mental Health Act 1959. HMSO, London

Mental Health Act 1983. HMSO, London

Mental Treatment Act 1930. HMSO, London

Ministry of Health and Department of Health of Scotland 1944 A National Health Service. The White Paper. Proposals in brief. Cmnd 6502, HMSO, London

Morris P 1969 Put away. Routledge and Kegan Paul, London

National Development Team 1977 Mentally handicapped children: a plan for action. HMSO, London

National Institute for Social Work 1988 Residential care – a positive choice. Report of the Independent Review of Residential Care (Wagner Report). HMSO, London

NHS and Community Care Act 1990. HMSO, London

NHS Executive/DoH 1994 Introduction of supervision registers for mentally ill people from 1 April 1994. Health Services Guidelines (94), HMSO, London

1978 The Future of Voluntary Organisations. Report of the Wolfenden Committee. Croom Helm, London

1987 Community care: developing services for people with mental handicap. HMSO, London

Police and Criminal Evidence Act (PACE) 1984. HMSO, London

Royal Commission 1908 Royal Commission on the Care and Control of the Feeble-Minded. London

Social Services Committee 1985 Community care: with special reference to adult mentally ill and mentally handicapped people (Short Report). HC 13.1, 1984/5 Session, HMSO, London

United Nations 1948 Universal declaration of human rights. Resolution 217 A(III), GAOR

Welsh Office 1983 All Wales strategy for the development of services for mentally handicapped people. Welsh Office, Cardiff

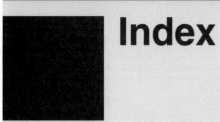

Index